Design That Cares

Planning Health Facilities for Patients and Visitors

Janet Reizenstein Carpman, Myron A. Grant, and Deborah A. Simmons

American Hospital Publishing, Inc.,
a wholly owned subsidiary
of the American Hospital Association

AHA ®

Library of Congress Cataloging-in-Publication Data

Carpman, Janet Reizenstein, date.
  Design that cares.

  Bibliography: p.
  Includes index.
    1. Health facilities—Design and construction.
2. Health facilities—Planning. 3. Hospitals—Design and
construction. 4. Hospitals—Planning. 5. Architecture—
Human factors. I. Grant, Myron A., date.
II. Simmons, Deborah A., date. III. Title.
RA967.C34   1986   725'.5   86–3445
ISBN 0-939450-80-1

Catalog no. 043180

Printed in the U.S.A.
2M-5/86-0094

Illustrated by Mary E. Yvon

Beryl Dwight, Editor
Peggy DuMais, Production Coordinator
Patrick J. Kane, Director, Graphic Design
Dorothy Saxner, Vice-President, Books

Contents

Foreword.. v

Acknowledgments vii

Introduction

Designing for Patients and Visitors 1

The Design Process.................................. 2

Organization and Scope of the Book 4

Part 1 The Need for Humanistic Design

Chapter 1. Current Trends and Their Impact
on Health Care 11

Part 2 A Journey through the Facility:
Achieving Design That Cares

Chapter 2. Arrival...................................... 25

Chapter 3. Wayfinding and the Circulation System 57

Chapter 4. Waiting and Reception Areas 101

Chapter 5. Diagnostic and Treatment Areas....................... 133

Chapter 6. Inpatient Rooms and Baths 155

Chapter 7. Gaining Access to Nature............................. 197

Chapter 8. Special Users 219

Chapter 9. Special Places and Special Services..................... 245

Part 3 Incorporating User Needs
and Preferences

Chapter 10. User Participation in Health Care
Facility Design.. 271

Conclusion 289

Bibliography 291

Index.. 305

About the Authors

Janet Reizenstein Carpman, Ph.D., is an environmental sociologist and a principal in Carpman Grant Associates, Behavioral Design Consultants, Ann Arbor. At the University of Michigan Medical Center, Ann Arbor, she directed the award-winning Patient and Visitor Participation Project for five years. Dr. Carpman has consulted widely with hospitals, design firms, and public agencies. She is the author of many publications, associate editor of the journal *Environment and Behavior*, and a former member of the board of directors of the Environmental Design Research Association.

Myron A. Grant, MLA, is a design researcher and designer and a principal in Carpman Grant Associates, Behavioral Design Consultants, Ann Arbor. At the University of Michigan Medical Center, Ann Arbor, he was the assistant project manager of the award-winning Patient and Visitor Participation Project for five years. Mr. Grant's work has concentrated on the design issues of health care environments and wayfinding systems. He specializes in developing processes and methods by which users can be involved in the design of both interior and exterior spaces.

Deborah A. Simmons, Ph.D., is assistant professor of environmental studies at Montclair State College, Montclair, New Jersey, and coordinator of school programs at the New Jersey School of Conservation, Branchville. In addition to her work in hospital design research, she has participated in research relating to hazardous waste management, national park planning, and energy conservation behavior.

Foreword

Individuals and their health care facilities have a long and varied relationship. The early hospitals of Europe were pesthouses serving more as places for dying than as places for healing. With the modern age of medical science and the twentieth century came the grand era of hospitals—clean, sterile, well-designed—serving as the community resource for healing all sorts of illnesses. Then came the age of technology, with elaborate health care facilities for diagnosis and therapy on a large scale. Through it all, the patient, as a human being, has been more an object on the scene than the focus of design. This book alters that perspective, permanently, we hope.

Even before the current period of intense competition for patients, some of us were wishing to place the patient as the top priority in facility design. Having seen hospital after hospital constructed primarily in the interests of physicians, trustees, administrators, staff, or government, we yearned to see a hospital constructed to serve the patient. So often communities and hospital staff members have eagerly awaited the opening of a spanking-new hospital only to find, once it is occupied, that patients and their families are inconvenienced, bewildered, or discomfited by a lack of sensitivity in design. How often have we all heard the lament, "Oh, if they had only asked me." Designing from the perspective of patients, their families, and visitors is what this book is all about.

The pathway from idea to practical application is tortuous. It is one thing to espouse the importance of sensitivity to patient concerns in health care facility design, but it is quite another to come up with practical ways and means for achieving it. This book grew out of the Patient and Visitor Participation Project at the University of Michigan Hospitals, whose mission was to take a large, complex teaching hospital construction project and influence its intractable design process to include the patient's needs and perspectives. The lessons learned from the Project's research, advocacy, and dogged perseverance have dramatically increased our design knowledge. As a result, this book is truly a breakthrough—the first of its kind and a real contribution to the field of health care facility design.

I offer one other thought to my colleagues in hospital administration, health care facility design, and health services delivery in general. If one wishes to feel the exhilaration of creative hospital design in the interest of the patients, two things are requisite. The first is a quality of leadership in one's governing body, medical staff, and senior management team that truly respects the patient and is willing to express that respect in tangible, specific allocations of funds, time, and energy. The second requisite is the presence of a talented, dedicated, and innovative core of professionals to lead and sustain the effort. Fortunately for us in our project in Ann Arbor, we have been blessed with both, the latter being the authors of this book.

Now, to all of you enthusiasts in health care facility design and activists in the interest of our raison d'etre, the patient, good reading!

Jeptha W. Dalston, Ph.D.
Chief Executive Officer
Hermann Hospital
Houston, Texas

Jeptha W. Dalston was executive director of the University of Michigan Hospitals, Ann Arbor, from 1976 through 1985.

Acknowledgments

This book is the result of interest, enthusiasm, and collaboration—all sustained by many persons over a period of years.

The initial concept of the Patient and Visitor Participation (PVP) Project was supported by Jeptha Dalston, Ph.D., then executive director, University of Michigan Hospitals, and was developed in conjunction with the staff of the Office of Hospital Planning, Research, and Development, under the direction of Douglas Sarbach, Ph.D. Judith Bernhardt, R.N., and Paul Couture, AIA, were responsible for developing the concept and the initial scope of work and worked hard to get the project off and running. The PVP Project's administration and research (the source of much of the material for this book) was funded by the University of Michigan Hospitals as part of the Replacement Hospital Program.

The PVP Project was successful, in part, as a result of the work of its research associates—a dedicated and hardworking group. Over the Project's lifespan, Susan Davenport Geer, Aura Glaser, David Hak, Yonit Hoffman, John Miller, Ph.D., Cheryl Norton, Marijean Price, Laurie Seuss, Deborah Simmons, Ph.D., and Kari Walker all contributed a great deal by gathering design-related information directly from several thousand patients and visitors. In addition to being a fine interviewer, Mark Vaitkus, Ph.D., worked with us to refine research designs and questionnaires and perform all the Project's data analysis.

Between 1980 and 1985, the PVP Project staff benefited from working closely with the staff of the University of Michigan Hospitals, especially the Office of Hospital Planning, Research, and Development (later, the Office of the Replacement Hospital Program). In addition to those mentioned above, Linda Ayers, Ted Belmore, Thomas Brubaker, Lynette Clark, Jody Cruden, Anne Dayanandan, J. Joseph Diederich, Dennis Dimoff, Cherie Donze, Richard Fritzler, Karen Frye, Rita Gibson, Todd Grant, Deborah Greene, Douglas Hanna, Pauline Hurst, Nancy Justice, Claudia Konrad, Barbara Kendall, Helen Kotlinski, Stephen Krebs, Valdemar Losse, Robert MacKenzie, Fatima Mosley, Kathryn Mull, Evelyn Neuhaus, Andrew Parker, Michael Pigg, Simon Ren, David Rogoff, Anne Schallhorn, Lois Solomon, Sandra Stone, Ken Thompson, Shirley Tommelein, Jill Van Cise, Beverly Walker, Michael West, Charlene York, and Mark Zimmerman all made contributions to the project, as did many of the Replacement Hospital Program consultants.

Throughout this time, the PVP Project staff were the recipients of the wise counsel of professors Stephen and Rachel Kaplan of the University of Michigan Department of Psychology and School of Natural Resources, in their role as methodological advisors.

As we explored the impacts of various design issues on patients and visitors, a number of health care facilities and other organizations were gracious enough to open their doors to us. Our thanks are extended to Bon Secours Hospital, Grosse Pointe, Michigan; Boston Floating Hospital, Boston, Massachusetts; Cedars Sinai

Hospital, Los Angeles, California; Chelsea Community Hospital, Chelsea, Michigan; Cottonwood Hospital, Salt Lake City, Utah; Detroit Receiving Hospital, Detroit, Michigan; Duke University Hospital, Durham, North Carolina; Gallaudet College for the Deaf, Washington, DC; Harper Grace Hospitals, Detroit, Michigan; Humana Women's Hospital, Indianapolis, Indiana; McMaster Hospital, Hamilton, Ontario, Canada; the Mayo Clinics, Rochester, Minnesota; the Michigan Commission for the Blind, Saginaw, Michigan; the National Center for a Barrier-Free Environment, Washington, DC; Nela Park (General Electric's lighting research facility), Cleveland, Ohio; Rochester Methodist Hospital, Rochester, Minnesota; St. Joseph's Hospital, Burbank, California; St. Joseph Mercy Hospital, Ann Arbor, Michigan; St. Margaret's Hospital for Women, Boston, Massachusetts; St. Mary's Hospital, Rochester, Minnesota; Shriners' Burn Institute for Children, Boston, Massachusetts; University of California at Los Angeles Medical Center, Los Angeles, California; University of Cincinnati Hospital, Cincinnati, Ohio; University of Utah Hospital, Salt Lake City, Utah; Walter Reed Army Medical Center, Washington, DC; Washington Hospital Center, Washington, DC; and the Women's and Infants' Hospital, Providence, Rhode Island.

During the course of our compiling materials for the book, several of our colleagues made contributions, including Joan Harvey; Jeff Hayward, Ph.D.; Anita Olds, Ph.D.; Richard Olsen, Ph.D.; Ronald Petersen, Ph.D.; Douglas Hamilton; and Robert Payne.

The idea for this book received strong backing from Dr. Dalston, who was then executive director of the University of Michigan Hospitals. His encouragement, coupled with that of Dr. Sarbach, gave us our initial start. The enthusiasm and support of the American Hospital Association (and later, its publishing arm, American Hospital Publishing, Inc.) provided the steam to keep us going. Suggestions by Joseph Sprague, AIA; Annette Valenta, Dr.P.H.; and Marjorie Weissman were particularly useful.

Successive drafts of the manuscript were ably reviewed for content by Judith Bernhardt, R.N.; Paul Couture, AIA; Jeptha Dalston, Ph.D.; J. Joseph Diederich; Rachel Kaplan, Ph.D.; Elliot Rothman, AIA.; and Herbert Sloan, M.D. Some architectural renderings were contributed by the Office of the Replacement Hospital Program. John Woodford and Diane Tremblay Tucker advised on syntax. Bridget Johnson word-processed the manuscript countless times, with great speed and competence. David Hak compiled the bibliography. Beryl Dwight, our editor, deserves special thanks not only for her skillful and sensitive editing but for seemingly boundless supplies of patience and tact as well.

Happily creating this book would have been impossible without staunch support at home. For this, our thanks go to Stephen Carpman, David Carpman, Christin Grant, Adrienne Grant, and Ron Widmar.

We would like to dedicate this book to the several thousand patients and visitors whose preferences and opinions shaped our work and to the millions more who we hope will experience design that cares in the very near future.

Janet Reizenstein Carpman
Myron A. Grant
Deborah A. Simmons

Introduction

This book is written for design decision makers—administrators, trustees, planners, architects, engineers, interior designers, landscape architects, members of citizens' committees, the health care delivery staff—those who fashion what a health care facility will be through policy-making, management, or planning. This book is for every decision maker, whether you are embarking on the construction of a multimillion dollar facility or simply planning to make a private clinic's waiting room more comfortable. The design issues discussed in this book apply to renovation and small-scale changes as well as to new construction.

Designing for Patients and Visitors

Patients and visitors represent particularly vulnerable user groups. They are virtually powerless in what they often perceive as an intimidating environment. They visit the health care facility under what are often emotionally stressful and physically debilitating conditions. At this time in their lives, they need a supportive, nonstressful environment, and they have little capacity to deal with a complex or confusing one.

It is also appropriate to focus on the design-related needs of patients and visitors because they are health care consumers. A large number of health care facilities are becoming concerned about their position in a competitive market. It is useful, therefore, to consider those aspects of health care delivery (such as the physical environment) that may provide a competitive edge when sensitively designed.[1]

Despite the compelling humanistic, marketing, and academic reasons for interest in the design-related needs of patients and visitors, this topic has not been widely addressed in either health care or design literature. However, the field is a growing one. This book attempts to bring together what is known about the design-related needs of patients and visitors and, in so doing, to provide a basis for future inquiry. The information in this volume is derived from both research-based and non-research-based sources. For the most part, the available literature on designing health care facilities is not research-based and is limited to descriptions of existing facilities. Whenever possible, we have drawn on information derived from research, such as that provided by the Patient and Visitor Participation (PVP) Project at the University of Michigan Hospitals.[2]

The Patient and Visitor Participation Project was a research and advocacy project that focused on the design-related needs of patients and visitors. It was created in 1980 as part of the design and planning process for the University of Michigan Replacement Hospital Program, a $285 million effort involving design and construction of a large adult general hospital, an ambulatory care facility, a parking structure, and other replacement and renovation projects. Completed in 1985, the PVP Project involved more than 3,200 patients and visitors and more than 1,200 staff members in

33 different studies ranging from schematic design issues like the layout of inpatient rooms to interior design issues like the location of signs.

The PVP Project, to our knowledge, produced the largest single body of research-based information on design-related needs and preferences of hospital patients and visitors. In addition, the PVP Project was the recipient of two national awards. In 1983 it was recognized as an outstanding example of environmental design research by the National Endowment for the Arts, and in 1985 it received an applied research award from *Progressive Architecture* for the report *No More Mazes: Research about Design for Wayfinding in Hospitals.*

The Design Process

Although no two design projects progress from abstract idea to concrete form in exactly the same way, there are predictable stages that every project goes through. During each stage, design decision makers make choices that determine what will be encased in bricks and mortar. It is important to understand the sequence of events and decisions that occur during a project before considering the specific design recommendations made in this book, because some decisions are appropriate only at specific times in the design process. Each stage is complex and time-consuming. For the sake of brevity we will only outline them here.

Predesign Programming

As soon as a project is shown to be needed and is deemed economically, socially, and politically feasible, the predesign programming stage begins. During the programming phase the basic parameters of the building, department, or room are decided upon, including its goals, its specific functions, the types of spaces it will contain, and the sizes of these spaces. Building programs vary widely in their comprehensiveness. Some provide only a list of spaces and their square footages, whereas others include performance criteria for how the space and systems of the departments will be used. The predesign programming stage usually results in a written document that serves as a set of instructions to the designer.[3]

Design Phase

Once the building's program requirements are set forth, the design phase can move ahead. The design phase is usually broken up into four subphases that coincide with the design's evolution from general to specific. These phases are block plans, schematic design, design development, and final construction documents.

Block plans show the building's configuration and its design concept in relation to a particular site. Departments, expressed as gross areas, are shown in their relationship to other departments, building entrances, vehicular traffic patterns, access points, and internal staff and patient movement patterns. Because block plans do not examine room-by-room detail and are relatively easy to prepare, alternative designs can be produced in a short time. They can be used to evaluate functional adjacencies as well as the flow of people and materials between departments. For example, in the case of a large hospital, the emergency department might be located where there is optimum access to the main road. In addition, surgery and radiology might be located adjacent to emergency, for ease of access to appropriate facilities and staff.

Schematic design goes one step further, showing every room that is functionally required, as well as corridors, mechanical spaces, stairs, elevators, and columns. The schematic design phase examines the relationship between all rooms within a department and formalizes the basic net and gross square footages of the building to confirm that the project can be built within budget. Its final stage is an evaluation of the relative merits of different heating, ventilation, air conditioning, plumbing, electrical, and fire protection systems.

Design development documents refine the schematic design even further. Drawings are prepared at a larger scale; instead of single line drawings, exact dimensions and thicknesses of walls are shown. All features of a room, including door swings, light fixture locations, counters and cupboards, medical equipment, and furniture, appear on design development drawings. All electrical, mechanical, and structural elements are defined.

Once the design development phase has been completed, the architect and engineers begin the *construction documents*. This detailed set of instructions for the contractor consists of working drawings and specifications—instructions about the quality of the materials and how to build the project. In addition, the construction documents include the Agreement between the owner and the contractor as well as forms that the contractor uses to bid the project. The owner is expected to sign off on all documents at the end of the construction document phase, as well as at each of the other phases. This sign-off means that the owner considers the plans complete.

Construction Phase

The construction work for most health care facility projects is awarded through a competitive *bid process*. During this phase, the owner (usually through the architect) responds to questions from potential contractors that may affect the quality or detail of the project. The contractor with the lowest bid price is usually awarded the contract, and the project then proceeds into construction.

During *construction*, the owner (again, through the architect or construction manager, if used) inspects the ongoing work in order to ensure compliance with the contract documents. Material substitutions, design modifications, and many other issues must be monitored in order to ensure that the final product is built to fulfill the program goals and operational requirements of its users, as ultimately defined by the construction documents.

Concurrent Planning

Interior design must progress concurrently with architectural design. Basic interior design services for health care facilities include space planning, which determines the layouts of rooms and achieves both aesthetic and functional goals; color coordination for all room finishes, furniture, and furnishings; and graphic design for signs and wall graphics. Interior design must work closely with architectural and engineering design to coordinate the compatibility of the sign system with the lighting, exposed air-handling diffusors, and devices of the fire-protection system. In addition, floor and wall materials and furniture layouts need to be compatible with other aspects of the design.

Landscape architecture also progresses concurrently as part of the total design work. Issues of site planning and exterior design, including vehicular and pedestrian circulation, parking, grading, drainage, exterior seating, selection of vegetation, and location of signs, are included as part of the site work.

Planning for medical equipment is also part of the design process. It begins at the same time as schematic design, expands into design development, and then continues through construction. During this phase, equipment is selected, its mechanical and electrical requirements are identified, and it is installed.

Design Review

Design review occurs throughout the design process, as the client evaluates the designer's progress by examining floor plans, equipment and specification lists, perspective drawings, three-dimensional models, and technical specifications. If parts of the design do not meet the performance criteria agreed upon earlier, alternative design approaches must be created.

Activation

Activation is the process of preparing to move into a new facility and the occupancy itself. Activation includes strategies for accomplishing the move, planning policies and procedures that will be used in the new facility, orienting staff to the new facility's layout and special features, and training staff to operate in the new surroundings.

Post-Occupancy Evaluation

Post-occupancy evaluation (POE), which is done after the environment has been occupied for a period of time, is the systematic assessment of how a particular environment actually functions in comparison to the design objectives.[4,5] If there are design-related problems, changes are recommended. POE findings can provide information that is valuable for other buildings, too. Because of the cumulative knowledge gained from this type of evaluation, a new design process can benefit from the experiences of previous ones.

Organization and Scope of the Book

This book has three parts. Part 1 provides background information on current societal and demographic trends and their impact on health care, leading to the growing emphasis on humanistic design. Part 2 contains the design chapters, with specific information on how the design of the facility can help to meet the needs of patients and visitors. Part 3 focuses on user participation in the design process, as a way for design decision makers to build on general principles by gathering information specific to the issues at hand.

The design chapters of part 2 are organized by health care facility spaces—waiting rooms, patient rooms, outdoor courtyards, and others. Each space is discussed according to relevant design and behavioral issues. The decision to structure these chapters in this way was made for two reasons. First, health care facilities are usually designed space by space, by designers and managers who determine the special needs of each functional unit. Thus, it may be more useful to present information about designing the emergency department or the lobby, rather than simply discussing an abstract behavioral concept such as privacy. Secondly, for the design decision maker interested in a specific area, such as the outpatient clinic or the admitting department, this space-by-space organization allows quick reference to relevant sections.

In addition, the design chapters are presented in an order that parallels the experience of a patient or visitor traveling through the facility. For each portion of the patient's or visitor's journey, we will discuss design-related issues in the same sequence as they would be experienced. This "flow scenario" of activities, spaces, and design-related needs is presented graphically and in the overall structure of the chapters.

The journey begins with arrival: finding the facility, parking, entering, and first destinations. The circulation system is next—how people find their way and how they use corridors, stairs, and elevators. We then discuss the outpatient's or visitor's use of waiting and reception areas, followed by the special concerns of designing diagnostic and treatment rooms. Our next stop is the patient room and bath. We then consider outdoor spaces that may be visited at various times—while waiting for test results, as a quiet place for lunch, or as a respite from the patient room.

Finally, we discuss patient and visitor needs with reference to special users, special places, and special services. First, we consider special user groups such as the elderly, the disabled, and the temporarily disabled, including those with mobility, hearing, and visual impairments. Next, we examine special uses of space: consultation, education, and grieving rooms; the emergency department; patient lounges; and child care facilities. Last, we include special policy considerations, such as providing overnight accommodations for visitors and outpatients.

Each design chapter contains three specific aids for the reader. **Design guidelines** provide suggestions on the design of the facility, with relatively detailed information about the issues under discussion. Whenever possible, the discussion draws directly on research findings. To highlight relevant research and to give examples of the potential role of research in design, **descriptions of research projects** and their results are provided in nearby boxes. Finally, specific **design review questions** relating to the issues discussed can be found at the end of the chapter. The design review questions, based on designers' recommendations as well as on research findings, are offered as a means of directly translating the information provided in this book into the design of a new or renovated health care facility.

As in any venture, there are limits to the scope of this book. Health care is an immense field encompassing scores of specialties, each with its own design requirements. Although each deserves attention, we have not attempted to cover the special design needs of such areas as pediatrics or psychiatric units. Instead, we have tried to cover the issues common to a range of uses. For example, we have discussed in detail the issues involved in designing a generic waiting room. Although some details may differ, the issues discussed should be appropriate to waiting rooms for a radiology department in a tertiary care hospital as well as to waiting rooms for a private physician's office.

Because each health care facility will differ from others in its requirements, we have not tried to make recommendations specific to such varied settings as a small clinic, a community hospital, a hospice, or a birthing center. Instead, we examine the generic issues involved in designing a circulation system, the patient's room and bath, diagnostic and treatment spaces, and other repeated or special spaces in a health care facility.

We offer this book as a place to begin, not as the final word in designing for patients and visitors. We offer what is known at present and, equally important, we offer a perspective on the relationship of design to high-quality care. We hope we have also provided a model of how to gain such information, so that our field can continue to grow and better serve patients and visitors and all health care facility users.

References _____

1. Falick, J. Humanistic design sells your hospital. *Hospitals.* 1981 Feb. 16. 55(4): 68-74.

2. Reizenstein, J. E., and Grant, M. A. *From Hospital Research to Hospital Design.* Patient and Visitor Participation Project, Office of Hospital Planning, Research and Development, University of Michigan, Ann Arbor, 1982.

3. Carpman, J. R. Influencing design decisions: an analysis of the impact of the Patient and Visitor Participation Project on the University of Michigan Replacement Hospital Program. Ph.D. dissertation, University of Michigan, Ann Arbor, 1983. Available from UMI, 300 N. Zeeb Road, Ann Arbor, MI 48106.

4. Zimring, C. M., and Reizenstein, J. E. Post-occupancy evaluation: an overview. *Environment and Behavior.* 1980 Dec. 12(4):429-50.

5. Zimring, C. M., and Reizenstein, J. E. A primer on post-occupancy evaluation. *American Institute of Architects Journal.* 1981 Nov. 70(13):52-58.

Part 1
The Need for Humanistic Design

Chapter 1

Current Trends and Their Impact on Health Care _____

Society is in transition. Although this is not a startling statement, it offers something to think about for designers of health care facilities. The nature and rate of future societal changes can only be speculated, but some of today's decisions must be based on speculations about our society in the year 2000 or 2020.

Mapping the future is, of course, an uncertain process. We may examine where we have been and where we are now, but that does not mean we can accurately determine where we are headed. Those who try to predict social uncertainties do not all see the same future, but they do agree that the issue of health care in the coming decades will be a primary concern.

Projections, Futurists, and the Direction of Health Care _____

One trend most likely to affect health care is the emergence of what futurist Alvin Toffler has dubbed the prosumer society, in which a greater proportion of a person's work will involve the production of goods and the provision of services for personal or family use.[1] Like the trends identified by Naisbitt in his book *Megatrends*, the evidence points to greater participation by individuals in everything from self-service gas stations to do-it-yourself divorces, with resulting changes in both personal and societal expectations.[2] As individuals become more involved in satisfying their own needs, they will gain skills and knowledge in areas that previously were mystifying. As they gain new skills, they will become more competent and demand greater participation in other areas, too.

In the health care field, Toffler points to the use of pregnancy test kits, self-examinations, coin-operated blood pressure machines, and the home use of such instruments as otoscopes as indicators of the rise of the prosumer society.

Linked to the emergence of the prosumer, do-it-yourself society is the increased importance of health as an indicator of overall quality of life. The popularity of jogging, meditation, and megavitamins shows that people have a strong interest in remaining sound and vital and in taking more responsibility for achieving and maintaining good health. As individuals become more knowledgeable and take more responsibility, their expectations of becoming full partners in their health care will grow. The result will be a society that demands a more active role in its health care.[3,4]

In addition to the less quantifiable trends proposed by Toffler, Naisbitt, and others, we can study changes documented by demographers and the U.S. census. Although less dramatic, the changes in age distribution, the fertility rate, urbanization, work status, and education will all profoundly influence the future of health

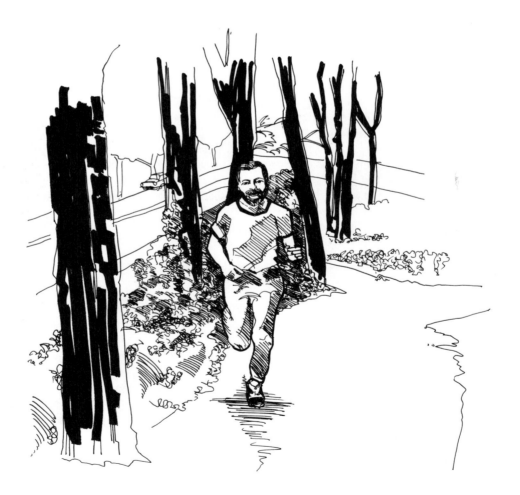

Increased participation in sports is one of the ways in which people are taking responsibility for their health.

care. What our society looks like, how we live, and how long we live will determine what demands are made on the health care field in the next few decades.

Perhaps the most significant demographic trend is the change in age distribution. Because we are living longer and our fertility rate is decreasing, the proportion of older citizens in the U.S. population will continue to grow. In fact, the distinction is now made between the "young old" in their 60s and the "old old" in their 80s. Whereas only 5.4 percent of the U.S. population was over 65 years old in 1930, the 1984 figure surpassed 12 percent.[5] In 1930, the median age of the population was 26.4, but by the year 2000 the median is expected to rise to 32.5.[6]

Our longer life span is due primarily to an improved standard of living and advances in health care. Yet, because of its unique needs, an older population will demand greater services from the health care system. Older people tend to have a greater number of chronic health problems, require more visits to the doctor, require a longer period of recuperation after an illness, and need more hospitalization than a younger population. As a patient grows older, the types of illnesses experienced often shift. And in addition to treating particular illnesses, doctors treating geriatric patients must be concerned with physiological and psychological changes directly related to the aging process.

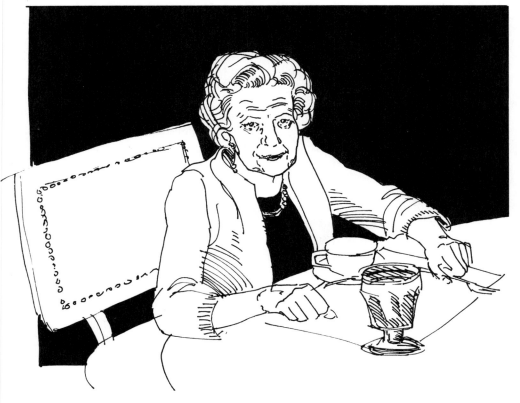

A healthier, longer-living society has a direct effect on the demand for health care.

However, health care will have to contend with more changes than just those related to serving an older population. Choices being made by couples across the country on how many children to have, or whether to have them at all, are profoundly affecting health care. In the post-baby-boom years between 1957 and 1973, there was close to a 50 percent decrease in the fertility rate (number of births per 1,000 women of childbearing age).[6] The conscious decision to have fewer children, to delay childbirth, or to have no children at all, aided by the availability of effective contraceptives, has already affected the demand for obstetric and pediatric units.

The number of infants born each year does not tell the whole story. Partly because childbirth is now more a matter of choice, it is reasonable to speculate that the parents-to-be will also want to make more decisions concerning the health care their child receives. Both parents already have become more involved in the delivery and in infant care. These shifts in parenting and the increased popularity of alternative birthing arrangements, such as midwives and birthing rooms, are reshaping obstetric and pediatric health care.

Other demographic trends, including the increased number of women in the work force, the continued urbanization of America, increased levels of education, and the changing occupational profile, will also put pressure on the health care system. With urbanization, not only is the geographical distribution of the population shifting but residents of urban areas tend to use doctors more often than do their rural counterparts. Changes in the work force, such as higher levels of education, will also put pressure on the health care establishment. As the level of education rises, basic knowledge about medical care also rises. A knowledgeable patient has greater expectations, which may alter the accepted definitions of high-quality care. Changes in these definitions—changes from the patient's point of view—may also result in a public reexamination of the basic policies and practices of health care.

Keeping a vigilant eye on lifestyle and demographic trends seems to be a prudent strategy for health care decision makers. Some of the shifts and their effects are easy to track and speculate about, but others are far from certain. Nevertheless, because society is unquestionably in transition and because its changes, the slow as well as the revolutionary, will affect health care, it is essential for health care leaders to plan for these shifts. Naisbitt, in *Megatrends,* suggests the need for long-term strategic planning to anticipate future conditions.[2] In making this argument, Naisbitt points to the failure of the more traditional short-term action plan as compared with the Japanese emphasis on goal-setting for the next decade.

In the health care field, where capital improvements and building costs are significant, planning for the long term is essential. Whether planning is for short-term or long-term goals, however, it must not be considered a static process. The long-term strategic plan must have enough elasticity to be altered as the need arises.[7] Likewise, even before this stage, the planning process itself must be a learning experience, because opportunities are available to learn from the process as well as from its results. Meeting the needs of consumers requires a dynamic approach to planning.

Health Care: Changing Within _____

Rapid developments in medical technology, changes in population and age distribution, and the increased role of government regulation are causing a revolution in the health care field.

"Old style" health care, dominated by the individual doctor's practice and the not-for-profit hospital, is rapidly becoming a thing of the past. Rising health care costs (at a rate of approximately 9 percent a year), an increasing supply of doctors, an uncertain future for Medicare and Medicaid, and diagnosis-related groups (DRGs) have transformed the health care field. The age of health care competition is upon us.[8] Birthing centers, health maintenance organizations, hospices, and big city hospitals must vie for a piece of the nearly $400 billion spent on medical care each year in the United States.[9]

In the race for patients and their health care dollars, the nature of the health care facility is changing, too. Throughout the nation, for-profit and not-for-profit hospital chains are springing up. Specialty facilities like drug-abuse centers, diagnostic clinics, outpatient surgery centers, and freestanding urgent care centers are providing services previously offered only at large hospitals. These changes have thrust health care into the world of big business and entrepreneurs. With intense competition for a market share that will sustain them, health care organizations are actively promoting themselves, and the patient is now the marketing target.[10] For-profit hospitals are introducing such amenities as restaurant-like menus and hotel-like furnishings.[11] Freestanding urgent care clinics are advertising their fast service ("In and out within 30 minutes"). To remain solvent and to keep patients coming back, health care organizations are beginning to nurture their "high-quality care" images in the media and in the minds of the public.

Design as a Component of High-Quality Care _____

Designing a health care facility is a complex process that must satisfy a multitude of competing criteria. The design must satisfy the demands of medical technology, that is, spaces must be flexible enough to accommodate complex equipment constantly being redesigned. Many facilities must also be flexible enough to handle a full range of activities, from a routine physical examination to a life-or-death emergency. The design must satisfy the medical staff, too. It must enhance the working efficiency of doctors and nurses who are dependent on the appropriateness of numerous elements such as ambient and task lighting, the size and configuration of each room, and the proximity of treatment rooms, ancillary services, and offices. With sanitary conditions so essential a factor, the needs of maintenance and housekeeping personnel must also be considered. And, in these days of fiscal constraint, the economic efficiencies of the design process, including life cycle costs of the building, must be factored into the design equation. Each of these demands on the design must be weighed against the other.

In the end, though, after all of the floor plans are drawn and the last coat of paint is on the walls, the health care facility will be a place where nurses, doctors, support service staff, patients, and visitors spend part of their lives. People will come to the hospital or doctor's office for a host of reasons. They will travel through the corridors, adjust the patient beds, drink from the water fountains, lie under X-ray machines, visit, and go about a variety of daily activities. The design must consider the many ways in which the facility will be experienced—what will be seen, heard, felt, and smelled.[12]

The technical design considerations, however, such as making room for a CT scanner or a crash cart, are of remote concern for many of the users of a health care facility. Of immediate concern is the availability of a comfortable place to wait, the accessibility of rest rooms for someone in a wheelchair, or the ability to find a particular destination easily. The design, therefore, must balance technological needs and human needs.

Designing for the human experience is essential. In choosing a health care facility, people consider a variety of factors that together help define the term "high-quality care."[13] Designing with the human experience in mind recognizes that people's images of health care facilities are multidimensional and that being technologically up-to-date may not be enough to satisfy patients and visitors.

The image people have of a facility concerns their relationships with the health care delivery staff, their belief in the effectiveness of the medical and nursing care being received, and their impression, good or bad, of the facility itself. The design of a health care facility reflects on the quality of care. Sending a "we care" message cannot stop with the staff. It must be designed into the facility itself.[3,4,13-15]

Developing a "we care" image has become as important in the health care field as it is in other service industries. Although the food in one restaurant may be virtually the same as in another, the service may be quite different. Likewise, from the moment the patient or visitor arrives at a health care facility, the design will convey certain symbolic messages. The nature of these messages is shaped through planning and genuine concern for the human experience. Humanistic design must be more than just an afterthought. It must move health facility design from its "hospital green" image to a sense of caring for the whole person.

The quality of the environment is important far beyond the image it presents of the health care facility, for the therapeutic aspects of design have to be considered also. The design of the facility, its color scheme, arrangement of furniture, availability of windows, and accommodation of family members are all part of the patient's movement toward recovery.[16-19]

Although the therapeutic aspects of design are not meant to be a substitute for medical and nursing care, they can enhance the efforts of health care professionals by creating a healthier setting for examination, treatment, and recovery. Just as the physical design can encourage or discourage the maintenance of sterile conditions and task efficiencies, design can encourage or discourage certain behaviors. Accordingly, the positive healing effects of design must be considered.

Focusing on Patients and Visitors

Try to remember the last time you waited to see a doctor or dentist. Did you glance through the magazines strewn on the waiting room table or shuffle the papers you brought from the office? Perhaps your heart beat a little more rapidly when you heard the dentist's drill, or you breathed a little more quickly when you smelled the antiseptic wafting in from the examination room. The simple, routine visit to a doctor's or dentist's office can be a profound and memorable experience. The physiological reactions (such as rapid heart beat or quickened breathing) that are experienced by many when visiting a health care facility may be accompanied by a host of psychological reactions as well.

If the goal is humanistic design, then the viewpoints of patients and visitors must be incorporated into the design process. It is not enough to have input from any single group of users at a health care facility. Medical and nursing staff can provide valuable insights about designing the environment so that it meets their needs, but even though their primary concern is patient care, their perspective on what is desirable design will not necessarily encompass the views of the patient or visitor.[20] In redefining the patient as a client and the visitor as a guest, health care facilities must begin to focus on patients' social and psychological needs, as well as their physical needs.

There are other, equally compelling, reasons for focusing on patients and visitors. Once they walk through the front door, these groups are virtually powerless.

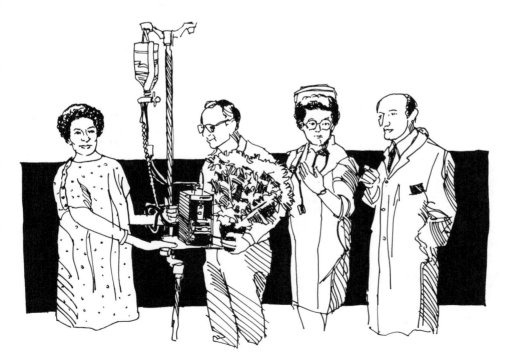

Decisions on health care facility design need to involve major user groups—medical staff, nursing staff, patients, and visitors—in a systematic way.

Under what are often crisis conditions, patients and visitors are vulnerable to demands on their physical or emotional capacities.[21] Yet, despite the impact of health care facility design and management on these users, few studies have examined these users or their needs. Of hundreds of articles published relating to the design of health care facilities, only a handful consider the patients' and visitors' perspectives in any detail.[22,23]

Designing for Patient and Visitor Needs

It is generally agreed that hospital patients and visitors are vulnerable groups and that the physical environment can be a source of stress. This stress can impede the ability of patients to recover from their illness. It can also increase hospital costs and decrease the quality of life for patients, visitors, and staff.

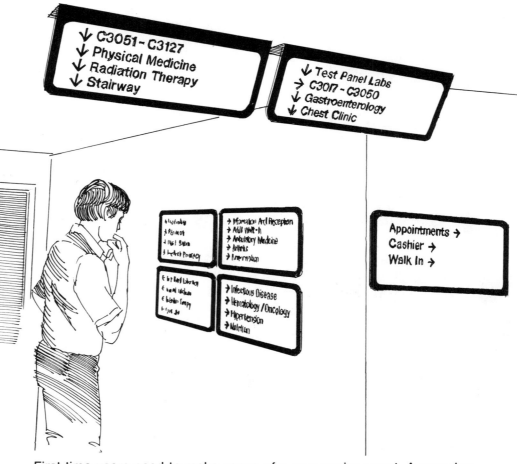

First-time users need to make sense of a new environment. A complex building layout and sign system can make finding one's way difficult.

Planners and designers can help reduce this stress, however, by taking into account the interaction between people and their environment. In particular, patients and visitors have needs with respect to wayfinding, physical comfort, the regulation of social contact (privacy and personal territory), and symbolic meaning.[24] These interactions must be a central concern when designing health care facilities.

Wayfinding. The ease with which people find their way around a building will affect their level of stress. Large, complex buildings such as hospitals are often like mazes, particularly for patients and visitors who visit them infrequently. Not being able to find one's way between various destinations leads to a sense of helplessness and frustration. Signage and graphics can help, but they need to work in conjunction with other features as part of a coordinated wayfinding system.

Physical Comfort. How individuals experience an environment is affected by noise levels, temperature, odors, and lighting, as well as by how successful those individuals are in manipulating their environment or comfortably positioning themselves within it. For example, the kind of noise that patients will hear if their room is located directly across the hall from a lounge will affect their comfort and ability to rest. Likewise, design issues—from the placement of bedside controls to the types of chairs available in waiting areas—will affect comfort levels, especially for someone with limited mobility.

Regulation of Social Contact (Privacy and Personal Territory). An essential need of patients and visitors is their ability to regulate the amount of interaction with others. Within the health care setting, a complex tapestry of social relations may be woven. The design must allow for visual privacy, acoustical privacy, social contact, and solitude. Patients wearing only a hospital gown should not feel as if they are on exhibit. Family members dealing with a tragedy should have an undisturbed place to grieve. Patients or visitors needing distraction should be able to find appropriate ways to focus their attention.

Symbolic Meaning. Beyond affecting physical comfort, the environment also transmits meaning. What patients and visitors see, hear, and smell blend into one image. The physical environment that supports the psychological needs of patients and visitors will be considered a positive, caring environment. On the other hand, physical arrangements that make the visitor or patient feel unimportant, or even forgotten, send a negative message.

Attending to the needs of patients and visitors will reduce their sense of helplessness and their sense of being adrift in a strange and complex environment. By attending to these behaviorally based design issues, the health care facility can make the experience of patients and visitors more positive and less stressful. Patients and visitors will have less trouble finding their way between destinations, will feel greater physical comfort, will be able to be social or private depending on particular needs, and will sense that someone cares.

References

1. Toffler, A. *The Third Wave.* New York: Bantam Books, Inc., 1981.

2. Naisbitt, J. *Megatrends: Ten New Directions Transforming Our Lives.* New York: Warner Books, 1982.

3. Panther, R. E. Hospital design in the year 2015. In: Lasdon, G. S., and Gann, J. S., editors. *The Future of Hospital Design: A Discussion Among Experts.* Washington, DC: U.S. Department of Health and Human Services, 1984.

4. Spreckelmeyer, K. F. Designing for health care in the twenty-first century. In: Heyer, O., and Graybow, S., editors. *Proceedings of the International Conference of the Association of Collegiate Schools of Architecture.* Washington, DC: ACSA, 1984.

5. Special Committee on Aging of the U.S. Senate. *America in Transition: An Aging Society,* 1984-85 edition. Serial no. 99-B. Washington, DC: U.S. Government Printing Office, 1985.

6. Cambridge Research Institute. *Trends Affecting the U.S. Health Care System.* Washington, DC: U.S. Dept. of Health, Education, and Welfare, 1975 Oct.

7. Michael, D. *On Learning to Plan and Planning to Learn: The Social Psychology of Changing Toward Future-Responsive Societal Learning.* San Francisco: Jossey-Bass Books, 1973.

8. Johnson, E., and Johnson, R. *Hospitals in Transition.* Rockville, MD: Aspen Systems Corp., 1982.

9. U.S. Department of Health and Human Services, Health Care Financing Administration. Telephone interview, Washington, DC, 1985 Mar.

10. Block, L. F., editor. *Marketing for Hospitals in Hard Times.* Chicago: Teach'em, Inc., 1981.

11. Johnson, B. Hospital "hotels": the time has come. *Michigan Hospitals.* 1985 Aug. pp. 5-11.

12. Lindell, M. The human hospital. *Dimensions in Health Service.* 1983 May. 60(5): 27-29.

13. Falick, J. Humanistic design sells your hospital. *Hospitals.* 1981 Feb. 16. 55(4): 68-74.

14. Tetlow, K. Healing research. *Interiors.* 1984 Oct. pp. 140-52.

15. Tetlow, K. New design for physical fitness. *Interiors.* 1985 Oct. pp. 168-76.

16. Canter, D., and Canter, S. Creating therapeutic environments. In: Canter, D., and Canter, S., editors. *Designing for Therapeutic Environments.* New York: Wiley, 1979.

17. Mathews, R. The psychological and social effects of design. *World Hospitals.* 1976 Mar. 12(1):63-68.

18. Petrie, R. E. Patient well-being is designers' first concern. *Michigan Hospitals.* 1980 Sept. 16(9):12-13.

19. Remen, S. Physical surroundings serve as therapeutic catalyst for patients. *Michigan Hospitals.* 1982 Apr. 18(4):20-25.

20. Parston, G. Hospital buildings and consumer needs. *Consumer Health Perspectives.* 1983 Sept. 9(5):1-7.

21. Burling, T., Lentz, E., and Wilson, R. *The Give and Take in Hospitals.* New York: G. P. Putnam's Sons, 1956.

22. Reizenstein, J. E. Hospital design and human behavior: a review of the recent literature. In: Baum, A., and Singer, J., editors. *Advances in Environmental Psychology.* Vol. 4, *Environment and Health.* Hillsdale, NJ: Erlbaum Press, 1982.

23. Reizenstein, J. E., Simmons, D. A., and others. *Hospital Design and Human Behavior: A Bibliography.* Architectural Series: A 673. Monticello, IL: Vance Bibliographies, 1982.

24. Shumaker, S., and Reizenstein, J. E. Environmental factors affecting inpatient stress in acute care hospitals. In: Evans, G. W., editor. *Environmental Stress.* New York: Cambridge University Press, 1982.

Part 2

A Journey through the Facility: Achieving Design That Cares_____

Chapter 2

Arrival

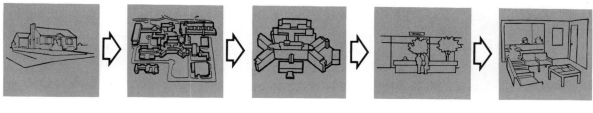

| Home | Complex | Building | Information Desk | Appointment |

The journey from home to the health care facility is a complex one for patients and visitors. It involves traveling to the facility, locating the entrance, becoming oriented once inside, and going to their first destination.

This chapter begins by looking at the needs of patients and visitors as they travel to the health care facility, whether arriving by car or traveling by public transportation. Next, it examines design issues related to making one's way from the parking lot or drop-off area to the entrance. The third section of this chapter examines the entrance area, a transition zone in which patients and visitors move from the out-of-doors into the complex activity of the health care facility. The final section describes four likely first destinations: an information desk, an area for storing outpatient and visitor belongings, the admitting department, and a visitor information center.

There is no typical experience shared by people traveling to a hospital or health care facility. Some patients and their companions will have visited the facility before. Others may be familiar with the general area but still have some difficulty finding their way. Still others will be making their first visit to the city or town. In addition, patients and visitors may differ in terms of how far they must travel. They may be traveling only a few blocks from home, from across town, from a nearby city, or from across the state.

Persons who travel great distances to get medical help are faced with special problems, such as staying overnight, being away from home, and missing work. They also bring a set of needs defined by their own personal situation. Someone with impaired mobility will have different needs from one who is unimpaired. An individual coming to the facility for a routine physical examination may find the trip less arduous than the patient coming in for a major operation. Finding the health care facility, making one's way to the entrance, and then proceeding to the admitting department or other destination—activities that are considered relatively simple tasks under normal circumstances—become anything but routine when complicated by emotional stress or physical duress.

Traveling to the Health Care Facility _____

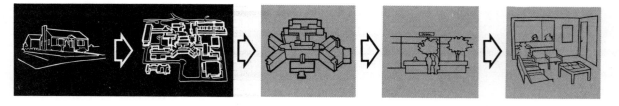

Home   Complex

In most areas of the United States the automobile is by far the preferred method of transportation to a health care facility. A small percentage of people, including trauma victims, the elderly, and the mobility-impaired, will arrive by ambulance. And, depending on the facility, some will arrive by bus or other public transportation. When a facility is designed, each of these modes of transportation should be considered, as well as the provision of parking areas, taxi stands, and bus stops.[1]

Arriving by Car

With such a large proportion of patients and visitors arriving by car, it is necessary to examine the range of their possible travel experiences to determine how to provide the environmental and operational support they need. Several issues will need to be addressed, including the ease with which drivers can find their way; the location, amount, and cost of parking; and the special parking needs of disabled people.

Wayfinding

Although the design of an orientation system often focuses on the interior of a building, finding one's way outside the health care facility may also be a problem for patients and visitors. The journey from home to registration desk is a multistage process. The typical patient or visitor may travel on a highway, as well as on a number of surface streets. They must locate the entrance drive, park their car in a parking area, and find their way to the entrance of the health care facility. Each step requires "reading" the environment, locating appropriate turning points, and finding the correct buildings. If useful environmental cues and orientation aids (such as signs and maps) are not available, there is a good chance they will become lost.[1,2]

Messages printed on interior and exterior signs are an important part of the experience. Signs direct, inform, and identify. Signs define appropriate behavior. Signs communicate. However, signs are only a limited form of communication. Because signs are not interactive, they cannot be asked a question or asked to rephrase directions. The message must be communicated easily without any need for further explanation or clarification.[3]

Messages on signs must be appropriately targeted to their audience, but selecting the most appropriate language may not be easy. The audience for any particular set of signs in or around a health care facility is quite broad, composed of persons with diverse backgrounds in terms of education, familiarity with the facility, and age. A further complication for a substantial number of hospital users is that English is their second language. Others may be functionally illiterate.

Understandable signs prevent confusion, unnecessary frustration, and loss of time. The following example illustrates the problem with signs that use language that is too formal or complicated for the reader:

> On a family swimming expedition as a child, I raced ahead of my parents only to return with the statement that we could not use that beach. "A large sign," I declared, "says 'Presbyterians only—vegetarians not allowed.' " My somewhat startled elders found upon inspection that it actually said "Pedestrians only—vehicles not allowed."[3]

The terms used on signs represent a major way in which a health care facility communicates with its consumers. Yet many of the terms commonly used may not be understood by all patients and visitors. When one first arrives at a medical complex, the sheer number of different buildings often proves very confusing. That's why it is important that buildings be given understandable names that make sense to patients and visitors (see Research Box #1). They are more likely to understand simple terms like *walkway* and *general hospital,* for example, than complex terms like *overhead link* or *medical pavilion.*[2]

Research Box #1:
Naming Hospital Buildings

Recognizing the importance of giving buildings and other facilities names that are understandable to patients and visitors, the Patient and Visitor Participation Project at the University of Michigan Hospitals conducted two studies to determine the most appropriate names for a series of hospital buildings.[2] In the first study, patients and visitors were asked to suggest terms for what was being called the *parking structure, hospital, ambulatory care facility, medical center,* and *pedestrian bridge.* In the second study, hospital visitors were asked to choose "best" and "worst" terms from a list of alternatives. This list was compiled from terms most frequently suggested in the first study and from alterna-

tives being considered by hospital planners.

Those interviewed were given a generic definition of each term (such as "building where people park their cars") and shown a page with a number of alternatives. They were asked to choose the best and the worst term.

As might be expected, the more simple and familiar terms were chosen best more often than the more complex or less familiar ones. Consequently, *general hospital* or *hospital* was preferred over *medical pavilion; outpatient clinic* was preferred over *professional office pavilion;* and *University of Michigan Hospitals* was preferred over *health sciences campus, health sciences center* or *health center.*

The design decision maker trying to develop an effective and understandable sign system is faced with a complex and often conflicting set of demands. These rules of thumb will help you design a successful exterior sign system:

● Once the wording for sign copy has been chosen, use it consistently throughout. For example, avoid using *outpatient building* on one sign and *clinics* on another.[3,4]

● Keep the message short enough (without losing meaning) so that a driver can read it quickly while driving. As a general rule, use no more than seven words in a message.[3,5]

● Keep the message clear enough to be interpreted similarly by all users.[3,5,6]

● Whenever possible, state the message in positive terms.[3,4]

● Use words and phrases that are well within a sixth-grade reading level.[4]

Exterior Sign Visibility

The text of a sign is not the only factor determining its adequacy. If the sign cannot be seen because of its location or cannot be read because of its color scheme or typeface, its usefulness is diminished. The sign that is obstructed by a tree or that seems to disappear into the wall will also be of little use. A number of factors can help ensure the sign's visibility:

● Mount signs so they face the driver directly and can be read easily from behind the steering wheel.[4,5]

● Locate signs so they can be easily seen and are within the viewer's 60-degree "cone of vision."[5]

● Because certain color combinations are more visible than others, consider the effect of the color scheme on the sign's visibility. The following list ranks color combinations from most visible to least visible: black on yellow, black on white, yellow on black, white on blue, yellow on blue, green on white, blue on yellow, white on green, white on brown, brown on yellow, brown on white, yellow on brown, red on white, yellow on red, red on yellow, white on red.[4,7-9]

● Avoid color combinations that rely on red and green because people who are color blind (approximately 10 percent of the male population) may not be able to distinguish these colors.[4,7-9]

- Consider the effect of letter size and typeface on sign visibility. Letters that are an appropriate size for a pedestrian who can stop and read a sign may not be appropriate for the driver going 30 to 35 mph. As a rule of thumb, use letters no smaller than 4 inches (10.1 cm) high where speed limits are 30 to 35 mph and no smaller than 5 inches (12.7 cm) where the speed limits are over 40 mph.[4]

- Provide outdoor signs that can be seen at night as well as during the day. Several options for lighting exterior signs at night are interior illumination, ground spot lighting, and reflective lettering.

Number of Signs and Sign Placement

As people drive to the facility, they will need specific directions at certain points along the journey. Signs direct the driver to the appropriate highway exit, through the city, and to the entrance of the health care facility. A hierarchical system of *major* and *minor* directional signs should be developed that provides an appropriate amount of information as it is needed, without causing confusion.[10] Major and minor signs should progress from general to specific information (for example, Medical Center, Metro-City Hospital, Patient Parking, Main Lobby, Admitting). On streets leading up to the facility, major directional signs point the driver to the facility. Major signs located at the edge of the site and the parking area provide the driver with information at crucial choice points. Minor directional and informational signs point to secondary entrances, call out special uses such as handicapped access or parking, and indicate traffic flow patterns around the facility.

Special Signs for Handicapped Persons

Clear signage that directs disabled persons to reserved parking areas and to specially designated routes and drop-off areas facilitates independent travel. To avoid unnecessary confusion, the international symbol of handicapped access should be used consistently.[11]

Environmental Cues

Visual cues created by buildings and their surrounding landscapes are important considerations in the development of an orientation system, because individuals will often rely on visual cues to make wayfinding decisions. If they see what they perceive to be an easy access to their destination, they will travel toward it. Unfortunately, this strategy may draw the individual into an inappropriate area (see Research Box #2). When the layout of a facility is being designed, the placement of buildings and other architectural features is an important consideration for alleviating potential congestion and confusion.

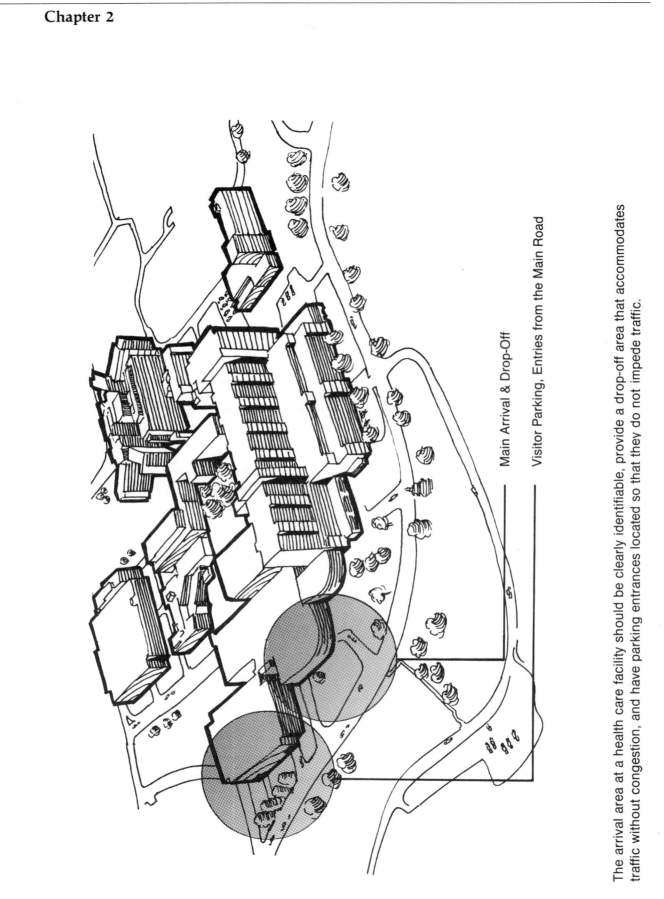

Main Arrival & Drop-Off

Visitor Parking, Entries from the Main Road

The arrival area at a health care facility should be clearly identifiable, provide a drop-off area that accommodates traffic without congestion, and have parking entrances located so that they do not impede traffic.

Research Box #2: Comparing Architectural and Verbal Wayfinding Cues

Designers at the University of Michigan Hospitals faced a potential wayfinding problem when they tried to determine where to locate the entrances to a new visitor parking structure.[12] The debate centered on the proposed relationship between the entrances to the parking structure and the circular drive for dropping people off at the hospital's main entrance. Because the drive and the parking structure need to be close to one another, one proposal was to construct an entrance to the parking deck accessed directly from the drop-off circular drive (see scheme A) with an additional entrance from the main road. Proponents of the scheme believed that this design would give drivers the option of entering the parking deck after dropping someone off in front of the main entrance. It was argued that people would read and follow signs and would turn into the circle only if they were dropping someone off.

Another proposal was to have both entrances to the parking deck accessed from the main road, away from the drop-off circle (see scheme B). Advocates of this scheme felt that having an entrance directly off the drop-off circle would lure drivers into the circle, causing needless traffic congestion.

Environment-behavior research was seen as a way in which these two differing views could be resolved. Rather than asking prospective drivers (in this case visitors to the hospital) which scenario they would prefer, researchers decided to ask them what they would actually do and how they would find their way given a certain situation.

Using a videotaped drive through a model of the entry area, the research simulated an automobile ride from the entrance of the medical campus to the drop-off circle and parking deck. With various scenarios simulated, hospital visitors could watch the television monitor and then tell the researcher where they would turn to park.[12]

The results showed that being able to see the entrance to the parking deck located adjacent to the drop-off circle lured a substantial percentage of drivers into the drop-off circle. Participants ignored the verbal cue of the signs that directed them to another entrance and instead followed the very powerful visual cue. However, if no entrance to the parking deck was visible from the drop-off circle, that is, if the visual cue was absent, they were more likely to follow directional signs and go straight to the more appropriate parking structure entrance, that is, bypass the drop-off circle entirely.

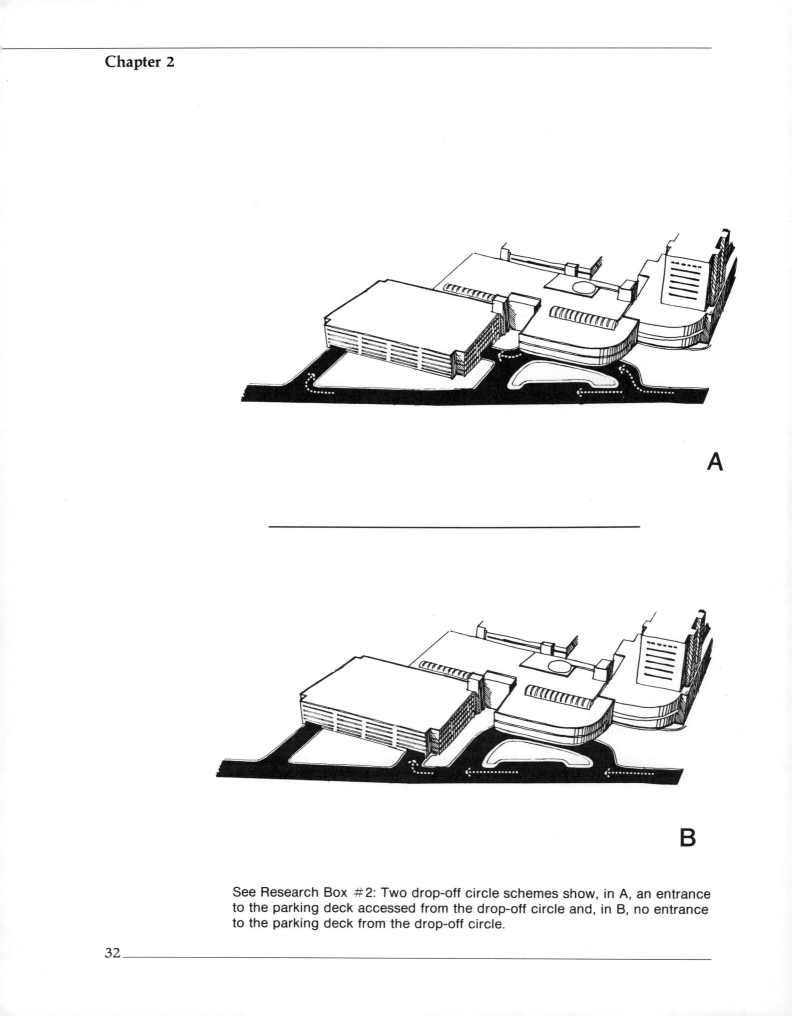

A

B

See Research Box #2: Two drop-off circle schemes show, in A, an entrance to the parking deck accessed from the drop-off circle and, in B, no entrance to the parking deck from the drop-off circle.

Drop-Off Area

Many health care facilities, especially hospitals, have a covered area at the main entrance where patients and companions can be dropped off and picked up. Such an area can make the main entrance easier to identify and also provides weather protection for people getting in and out of their cars. An attendant may be posted there to offer assistance. Drop-off areas are often accessed by circular drives, to allow for smooth transition to and from the main road. Parking is usually available nearby.

When designing a drop-off and pick-up area for a health care facility:

- Provide easy access to the drop-off area from major roads leading to the facility. A circular drive is one alternative.

- Locate the drop-off area immediately adjacent to the front door.

- Provide sheltered access to the building.

- Provide barrier-free access between the drop-off area and the area inside the main entrance.

- If the volume and the mobility characteristics of patients and companions warrant it, provide an attendant on duty throughout the day to assist people in making their way between their car and the building entrance.

- Design the drop-off area so that there is ample room for cars that are dropping off and picking up patients and for those that are driving through.

- Provide parking nearby and identify the route with clear signs.

- Provide a taxi stand nearby that will not create congestion in the drop-off area, or provide a system by which taxis can be called when needed.

Parking

Providing parking for visitors, patients, and staff often proves to be a complex problem. The design of the parking system needs to include safety, physical comfort, convenience, and accessibility features. Policy issues, such as parking rates and whether or not to make valet parking available, also must be factored in.

Long-Term Parking Rates

To recover the costs of providing a parking facility, many health care organizations charge for the use of the parking area. For the patient or companion visiting the facility for a short time, a standard parking fee may seem quite reasonable. On the other hand, for the patient or visitor spending several hours a day over a period of weeks or months, the standard parking fee may be seen as an unnecessary burden. Antagonism toward the daily cost of parking may foster an image of the facility as uncaring and unresponsive.[1]

In setting a parking fee policy, the facility sends a symbolic message. Depending on that policy, long-term patients and visitors may believe either that the facility is taking advantage of them or that the facility recognizes their hardships and the importance of visitors to the patient's recovery process.[1] Lowered long-term fees or free parking for patients and visitors, subsidized by rates charged to other users, might be a useful marketing strategy.

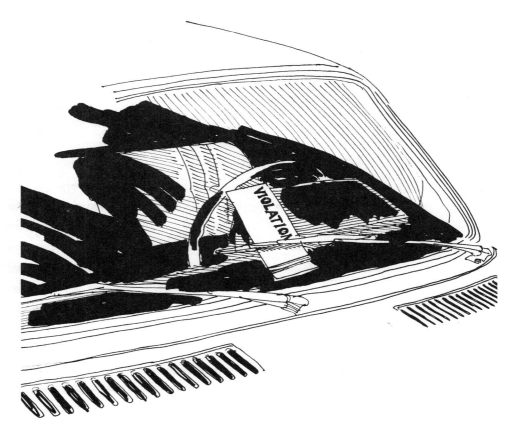

Parking violations, high fees, and too few parking spaces are common complaints of health care facility patients and visitors.

Park and Ride Options

In many urban areas, finding enough space for parking is a perennial problem. With construction programs that turn parking spaces into the "new wing," patients' and visitors' parking areas may end up some distance from the main facility. Although perhaps not an optimum solution, a remote parking lot with a frequent shuttle bus may be an acceptable option if visitor parking cannot be provided closer to the health care facility. For example, when visitors to the University of Michigan Hospitals were asked if they would be willing to park their cars in a parking lot one mile away if it was served by a shuttle bus leaving every 15 minutes, two-thirds said they would be willing to do so.[1] Other considerations when developing a shuttle bus system include security (especially at night), adequate signage, and weather-protected bus shelters with comfortable seating.

Parking for Permanently Disabled Persons

In many states, providing for the transportation needs of the disabled has been incorporated into public policy. Whether mandated by law or not, a sufficient number of handicapped-accessible parking spaces should be reserved, clearly marked with the international symbol of access. These spaces should be in close proximity to the facility, so that the distance from these parking spaces to the health care facility is kept to a minimum.

Parking for Temporarily Disabled Persons

Although the needs of the permanently disabled are now beginning to be recognized and met by both policy and environmental design, persons who are temporarily disabled (such as those on crutches, with casts, with bad backs, or those who have had recent surgery) traditionally have had to "make do." For permanently disabled persons, there are an increasing number of mechanisms for identifying vehicles so that special parking can be offered close to their destination. However, those who are temporarily disabled may have no way of obtaining the special parking or assistance they need. Because many patients fall into this category, a health care facility should be particularly sensitive to the needs of this group. There are several possible solutions to this problem.[13] For example, a number of spaces on the ground level of the parking structure could be designated for the temporarily disabled. Forms establishing the person's "temporarily disabled" status could be time-limited, signed by a physician, and mounted on the dashboard of the patient's car. If valet parking is available, the health care facility could reduce the fee for handicapped and temporarily-disabled persons.

Arriving by Public Transit

The majority of patients and visitors travel by private auto, but many may use the local public transit system.[1] Although this section focuses on buses, the guidelines could also apply to a rail system.

People who live in the area may use the bus system as a regular means of transportation, and visitors from out of town may find it more convenient to use the bus for their daily trips from the hotel rather than fighting traffic and parking in an unfamiliar city.

Whether or not travelers are familiar with the local bus system, they need information about schedules, pick-up and drop-off points, and fares. Once they arrive at the bus stop closest to the health care facility, they need to be able to find their way to the facility's entrance.

Having a bus stop adjacent to the main entrance of the health care facility will aid the users' wayfinding and decrease the distance they have to walk. The bus stop should be in an obvious location, with good visibility to and from the main entrance so that the patient or visitor will know where to go, where to wait, and where to get assistance. Directional signs and maps, including audible and tactile messages, will also aid wayfinding.[4,11]

When patients and visitors leave, they need a comfortable, accessible, weather-protected, safe place to wait for their bus to arrive. They may have a lengthy wait, and the aggravation of waiting is heightened during cold or rainy weather. A comfortable and safe place to sit may relieve some of the aggravation. Ideally, the shelter would provide not only seating, protection from the weather, and heat, if possible, but also a sense of security, especially for those traveling at night. It should be placed within full view of the main entrance and have adequate evening lighting.

Patients and visitors using the bus system should be able to go to a central location to obtain information. Bus schedules, route maps, the fare schedule, and appropriate phone numbers should be made available at the health care facility's information desk, as well as within the bus shelter.

Making One's Way to the Entrance Area

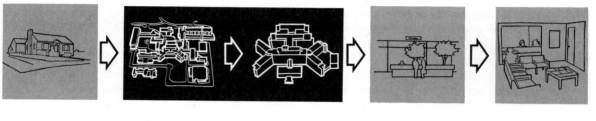

Complex   Building

Patients and visitors face a transition period when they move from the car, taxi, or bus to the main entrance. They need to orient themselves to where they are and where they wish to go. They should feel safe, knowing that if there were an emergency, they could obtain help. In addition, the journey to the entrance should be a comfortable one.

Wayfinding

Wayfinding problems may not disappear when the patient or visitor arrives at the parking area or is dropped off by a taxi or bus. Although most patients and visitors have little or no trouble finding their way, those who are unfamiliar with the facility may easily become lost.[1,2,14] A wayfinding system consisting of signs, color coding, You-Are-Here maps, and other elements can help direct visitors and patients from their parking spot or other drop-off point to their destination. Within a parking structure, clearly marked floor levels, identification signs, and major directional signs that are visible from every section of the structure can become integral parts of this system.[2] Within a parking lot, too, section signs and major directional signs should be visible throughout the lot.

You-Are-Here Maps

You-Are-Here (YAH) maps greatly aid orientation in a large health care facility, when patients and visitors leaving the parking area are going to a number of different buildings. Placing a map at the pedestrian exit of a parking area will allow people to gain an overall understanding of the layout of the facility and to plan the most direct route.

Because the purpose of a You-Are-Here map is to orient, it is essential that the information be presented clearly.[15] The map should be oriented so that "forward is up," that is, if the visitor is facing east while looking at the map, the map should be oriented so that east is at the top of the map. The map's location should be selected thoughtfully. Mounting the map near an identifiable object or structure that is shown on the map will help persons locate their position on the map. Because the viewer needs at least two points on the map for reference, the You-Are-Here symbol should be combined with at least one other point of reference, such as a prominent landmark. Labeling the objects or buildings will provide additional reference points.

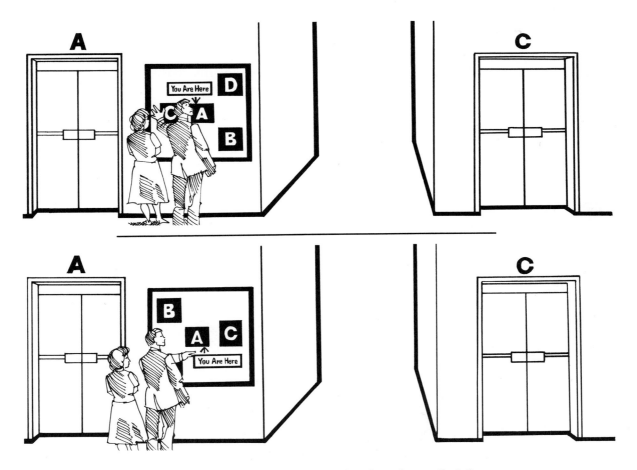

In these examples of You-Are-Here maps, the top drawing shows that the viewer is forced to mentally realign the map, whereas the bottom drawing shows the correct orientation of the map: forward is up.

Source: Levine, M. You-are-here maps: psychological considerations. *Environment and Behavior.* 1982 Mar. 14(2):221-37. Copyright 1982 Sage Publications, Inc. Reprinted, with changes, by permission of Sage Publications, Inc.

Safety and Security

Patients and visitors will find themselves in the parking structure at various times throughout the day and night, some while traveling alone, others while experiencing illness. If a person requires medical or other emergency attention within the parking area, design, security staff, and systems should guarantee that help is available. For example, the parking structure floor-to-ceiling height must allow ambulance access. The installation and maintenance of an emergency audio communication system, video cameras, and appropriate lighting within the parking area will provide an extra measure of security. Security guards or attendants should be available to help individuals in need.

Access for Disabled Persons

Entering the health care facility may be anything but easy for permanently or temporarily disabled persons trying to make their way from the parking area or drop-off point to the appropriate entrance.[4,11,16,17] In some instances, the journey may require travel from an upper floor of a parking structure, along sidewalks, and across a number of streets. At each of these points in the journey, the disabled person may find travel difficult. A number of design features should address this problem, including parking place width, location within the structure or lot, and grade level.

The disabled person may need to transfer from a car to a wheelchair. This process is greatly aided if the parking space is on a level grade and if the space is

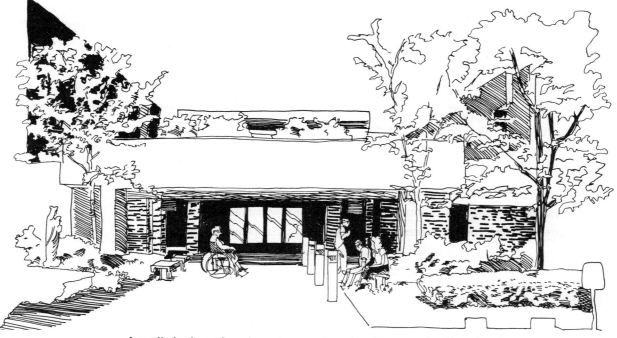

A well-designed main entrance to a health care facility should provide outdoor seating for people waiting for rides, be wheelchair-accessible, and have clear visual access between the drop-off area and the main entrance.

wide enough to open the car door to its fullest position (12 feet/3.6 meters). Vans equipped with a side wheelchair lift need 16 feet (4.8 meters). Safety within the parking structure can be maximized by providing a snow-free route that will not conflict with auto traffic.[11]

Because disabled or temporarily disabled individuals may be parking in the upper levels of a parking structure, it is important that a wheelchair user be able to enter the elevator lobby and elevator easily. If there is a curb, access ramps should be provided. The elevator should be at least 4'3" by 5'8" (1.3 meters by 1.7 meters) to accommodate a wheelchair. The elevator controls should be placed within reach, at a maximum height of 48 inches (1.2 meters).[4,11,16,17]

Once disabled persons have traveled to street level, barriers may still face them. Vision-impaired persons need to be able to follow the desired route and to avoid physical obstacles in the path. They also need to determine the proper route and must be able to walk along that route safely. Design considerations such as signage with raised lettering or braille symbols, sidewalks that are free from obstructions, such as street furniture and equipment, and changes in the texture of the sidewalk indicating entrances, streets, and so forth, will give visually-impaired people greater independence.

Hearing-impaired individuals need to be able to follow the desired route safely without requiring spoken directions. It is particularly important that signs and maps be available to direct hearing-impaired persons to their destinations. Warning signals like those used on emergency vehicles should provide visual as well as auditory cues.[18]

For mobility-impaired people, both ambulatory and chairbound, the design of sidewalks is particularly important if they are to travel unassisted. Several criteria are important:

- Build sidewalks wide enough to allow two wheelchairs to pass easily, at least 5 feet (1.5 meters) wide.[4,11,16,17]

- Eliminate obstructions (such as grates) that may catch wheels or crutches; keep benches or other street furniture that may make maneuvering difficult away from the circulation path.

- Provide curb cuts at all street crossings at a low enough grade to be wheelchair accessible, that is, not more than a 16.6 percent grade, and preferably at an 8.3 percent grade.[4,11,16,17]

- Design grades to be flat enough to allow easy movement. If grades must be greater than 5 percent, provide handrails.

- Avoid the use of brick and other uneven paving materials that might create a bumpy ride for patients in wheelchairs.

Entrance Area

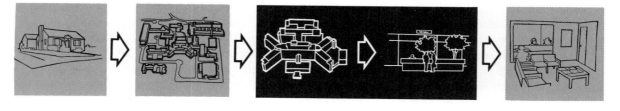

Building   Information Desk

In many ways the entrance sets the tone for the health care facility.[19] It makes an initial statement about the facility and welcomes the user. It provides a transition zone from the outdoors to the interior environment, a place where people put out cigarettes, kick off mud, and take off coats and hats. The entrance is also a place for people to wait for transportation, to communicate with others, and to become oriented to the layout of the facility.

Introducing the Interior Wayfinding System

Upon entering the facility, patients and visitors want to know where they must go. A well-designed set of signs and maps in conjunction with an information desk located near the entrance can help orient them to the facility and introduce its wayfinding system. Consequently, users will know where to look for additional directional information as it is needed.

Providing for Special Users

Sometimes the main entrance can become congested and confusing. Special consideration should be given to those who have difficulty moving about, finding their way, or handling their belongings. Older persons may need special help, and disabled persons may have special needs that should be attended to immediately upon entering. An attendant or a volunteer may be able to supply some of these needs—directing users to various services, helping them with their belongings, providing needed information, and simply being available for assistance.

    To accommodate these special users, designers of an entrance area need to consider the following:[11,17]

- Make the doorway passable by someone in a wheelchair or by someone who is vision-impaired. Turnstiles and revolving doors, for example, may prove hazardous to those who move with some difficulty and may be inaccessible for someone in a wheelchair or pushing a baby stroller.

- Provide doors that can be easily opened by people with little upper body strength. The force needed to open a door should not exceed 8 pounds. Automatic doors that open with a pressure-sensitive mat or an electronic eye may be a good trade-off between ease of accessibility and a door that will not blow open in the wind.

- Avoid obstructions at the entrance way. For example, mud walk-off mats and pressure-sensitive mats should be flush with the floor. This will allow a wheelchair to maneuver more easily.

- Provide space out of the flow of traffic for storing wheelchairs.

Waiting in the Entrance Area

Patients and visitors waiting to be picked up by a companion, taxi, or bus need a comfortable and safe place to wait. The main entrance often becomes an official waiting area because its location allows observation of traffic in front of the facility. Consequently, the entrance area needs to be large enough to accommodate both through traffic and those who are waiting. Rest rooms, comfortable places to sit, and convenient places to put belongings should be provided. In addition, services are needed to support the transition between the facility and the outdoors—taxi phones, maps (how to get back to the freeway), bus schedules, and signs directing the users out of the building and back to the bus stop or parking lot. Finding one's way back to the parking area may be as difficult as making one's way from it to the entrance, but confusion can be reduced if appropriate "reverse" signs and maps are available.

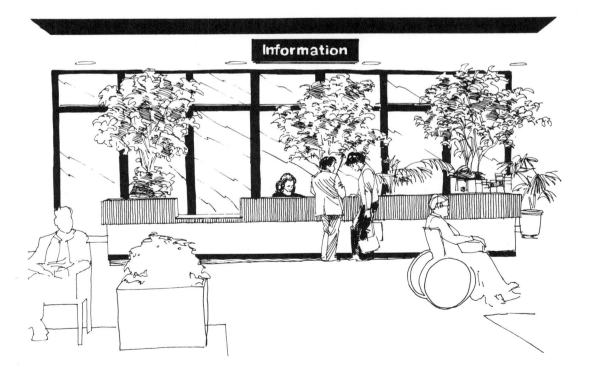

A large, clear sign and an obvious counter will draw patients and visitors to the facility's main information desk.

First Destinations

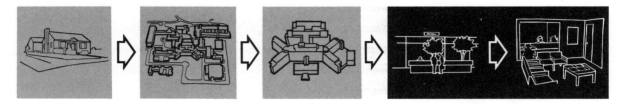

Information Desk   Appointment

Patients' and visitors' first official contacts with health care personnel are often at an information desk or some area, such as a security booth or reception desk, that serves the same purpose.

Information Desk

An information desk often serves a variety of functions. It provides a clearly identifiable place for patients and visitors to have questions answered, where they can find out about hours of operation, availability of services, and bus schedules. It officially, yet informally, welcomes people. Attendants at the information desk can help orient patients and visitors to the facility by providing clear directions. Yet, whether or not the information desk is able to serve these functions may depend on its location and design:

- Provide direct visual access to the information desk from the patients' and visitors' entrance. Provide highly visible signage identifying the information desk.

- Provide visual access from the information desk to the entrance so the staff has a clear view of people as they enter the facility.

- Design the information desk so those entering the facility can distinguish it from other counters or windows in the entrance area, such as the cashier, a security desk, or reception area for the admitting department.

- Make the information desk accessible and welcoming to all users. As patients and visitors stop, the area surrounding the desk may become crowded. Thus, the surrounding circulation area needs to be generously designed to prevent congestion. The desk should have a portion of the counter low enough—30 to 33 inches (76 to 83 cm) high—for the wheelchair user to talk comfortably with an attendant or to fill out forms.[11]

- Provide special training to staff at the information desk in giving directions. The Bellevue Hospital experience (see Research Box #3) shows that a percentage of those stopping at the information desk will receive what they consider to be misinformation. Although some of the problem may be due to the sign system or to forgotten or misinterpreted instructions, a uniform way of giving instructions will still be helpful. One approach is the use of customized maps that patients and visitors can take with them.

Research Box #3: Using the Information Desk as a Wayfinding Aid

As part of an evaluation of a major renovation of their entry area, researchers at Bellevue Hospital in New York City examined the relationship between use of the information desk and wayfinding problems.[19] Through interviews, they found that 74 percent of patients stopped at the information desk before proceeding to their various destinations, and 80 percent of this group thought they were given accurate directions. The important role played by the information desk in orientation is shown by the fact that the vast majority of those who thought they were given accurate directions experienced no major problems finding their destination. Unfortunately, 20 percent of those stopping at the information desk thought they had been given misinformation. As a result, most of these individuals experienced a major problem in finding their way. Obviously, not all of those who enter the facility will feel it is necessary to stop at the information desk, but its availability is crucial for those who are not familiar with the facility.

Storing Belongings

During the colder months in northern regions, people are bundled up with overcoats, hats, scarves, and mittens. For the outpatient who may be visiting a number of different clinics or the visitor who may spend several hours moving back and forth between the patient's room, the waiting room, and the cafeteria, keeping track of personal belongings may become a nuisance.[1] A simple solution to this problem would be to provide coin-return lockers or a coatroom where belongings could be checked and safely stored during the outpatients' or visitors' stay in the building.

Admitting Department

The admitting department is often the second destination for inpatients coming to the health care facility. Typical admissions procedures require patients and their companions to wait, to fill out forms, to have interviews with staff, and probably to visit one or more ancillary services before settling in the patient room. During this process, patients and companions need a comfortable place to wait and a private place to carry on confidential conversations with hospital personnel. The ability of the facility to meet these needs is linked with environmental design (see Research Box #4):[20]

- Because of the personal nature of much of the information discussed in the admitting department, patients should be able to feel that their conversations with the admitting staff will not be overheard. To help ensure acoustic privacy, provide private offices, tall partitions, or spatial separations of task areas.

- Store written records in such a way that patient confidentiality is ensured.

- Staff and patients need a comfortable conversational distance between one another. Avoid obstructions, such as computer terminals.

- Patients and their companions need to move about the admitting area safely. Keep passageways clear of obstructions, provide chairs that will not tip over easily, and eliminate furniture with protruding or sharp edges.

- Because many patients who are soon to be admitted are in wheelchairs, provide wheelchair access to desks, seating areas, and circulation paths.

Patient Registration

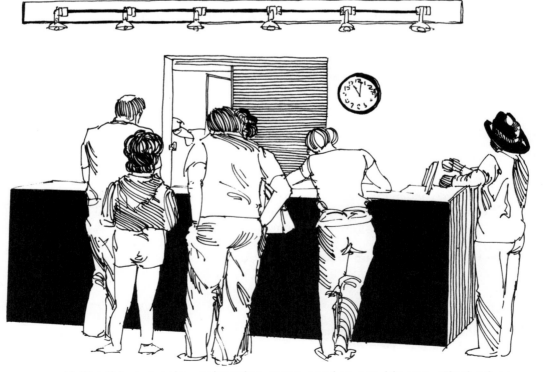

Unlike this example, registration areas need to provide acoustical privacy because patients may need to discuss personal information. Wheelchair access is also an important design criterion.

Research Box #4: Designing an Admitting Department

The relationship between behavioral needs and design in 26 different admitting departments was explored in a detailed study.[20] Four design-related needs were examined: confidentiality (privacy), communication, safety and security, and reduction of stress. Although this study examined only the admitting staffs' *perceptions of patient needs* and how well they were being met by the existing environmental conditions, it provides some valuable insights into links between environment and behavior:

Confidentiality (Privacy): Admitting staff considered confidentiality to be the patient's most urgent need. While being admitted to the hospital, patients must report, both verbally and in writing, a wide range of personal information concerning their health history and financial status, as well as their current health problems. The researcher found that the overall design of the department and the proximity of spaces within the department affected perceived confidentiality and privacy. An open plan, where visual and acoustical privacy was limited, was generally disliked by the staff. They believed that it intruded not only upon the patient's privacy but on theirs as well. Partitions and private offices, however, seemed to give a symbolic sense of confidentiality even though acoustic privacy was not appreciably increased. The spatial "buffering" of work, waiting, and interview areas increased the perception of visual and acoustical privacy.

Communication: Communication refers to those design features that increase or decrease the ability to have successful conversations. Increasing communication was seen by the staff as the patient's second most urgent need. Reduction of noise levels and other distractions increased communication. Interestingly, symbolic aspects of the design also were considered important. Furniture arrangements (such as the spatial arrangement and proximity of chairs and the use of a desk as a potential barrier) were seen as indicators of communication. Other symbolic factors, such as whether patients and staff were supplied chairs of equal quality, were also linked to communication.

Safety and Security: Although admitting staff were concerned about their own security and the security of their belongings, they were more worried about the patient's safety while in the admitting department. In particular, they felt that some chairs could easily be tipped over, that some spaces were too small to allow safe wheelchair access, and that some surfaces had dangerously protruding sharp edges.

Reduction of Stress: Being admitted to a hospital is a stress-inducing experience. However, design elements can be used to reduce stress.

Admitting staff taking part in this study believed that the reduction of stress was the patient's least urgent need, whereas they rated it as their own second most urgent need (behind communication). Ambient factors seemed to be particularly important to stress reduction: the ability to control noise, thermal comfort (both temperature and humidity), and lighting. The availability of natural lighting from windows was particularly enjoyed. In addition, the ability to find one's way easily was considered an important stress reducer.

Visitor Information Center

Hospitals and other long-term care facilities often receive visitors who are feeling stressed because of the hospitalization of a loved one and also because of the unfamiliar setting. Visitors tend to be strangers in a technical and seemingly threatening environment.

Unfortunately, visitors are often the forgotten people of the hospital or long-term care facility. Even though they are present in large numbers, visitors typically have no official role, no connection with the administration, and no space of their own. Their need for basic information about services, procedures, or even the location of a suitable place to eat are often not met.[13]

Visitors seem to be caught in an information dilemma. They need information, but their greatest contact with people in the hospital other than the patient is with other visitors. Any true exchange of information tends to be informal and accidental. Visitors often share the same waiting space, but communication between them is limited by a reluctance to bother someone else who is worried. Visitors are also reluctant to approach the medical staff for information, fearing that time spent with them is time taken away from the patient. This isolation leads many visitors to perceive their concerns as insignificant and results in their acting quite passively about finding solutions.[1]

One approach to relieving the invisible visitor syndrome is to provide a central area where visitors can bring their questions and problems and, perhaps most important, come in contact with each other. The health care facility has an opportunity to demonstrate its concern for the stress most visitors are experiencing by anticipating the visitors' need for information. Visitors would greatly appreciate some center where they could easily get information about hospital policies, overnight accommodations, food, shopping, parking, and social services. A message board and a ride board for arranging carpools are additional services that would be welcomed.[1,21]

Conclusion

The arrival process is quite complex, involving such diverse issues as access, orientation, and physical comfort. This chapter has outlined some of the design-related needs of patients and visitors that will make the transition from home to first destination as comfortable as possible. But arriving is only the first stage of the patients' and visitors' journey. After arriving, they may visit various public spaces (for example, the cafeteria, chapel, gift shop, or main lobby), they may be headed toward a diagnostic or treatment clinic, or they may be going to an inpatient room. The chapters that follow trace each of these journeys.

Design Review Questions

Traveling to the Health Care Facility

Arriving by Car

Wayfinding
- ☐ Do all building names make sense to the general public?[2]
- ☐ Is the sign copy consistent in using the same term when referring to the same destination?[3,4]
- ☐ Is the sign copy short enough so that a driver can read it quickly?[3,5]
- ☐ Are directional signs worded in such a way that the message is communicated clearly to all users?[3,4]
- ☐ Whenever possible, have messages been stated in positive terms?[3,4]
- ☐ Are the words and phrases used within a sixth-grade reading level?[4]

Exterior Sign Visibility
- ☐ Does the sign face the driver directly and can it be easily read from behind the steering wheel?[4,5]
- ☐ Is the sign located so that it is easily seen? Is it within the viewer's 60-degree "cone of vision"?[5]
- ☐ Does the color combination of letters and background provide enough contrast?[4,7-9]
- ☐ To accommodate persons who are color blind, does the color scheme avoid relying on red and green?[4,7-9]
- ☐ Are the letters on the sign large enough to be read while driving the posted speed limit?[4]

  Are exterior signs visible at night as well as during the day?

Number of Signs and Sign Placement[10]
- ☐ Is the sign system designed so that the driver is given appropriate information as it is needed?
- ☐ Has a hierarchical system of major and minor signs been developed?
- ☐ Do major directional signs point the way to the facility from adjacent streets and the parking area?

Notes

Design that Cares: Planning Health Facilities for Patients and Visitors, by Janet R. Carpman, Myron A. Grant, and Deborah A. Simmons. ©1986 by American Hospital Publishing, Inc.

☐ Do minor directional signs point the way to secondary entrances, staff or delivery entrances, and other special entrances?

☐ Do minor directional signs indicate traffic flow for people, cars, and bicycles?

Special Signage for Handicapped Persons
☐ Is the international symbol of access used consistently?[11]

Environmental Cues
☐ Are buildings and the adjacent landscape designed to provide easily identifiable orientation cues?[12]

Drop-Off Area
☐ Has easy access been provided to the drop-off area from major roads leading to the facility?

☐ Is the drop-off area located immediately adjacent to the front door?

☐ Is there sheltered access to the building?

☐ Is there barrier-free access between the drop-off area and the area inside the main entrance?

☐ If the volume and characteristics of patients and companions warrant it, is there an attendant on duty throughout the day to assist people in making their way between their car and the building entrance?

☐ Is the drop-off area designed so that there is ample room for cars dropping off and picking up patients and for those that are driving through?

☐ Is parking provided nearby, and is the route clearly identified with signs?

☐ Is there a taxi stand nearby that does not create congestion in the drop-off area? Or, is there a system by which taxis can be called when needed?

Parking

Long-Term Parking Rates
☐ Has the facility developed a long-term parking fee schedule that takes into consideration financial hardships faced by long-term patients and visitors?[1]

Park and Ride Options
☐ If patient and visitor parking is not within easy walking distance of the facility, are shuttle buses available at frequent intervals?[1]

☐ Is a comfortable, safe, weather-protected place with seating available for those waiting for the shuttle bus?

Notes _____

Design that Cares: Planning Health Facilities for Patients and Visitors, by Janet R. Carpman, Myron A. Grant, and Deborah A. Simmons. ©1986 by American Hospital Publishing, Inc.

Parking for Permanently Disabled Persons
- [ ] Has the facility developed a parking policy that meets the special needs of permanently disabled persons?
- [ ] Are there handicapped-accessible parking spaces reserved in close proximity to the facility entrance?
- [ ] Are all spaces that are reserved for handicapped use clearly marked with the international symbol of access?[11]

Parking for Temporarily Disabled Persons
- [ ] Has the facility developed a parking policy that meets the special needs of temporarily disabled persons (such as those on crutches, with casts, with bad backs, or those who have had recent surgery)?[13]

Arriving by Public Transit
- [ ] Is a city bus stop adjacent or easily accessible to the facility?
- [ ] Is the bus stop in an obvious location with good visibility to and from the main entrance?
- [ ] Are signs and maps (including audible and tactile messages) available to aid people in finding the bus stop?[4,11]
- [ ] Is the bus shelter a comfortable, adequately-sized, and weather-protected place, with adequate lighting at night and plenty of seating?
- [ ] Are bus schedules, route maps, and fare schedules available to the patients and visitors at a central location?

Making One's Way to the Entrance Area

Wayfinding
- [ ] Has a wayfinding system been developed to guide patients and visitors from the parking area and drop-off area to the entrance?[2]
- [ ] Within a parking structure, are floor numbers visible from every section of the structure?[2]
- [ ] Within a parking lot, are section identification signs and major directional signs visible throughout the lot?

You-Are-Here Maps[15]
- [ ] Are interior and exterior You-Are-Here (YAH) maps available to orient people to the layout of the facility?
- [ ] Are YAH maps placed at the pedestrian exits of a parking area?

Notes

Design that Cares: Planning Health Facilities for Patients and Visitors, by Janet R. Carpman, Myron A. Grant, and Deborah A. Simmons. ©1986 by American Hospital Publishing, Inc.

☐ Are names shown on the buildings of the YAH map?

☐ Are YAH maps placed near identifiable points in the environment so that people will have a unique feature to orient themselves to?

☐ Are YAH maps oriented so that forward is up?

☐ Do the YAH maps include memorable features of the exterior environment?

Safety and Security

☐ Does the parking structure floor-to-ceiling height allow ambulance access?

☐ If someone experiences an emergency within the parking area, are security measures adequate to guarantee that help is available?

☐ Has an emergency audio communication system been installed and maintained?

☐ Are security guards or attendants available to help individuals in need?

☐ Are video cameras available to provide surveillance of the parking area?

☐ Does the parking area have adequate lighting?

Access for Disabled Persons

☐ Are handicapped-accessible parking spaces located on a level surface?[11]

☐ Are the handicapped-accessible parking spaces wide enough to accommodate cars with the car door open to its widest position and for vans equipped with a side wheelchair lift?[11]

☐ Within the parking structure or lot, is a wheelchair route available that will not conflict with auto traffic?[11]

☐ Are elevators available within the parking structure if it is two or more stories high?[11]

☐ Are elevator lobbies easily accessible? If there is a curb, is an access ramp provided?[11]

☐ Are elevators wide enough to accommodate a wheelchair?[4,11,16,17]

☐ Are elevator controls within easy reach of someone who is seated?[4,11,16,17]

☐ Is the route from the parking or drop-off area accessible to disabled people during all seasons?[11]

☐ Are sidewalks wide enough to allow two wheelchairs to pass easily?[4,11,16,17]

Notes _____

Design that Cares: Planning Health Facilities for Patients and Visitors, by Janet R. Carpman, Myron A. Grant, and Deborah A. Simmons. ©1986 by American Hospital Publishing, Inc.

☐ Have obstructions such as benches or other street furniture and drainage grates been eliminated from the circulation path because they may make maneuvering difficult for those in a wheelchair or on crutches?[11]

☐ Are curb cuts available at all street crossings?[4,11,16,17]

☐ Are the curb cuts at a low enough grade to be wheelchair accessible?[11]

☐ Are circulation areas free of surfaces that create a bumpy ride?

☐ Are paving materials selected that will not be slippery when wet?

☐ Are grades flat enough to allow easy movement?[11]

☐ Are handrails provided on grades greater than 5 percent?[11,17]

☐ Is signage with raised lettering or braille symbols available for vision-impaired users?[16]

☐ Are changes in sidewalk texture (such as a broomed finish) provided to indicate entrances, streets, and the like to visually-impaired people?[11,17]

☐ Do all warning signals provide visual as well as audible cues?[18]

The Entrance Area

☐ Does the drop-off and entrance area provide sufficient weather protection for the local climate?

☐ Are ashtrays available?

☐ Is there a mud walk-off mat?

☐ Is the entrance area spacious enough to minimize congestion?

Introducing the Interior Wayfinding System

☐ Is there a well-designed and optimally located set of interior signs and maps placed near the entrance, in conjunction with an information desk, to help orient patients and visitors to the facility?

Providing for Special Users[11,17]

☐ Is the entrance area accessible to handicapped persons as well as to persons with baby strollers?

☐ Is the doorway passable by someone in a wheelchair or someone who is vision-impaired?

☐ Have automatic doors been considered at major entrances and other places frequently used by permanently or temporarily disabled persons?

☐ Can the door be opened by someone without much upper body strength?

Notes

Design that Cares: Planning Health Facilities for Patients and Visitors, by Janet R. Carpman, Myron A. Grant, and Deborah A. Simmons. ©1986 by American Hospital Publishing, Inc.

☐ If the force needed to open the door must exceed 8 pounds (to avoid having it blown open by the wind), has an automatic door activated by an electric eye or pressure-sensitive mat been installed?

☐ Is the entrance area free of obstructions?

☐ Are mud walk-off mats and pressure-sensitive mats flush with the floor?

☐ Are ashtrays, newspaper machines, chairs, and other pieces of furniture out of the circulation path?

☐ Is there a place to store wheelchairs out of the flow of traffic?

Waiting in the Entrance Area
☐ Is there sufficient room in the entrance area for people to wait for their transportation?

☐ Are there comfortable places to sit, and is there room for belongings?

☐ Are rest rooms available nearby?

☐ Are taxi, house, and public phones available?

☐ Are signs and maps available to direct people out of the facility, back to parking, and out to major roads?

First Destinations

Information Desk
☐ Upon entering the facility, can patients and visitors clearly see where they should go for information or assistance?

☐ Can patients and visitors distinguish the information desk from other counters or windows that may be located in the entrance area?

☐ Is the information desk identified by highly visible signage?

☐ Does the staff at the information desk have a clear view of the entrance? Can they see who may need assistance?

☐ Is there sufficient room surrounding the information desk so the circulation area does not become congested?

☐ Does at least some portion of the information desk accommodate the needs of a person seated in a wheelchair?[11]

☐ Has the staff been trained to give directions in a uniform way?[19]

Notes _____

Storing Belongings

☐ Have lockers or a coatroom been provided so that belongings can be checked and safely stored during the outpatients' or visitors' stay in the building?

Admitting Department[20]

☐ Has a comfortable place been provided for patients and companions to wait?

☐ Are interview areas in the admitting department designed to ensure patients' acoustical privacy?

☐ Are written records stored so that confidentiality is ensured?

☐ Are interview areas designed to facilitate conversation and self-disclosure?

☐ Is furniture arranged so those having conversations face one another and are not obstructed by equipment?

☐ Have private offices, tall partitions, or spatial separation of work areas been provided to reduce noise and increase privacy?

☐ Are desks, seating areas, and circulation routes within the department handicapped-accessible?

☐ Are passageways kept clear of obstructions?

☐ Has the furniture been selected with safety in mind?

☐ Are chairs and other furnishings stable?

☐ Has furniture with sharp or protruding edges been avoided?

☐ Can the staff adequately control both temperature and humidity within the admitting department?

☐ Can the staff adequately control the lighting within the admitting department?

☐ Is natural lighting available?

☐ Does the wayfinding system guide patients and their companions from the admitting department to other areas of the facility?

Visitor Information Center

☐ Is there a place for visitors to obtain basic information about services and procedures within the health care facility and other relevant services within the surrounding community?[1,13]

☐ Is there a place where visitors can communicate with other visitors?[1,13]

☐ Are information exchange systems provided, such as a message board or ride board?[1,21]

Notes

References

1. Reizenstein, J. E., Grant, M. A., and Vaitkus, M. A. Visitor activities and schematic design preferences. Unpublished research report #4, Patient and Visitor Participation Project, Office of Hospital Planning, Research and Development, University of Michigan, Ann Arbor, 1981.

2. Carpman, J. R., Grant, M. A., and Simmons, D. A. *No More Mazes: Research About Design for Wayfinding in Hospitals.* Patient and Visitor Participation Project, Office of the Replacement Hospital Program, University of Michigan, Ann Arbor, 1984.

3. Marks, B. The language of signs. In: Pollet, D., and Haskel, P., editors. *Sign Systems for Libraries.* New York: R. R. Bowker Co., 1979.

4. American Hospital Association. *Signs and Graphics for Health Care Facilities.* Chicago: AHA, 1979.

5. Follis, J., and Hammer, D. *Architectural Signing and Graphics.* New York: Watson Guptill, 1979.

6. Passini, R. Wayfinding: a study of spatial problem-solving with implications for physical design. Ph.D. dissertation, Pennsylvania State University, University Park, 1977. Available from UMI, 300 N. Zeeb Road, Ann Arbor, MI 48106.

7. Institute for Signage Research. Technical and psychological considerations for sign systems in libraries. In: Pollet, D., and Haskel, P., editors. *Sign Systems for Libraries.* New York: R. R. Bowker Co., 1979.

8. Wechsler, S. Perceiving the visual message. In: Pollet, D., and Haskel, P., editors. *Sign Systems for Libraries.* New York: R. R. Bowker Co., 1979.

9. Weisman, G. D. Way-finding and architectural legibility: design considerations in housing environments for the elderly. In: Regnier, V., and Pynoos, J., editors. *Housing for the Elderly: Satisfaction and Preferences.* New York: Garland Publishing, Inc., 1982.

10. Selfridge, K. M. Planning library signage systems. In: Pollet, D., and Haskel, P., editors. *Sign Systems for Libraries.* New York: R. R. Bowker Co., 1979.

11. Harkness, S. P., and Groom, J. N. *Building without Barriers for the Disabled.* New York: Watson Guptill, 1976.

12. Carpman, J. R., Grant, M. A., and Simmons, D. A. Hospital design and wayfinding: a video simulation study. *Environment and Behavior.* 1985 May.

13. Reizenstein, J. E., and Grant, M. A. Patient and visitor issues: currently unmet needs and suggested solutions. Unpublished research report #4a, Patient and Visitor Participation Project, Office of Hospital Planning, Research and Development, University of Michigan, Ann Arbor, 1981.

14. Shumaker, S., and Reizenstein, J. E. Environmental factors affecting inpatient stress in acute care hospitals. In: Evans, G. W., editor. *Environmental Stress.* New York: Cambridge University Press, 1982.

15. Levine, M. You-are-here maps: psychological considerations. *Environment and Behavior.* 1982 Mar. 14(2):221-37.

16. Kamisar, H. Signs for the handicapped patron. In: Pollet, D., and Haskel, P., editors. *Sign Systems for Libraries.* New York: R. R. Bowker Co., 1979.

17. English Tourist Board. *Providing for Disabled Visitors.* Pamphlet, English Tourist Board, 1983.

18. Carpman, J. R., Grant, M. A., and Norton, C. Needs of the hearing impaired in a hospital setting. Unpublished research report #30, Patient and Visitor Participation Project, Office of the Replacement Hospital Program, University of Michigan, Ann Arbor, 1984.

19. Olsen, R. V., and Pershing, A. Environmental evaluation of the interim entry to Bellevue Hospital. Unpublished report, Environmental Psychology Department, Bellevue Hospital, New York, 1981.

20. Valenta, A. L. Human behavioral needs in hospital admissions management: some architectural implications. Ph.D. dissertation, University of Illinois at the Medical Center, Chicago, 1981. Available from UMI, 300 N. Zeeb Road, Ann Arbor, MI 48106.

21. Zimring, C. M., Carpman, J. R., and Michelson, W. Designing for special populations: mentally retarded persons, children, hospital visitors. In: Stokols, D., and Altman, I., editors. *Handbook of Environmental Psychology.* New York: John Wiley and Sons. In press.

Chapter 3

Wayfinding and the Circulation System

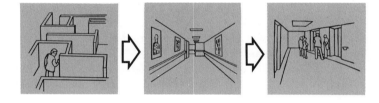

Making One's Way   Corridor Design   Unplanned Uses

The circulation system of a facility consists of passages—corridors, elevators, and stairways—full of movement by both people and materials. These passages tie the facility together. But even though the prime function of the circulation system is to get people and materials to their destinations, circulation needs to be thought of in much broader terms. Circulation passages are also places where patients and visitors spend time waiting, gathering information, and talking. They are places where equipment is stored. They are places where members of the medical staff confer. They are also places where people can become confused or lost.

This chapter begins by examining how people find their way around large, complex buildings—the kinds of buildings that often house health care services. We will describe various components of a "wayfinding system," such as floor numbering, sign terminology and You-Are-Here map design, while emphasizing that these elements need to work in a mutually reinforcing way to make sense to first-time users. We then look at major design features within the circulation system of corridors, stairways, and elevators, emphasizing how these can be designed to meet the needs of patients and visitors.

Making One's Way through the Facility _____

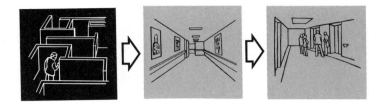

For patients and visitors, time spent in a health care facility is often filled with anxiety over a threatening illness. With the demands of illness or a family crisis occupying their minds, these people may not pay attention to their route in the corridors of a complex and unfamiliar environment. When under stress and preoccupied with their own concerns, they cannot necessarily rely upon previous knowledge about how to make their way through the facility. Consequently, what might otherwise be considered little inconveniences, such as maze-like and cluttered corridors, may tax the emotional strength of a patient facing surgery or a visitor concerned about a critically ill relative (see also chapter 8).[1,2]

Unfortunately, many health care environments are not designed so people can find their way easily. Health care facilities are often housed in large and complex buildings. They are often built incrementally, with the inadvertent result that common patient and visitor destinations are not necessarily near one another. A single trip to see a doctor, with its associated diagnostic tests, may seem like a tour of the entire medical complex. The difficulties patients encounter are complicated by the physical limitations of illness, such as increased stress and a lack of visual acuity or stamina. Confusing signs that use medical terminology make their experience even more difficult.

As individuals make their way through the environment, they are hindered or helped by the availability of a variety of environmental cues. In a successful wayfinding system, specific orientation aids, such as signs, maps, colored lines, directories, landmarks, and the site and building layouts themselves, combine to help guide people to their destinations. The close proximity of common destinations, availability of visual cues that provide landmarks (such as windows, plants, artwork, changes in floor covering), easily understood terminology, clear floor and room numbering systems, availability of well-trained staff for giving directions, and the signage system should all work together as an integrated system. No one element can work in isolation. Because the emphasis is on the development of a clear, efficient, and nonstressful wayfinding system, there should be a number of guiding and reinforcing cues.[3]

Costs of Unsuccessful Wayfinding

Successful wayfinding experiences, those occasions when everything goes well, are seldom thought about. On the other hand, an unsuccessful wayfinding experience is

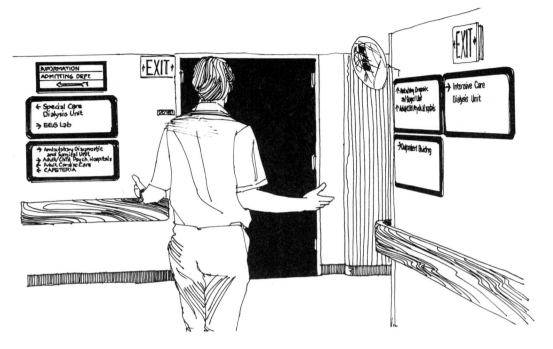

First-time users of large health care facilities like hospitals are often overwhelmed by the complexity of the building, the quantity of signs, and the unfamiliar language used on those signs.

not soon forgotten and may incur both direct and indirect costs. For people having trouble finding their way, time may be lost or appointments missed. For employees in a particularly confusing building, work time may be lost by frequently giving directions and having to learn new routes.[5-8]

And there are other costs associated with disorientation. There is considerable evidence to support the notion that a spatial disorientation is disruptive and causes stress.[9-11] The amount of stress produced by disorientation depends on the individual's ability to cope with uncertainty and varies with specific situations, such as the need to be on time for an appointment. However, in analyzing the relationship between disorientation and design, it is important to consider that wayfinding problems have their own particular costs in the health care environment. Stress caused by disorientation may result in feelings of helplessness, raised blood pressure, headaches, increased physical exertion, and fatigue.[2] In addition, patients may be affected by the wayfinding troubles of visitors who, because they became lost, may have less time to spend with patients. In one study of visitor stress, it was found that the largest source of stress for visitors was trying to find their way around the hospital.[12]

The wayfinding problems faced by a visitor or patient are graphically outlined in the following "typical trip" to a hospital clinic:

Parked in level "B" (remember Green Area), take elevator to plaza, take bus to hospital entrance (sign reads Outpatient Department); inside to floor 1, corridor 2, turn left on corridor 7 to large directory (information booth was unattended); directory not helpful; told of another information booth down the corridor in the lobby; long walk past corridor 4 to information booth, told, "The clinic is on the second floor; take this corridor (7) to "0" elevator, follow orange tape." Sent from the clinic to the cashier on the first floor. Stepping from the elevator, see sign saying "cashier" but the window is closed. Ask the pharmacist, who says, "Down this corridor and on your left." In transit, see signs for parking, pay cashier and ask directions: "Walk right through the lobby to the elevator and down." At the elevator the sign reads, "Elevator to Brown level." A bus arrives to take to car in the Green level? "B" level? "B" Area?. . .[10]

The stress brought about by disorientation may also express itself in anger, hostility, discomfort, indignation, or even panic. The disorientation felt by those visiting a particular facility may surface as a generalized hostility toward the organization.[13] Finally, an employer may experience indirect wayfinding costs such as high rates of personnel turnover and absenteeism due to the stress brought about by employees continually trying to find their way.[5,7]

For the elderly and other particularly vulnerable populations, problems with spatial orientation may have a significant, long-term impact. One study suggests that problems with wayfinding may affect the older person's sense of control.[3] Special simulation techniques have been developed to familiarize older people about to move to a care facility with a layout of the new environment. The premise for this work is that having wayfinding information prior to moving may somewhat diminish negative effects of relocation, such as increased incidence of illness and even death.[14]

The importance of this link between stress and wayfinding is reinforced by additional empirical evidence. One study of the relationship between stress and the availability of orientation aids found that when additional wayfinding aids such as directional signs were provided, there was a decrease in reported levels of stress.[11] However, another study points out that the use of a lot of signage may be an indication of an environment that does not enable people to find their way easily. In this case, signs are used as an attempt to remedy a confusing building.[15]

Landmarks and Building Layout

Trying to find a particular destination involves a complex interaction between a person and the environment. In essence, making one's way through the "maze," moving from here to there, involves a spatial problem-solving process.[16] To find their way, individuals use their previous knowledge of the building or of buildings in general, in conjunction with cues "read" from the environment. Along the path, wayfinders must constantly make choices—a right turn here, continue straight there—based on these cues.[9,17,18] However, to make the necessary choices, to solve the "maze," wayfinders must continually know where they are in relation to their final destination. Without this sense of location, the individual may feel lost and become disoriented.

It is easy to assume that signs and directories are the most effective elements of a wayfinding system. But in a study of orientation in university buildings, it was

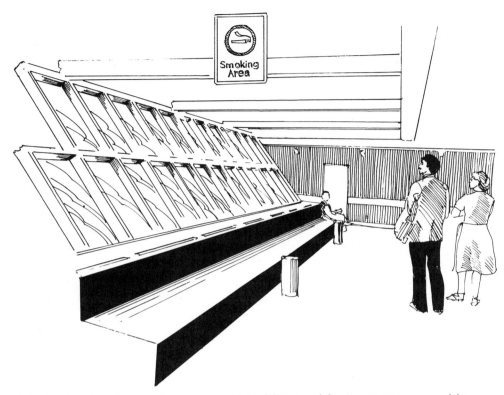

Interior landmarks, such as unusual architectural features or memorable artwork, can help people make sense of a complex environment.

found that the "form" of the building (including the number of corridors, the placement of points where a directional choice must be made, and the building's symmetry) constituted the strongest predictor of successful wayfinding.[15] The availability of environmental cues and architectural features like visual distinctiveness, well-differentiated spaces, and easily recognized landmarks (such as plants, artwork, and furniture arrangements) all give wayfinders useful information about their location.[9,18,19] Instead of simply moving sequentially from one sign or spot along the path to another with no idea of how it all fits together, moving through a building that has a sufficient number of landmarks, views to the outside, and easily differentiated spaces can result in an understanding of the overall structure of the building and the interrelationship of its constituent spaces. Such an overall understanding allows the individual to move freely and easily throughout the building, without becoming lost.

General considerations for developing a coherent wayfinding system include:

- Consider first-time users of the health care facility as the "least common denominator" for decision making regarding wayfinding. These are the people who will be most unfamiliar with every aspect of the setting and, correspondingly, those likely to experience the most wayfinding-related stress. If the wayfinding system works for the first-time user, it will work for all users.[1]

- Keep in mind that the way to reduce the maze-like quality of health care facilities is not to rely on a single device like signs, but to design or implement a mutually reinforcing group of aids—a wayfinding system. Such a system may include, but not be limited to, the basic layout of the building and site, interior and exterior landmarks, signs, maps, terminology, color coding, floor and room numbering systems, and verbal directions.[3]

- When possible, locate related functions that patients and visitors will be using in close proximity to one another. (For instance: admitting, laboratory, and X-ray.)[1]

- If a new health care facility is being designed, consider the impact of the building's form (including the number of corridors, views to the outside, location of decision points such as corridor intersections, and building layout) on wayfinding for first-time users.[15]

- Develop interior landmarks by using such elements of design as the architecture, lighting, color, texture, artwork, and plants to make different parts of the hospital as unique, noticeable, and memorable as possible.[1]

Floor and Room Numbering Schemes

The patient's and visitor's arrival at a health care facility requires negotiation of city streets, parking areas, and pathways to the facility's entrance. For the most part, their travel remains within the same plane; route decisions primarily involve which way to turn. But once inside the facility, an additional level of complexity is added: floor choice. Floor choice is made more complex if potential destinations are found below grade level (see Research Box #1), if buildings are linked together by corridors or "skyways," and if floors are labeled in ways not understandable to first-time users.

From the user's point of view, being able to find the right floor may be more problematic than finding a destination on a particular floor. This was illustrated by one study that showed a majority of the wayfinding errors made by people trying to find their way in a town hall related to floor choice.[10] Likewise, for an elderly population, getting off on the wrong floor has been found to be a common and frustrating experience.[20] Floor number confusion can be reduced in several ways:

- Floor number designations should logically relate to the main entry floor and should indicate whether floors are above or below grade.

- Consider the relationship among floor numbers of buildings that are linked together; avoid situations where floor 2 of one building links to floor 4 of another.[1]

- Design floor designations so that they can be easily used in the room numbering system for each level (for example, rooms in floor 5 would all begin with the number 5).[6]

- Begin rooms on floors below the entrance level with a prefix likely to be widely understood by first-time users (see Research Box #1).[6]

Research Box #1: Numbering Floors

With construction of a new adult general hospital by the University of Michigan, a need arose to examine floor numbering options and to select the most effective system. The new hospital would have two floors below the main entry level, one of which would continue into the new outpatient building. Given this spatial arrangement, the task was to develop a floor numbering scheme that would be understandable.

Researchers conducted a study of the advantages and disadvantages of various floor numbering options.[6] The study was designed to discover which of several feasible and conventional floor numbering alternatives would be most comprehensible to hospital inpatients, outpatients, visitors, and staff. Because floor numbers would have to be abbreviated to fit on elevator buttons, no more than four characters were used for any of the options. The five floor numbering options tested for the floors below the main entry level were *A, B; B1, B2; Sub 1, Sub 2; 1, 2; and LL1, LL2.*

Participants were asked a series of questions concerning (1) the clarity of various options in relation to a simple wayfinding task (2) their rating of each option regarding its overall desirability, and (3) their choice of the "best" and "worst" options. From the results of these interviews, the option that was interpreted clearly most often and was highly preferred by patients and visitors was *Sub 1, Sub 2.*

Sub 1 and *Sub 2* give the user a clear point of reference and a clear distance to travel. To most people, the term *Sub* designated something that might be found below; *Sub 1* meant one floor below entry, and *Sub 2* meant two floors below entry. None of the other alternatives provided as clear a point of reference. With *A, B* and with *B1, B2* the users did not know which was the lowest level; with *LL1, LL2* the participants found it difficult to interpret *LL,* and with *1, 2* there was confusion about where floor counting began, at the lowest level or at the entry floor.

However, while the staff saw wayfinding as an important patient and visitor criterion for deciding on a floor numbering scheme, they also considered the image projected by the numbering options. Many of the staff reported that any alternative that suggested that the floors were in the basement (that is, *B1, B2* and *Sub 1, Sub 2*) produced a bad image. They felt that it might be demoralizing and feared that patients would not want to be treated in a basement.

The ability of a floor numbering scheme to project an image is interesting, if not directly related to wayfinding concerns. However, in selecting an alternative that seems to best meet the wayfinding needs of patients and visitors (for example, *Sub 1, Sub 2*), some methods of moderating the "basement" image of the space need to be addressed.

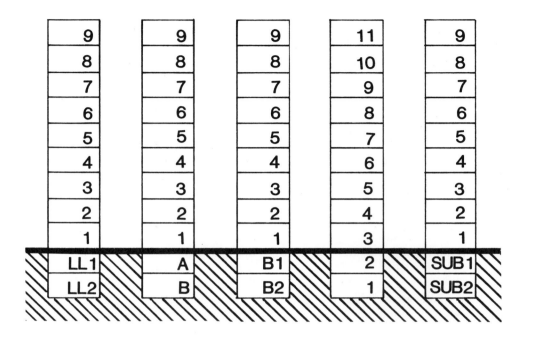

9	9	9	11	9
8	8	8	10	8
7	7	7	9	7
6	6	6	8	6
5	5	5	7	5
4	4	4	6	4
3	3	3	5	3
2	2	2	4	2
1	1	1	3	1
LL1	A	B1	2	SUB1
LL2	B	B2	1	SUB2

See Research Box #1: These five floor-numbering options were evaluated for a building with two floors below the entry level.

Once patients and visitors reach the appropriate floor, they continue to search for their destination. Although some rooms will be identified by name (such as *Surgery Waiting Area*), they may need to find a room or office with only a room number to guide them. The logic and placement of room numbers along the corridor will aid their search. At corridor intersections, room numbers will help them select whether to turn left or right and, of course, watching for the specific room number will tell them when they have reached their proper destination.

Although there is no foolproof way to ensure usefulness of a room numbering system to first-time users, there are ways to make the system effective. Simplicity, consistency, flexibility, and visibility should be major criteria.

A numbering scheme should be simple. For instance, rooms could be numbered in a continuous series with odd numbers on the left side of the hall and even numbers on the right. Or, patient rooms could be numbered consecutively and separately from staff rooms. Simplicity might also suggest a correspondence between the room number and floor number, for instance, all rooms on the fifth floor would begin with the number 5. Another consideration related to simplicity is to avoid using a combination of letters and numbers to identify a space (such as *NIB416*), because sequences like this are difficult to read and remember. There is also the potential for confusion between letters and numbers (such as the letters *I, O, Q*, and the numerals *1* and *0*).

If at all possible, room numbering schemes should be used consistently from floor to floor when floors have similar layouts. Again, they should begin with the floor number and progress in the same direction on each floor.

One seemingly pervasive characteristic of hospital buildings is that they undergo almost constant renovation.[21] A side effect of renovation is that corresponding room numbers will come and go. Consequently, the room numbering system needs to be flexible enough to allow for future renovation without unduly disrupting its logic. Leaving out a few numbers at planned intervals is one approach.

Efforts to produce a room numbering system that is simple, consistent, and flexible should be supplemented by attention to the numbers' visibility. For those rooms that patients and visitors will identify primarily by number, the numbers need to be large and graphically contrasting enough to be easily recognized. The requirements of elderly users and people with vision impairments also need to be carefully considered.

In designing a room numbering system, consider these points:

- Design the room numbering system to be flexible enough to allow for future expansion and renovation without undue disruption of the sequence.[1]

- Use the numbering system consistently on floors having similar use and layout.[1]

- Within the numbering system, differentiate between those numbers needed by patients and visitors and those used only by staff. One way is to use a larger size number on signs indicating patient or visitor destinations than on signs directed only at staff.[1]

- With the exception of inpatient rooms, identify by name those rooms that will be primary patient and visitor destinations. Use numbers or numbers and names for rooms used primarily by staff.[1]

- If a room's number is its primary means of identification by patients and visitors, make the number large enough to be easily seen.[1]

- Place patient room numbers so that they are visible when the door is open.

- If possible, avoid using a combination of letters and numbers to identify a space, such as NIB407.[1]

- If letters and numbers must be used in the same sign, avoid those letters that may be interpreted as numbers, such as I, O, and Q.[1]

- Start numbering systems as close as possible to the main entry point for that floor—such as the lobby, outpatient entrance, or elevators.[22]

- Whenever possible, use a simple numbering system, such as numbering rooms in a continuous series with odd numbers on one side of the hall and even numbers on the other.[22]

- Use sign materials that will resist damage and are easily stocked and replaced.[1]

- Consider coordinating inpatient room and telephone numbers.[1]

Terminology

Signs are intended to communicate. As in any form of communication, however, the messages on signs must be appropriately targeted to their audience. Unfortunately, selecting the most appropriate words may not be easy. As described in chapter 2, the audience for any particular set of signs in a health care facility is quite broad, including medical staff, patients, visitors, and service personnel. A further complication for a substantial number of users is that English is their second language.

Health care facilities with large numbers of consumers who speak a language other than English may need to consider the benefits and costs of bilingual or multilingual signs and other information materials. It is certainly preferable to direct information to people in ways they can best understand. In fact, a health care facility that provides information in the consumer's native language also conveys an important symbolic message of sensitivity and respect for the user's ethnic heritage—something that may be an important marketing advantage. However, multilingual signs imply more words per sign or more signs per location and risk a situation of information overload where signs are not heeded at all.[23]

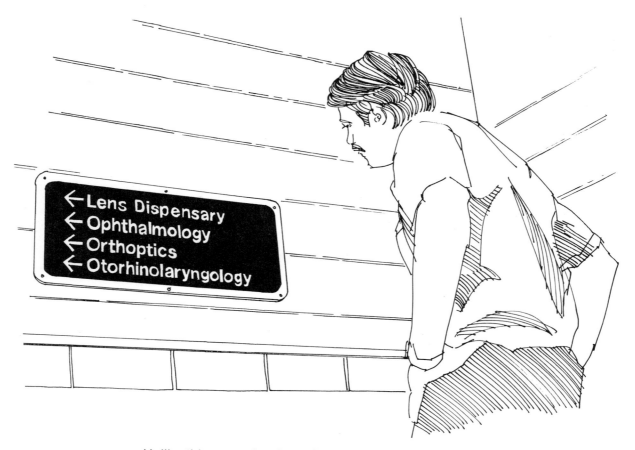

Unlike this example, signs directed at patients and visitors should use terminology they can understand.

Although the terms used on signs and in verbal directions represent a major way in which the health care facility communicates with its consumers, many of the technical and medical terms used may not be widely understood by patients and visitors (see Research Box #2). Developing a terminology system comprehensible to all users avoids the risks of increasing the number of misunderstandings and the number of patients or visitors having trouble finding their way. The problems stemming from use of overly technical terminology are illustrated by the following incident:

An elderly woman was spotted in the hospital by a hospital staff member who thought she looked lost. He asked the woman where she was trying to go and she said, "Gerontology." The staff member started to give detailed directions, but because the Institute of Gerontology was located several blocks away, he asked if she was sure that this was her destination. "Oh yes," she said, "I have it right here on this slip of paper." On the slip of paper was written *gastroenterology.*

Confusion caused by misreading or misunderstanding technical or medical terminology increases the likelihood that some persons, like the elderly woman in the example, will have a difficult time finding their way and will wind up being late for, or perhaps missing, an appointment. Patients or visitors may refrain from asking questions because they think they understand a term when they really do not. Or, the term may cause needless worry about their illness:

A patient told one hospital staff member that earlier in his treatment he had been scheduled to go to nuclear medicine for some tests. He became so frightened at the thought of being bombarded with radiation that he almost canceled his appointment. To him, *nuclear medicine* meant *radiation.* He also assumed it meant that he had a terminal disease for which there would be little hope. To his surprise and joy, his fears on both counts were unfounded.

Any such difficulty represents far more than a mere inconvenience. Being lost or confused can result in anger, stress, and missed appointments. It may also cause some people to choose another health care facility, where they feel more confident about finding their way. People dislike showing ignorance, and a signage system that is misunderstood may cause people to feel incompetent. Although patients interviewed in one study did not think there would be a difference in the quality of medical care at a hospital using lay terms as compared with one using medical terms, they said the terminology used would influence their choice of a hospital. In other words, all things being equal, the majority of these patients would choose to go to a hospital using lay terms.[1] The use of an inappropriate signage system, one that relies too heavily on unfamiliar medical or technical terms, runs the risk of alienating visitors and patients.

Research Box #2:
Selecting Terms to Use on Signs

Although general guidelines for writing sign copy exist, it has not been clear how these guidelines should be translated for use in a health care facility. Little information was available to planners at the University of Michigan to guide them in determining those terms that were most appropriate and would be best understood. As part of the Patient and Visitor Participation Project, studies were conducted to help guide the selection of appropriate hospital signage terminology.[1] Medical terms conventionally used for hospital departments and procedures (such as *Otorhinolaryngology, Cardiology*) were tested along with common language terminology (such as *Ear, Nose, and Throat; Heart*). To gather information on the comprehension of various medical terms, 240 randomly sampled patients and visitors were interviewed.

In all, 67 terms were tested. Each term was tested in at least two ways: (1) presenting the respondent with the technical term and (2) giving the respondent a description or lay definition of the term. In testing each term, the objective was to see if there was a difference in the participant's understanding of lay terms versus technical or medical terms. When testing the technical terms, participants were shown the printed word (for example, *thoracic surgery*) while the interviewer pronounced it clearly. Consequently, participants were given both visual

and aural cues. They were then asked if they felt they knew what the term meant. If they said yes, they were asked what they thought of when they heard that term. For an additional set of terms, participants were given a lay definition (such as, "where people who do not need to be hospitalized receive medical care") and then were asked to give an appropriate term.

The results of the study were not necessarily predictable. Overall, the participants understood a greater number of the technical terms than the researchers originally estimated. However, it cannot be said that the participants consistently favored either the technical or the lay terms. Examples of comprehension include:

Commonly Understood Terms	Commonly Misunderstood Terms
Admitting	Ambulatory Care
Dermatology	Internal Medicine
Cardiology	Endocrine and
Diagnostic Radiology	Metabolism
Intensive Care Unit (ICU)	Neonatal
Ophthalmology	Nuclear Medicine
Pediatrics	Otorhinolaryngology
Psychiatry	Walk-in Clinic

An unexpected finding of the research was that patients and visitors often thought they knew what a term meant when, in fact, they did not.

The following are some suggested guidelines for the development of an understandable signage system:

- Decide separately for each department what terminology is to be used for naming the department and base each decision on patients' and visitors' abilities to understand the term.[1]

- Encourage each department to use consistent terminology on its signs and in its written and verbal communications with patients and visitors.[22,24]

- Develop messages that will be interpreted similarly by all users. Avoid using ambiguous terms like *child care,* which could be interpreted as a nursery or babysitting center or as a pediatric medical care area.[24,25]

- Use consistent terminology on signs throughout the facility. For instance, avoid using *X-ray* on one sign and *radiology* on another.[22,24]

- Whenever possible, state the message in positive terms.[22]

- Avoid using words and phrases on signs that are beyond a sixth-grade reading level.[22]

Symbols and Pictographs

It appears that symbols or pictographs are increasingly being used in conjunction with verbal messages on signs. Symbols for wheelchair access, rest rooms, and telephones have become commonplace in many public buildings. They provide an easily recognizable form of information that requires neither the ability to read nor knowledge of a particular language. Also, when properly designed, symbols can reiterate the message, thus aiding individuals in their task of interpreting sign messages.

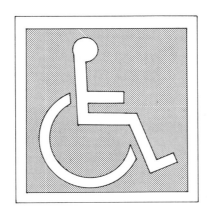

Some symbols used in health care facilities are widely understood, such as this symbol for barrier-free access. Other symbols may not communicate as well.

However, symbols are not a panacea. Many hospital terms do not translate easily into symbols, and a symbol system can quickly become contrived. For those symbols that are used in the health care facility setting, the following considerations are important:

- Before the decision to use symbols is made, test each one for comprehension by patients and visitors.
- Coordinate the entire symbol system so that the styles, colors, shapes, and backgrounds remain consistent.[25]
- Limit the number of symbols used.[25]
- Use only one symbol per message.[25]
- Unless symbols are widely used and recognized, use them only as a supplement to verbal information.[25]
- Avoid using arrows for nondirectional signs.[23]

Signs

In addition to the message itself, in words, symbols, or pictographs, a number of other considerations are necessary in planning a successful sign system.

Mounting and Typeface

The usefulness of any sign system is limited by the ability of patients and visitors to see the information. Signs may be difficult to read if they are mounted too high, located behind another sign, or in a position that reflects glare. In addition, the positioning and construction of signs require safety considerations. The safety and usefulness of signs can be facilitated in the following ways:

- Mount signs with a bottom edge at least 7 feet (2.1 meters) above the floor if they project from the plane of the wall or hang from the ceiling.[22]
- Avoid sharp edges or exposed fasteners on signs.[27]
- Design lighting that does not cause glare on nearby signs.
- Place signs to provide maximum visual exposure, particularly along routes of travel.[28]

Typeface style and size are important in designing a sign system. Although a vast array of typeface styles is available, many are not appropriate for the health care environment, where patients' visual acuity may be poor. Both letter size and style should contribute to easy reading for patients and visitors whose attention span or physical capabilities may be limited:

- Use a combination of upper-case and lower-case letters.[22,28]
- Use sans serif typefaces, that is, those without short cross lines at the end of the strokes.[22]

- Align words at the left margin.[22]

- Use letters that are two to three times larger than the minimal size necessary for reading by a person with normal vision.[29]

- Base minimum letter size on a ratio of 1 inch (2.5 cm) of letter height for each 25 feet (7.5 meters) of distance.[28]

System Maintenance

Health care facilities, especially hospitals, undergo renovations and relocations almost continually.[21] Such changes can play havoc with an otherwise finely tuned sign system. Each time a public destination is moved, many signs must be changed.

There are several ways a health care organization can respond to the ongoing need to update signs. To facilitate consistency and accuracy, sign-related information and decisions should be the responsibility of a single individual. Ideally, data pertaining to each sign in the facility should be stored in a computer system that is easy to manipulate. In this way, when a public destination moves, all the signs that mention that destination can be identified and subsequently altered.

The signs themselves should be fabricated in a way that allows message changes to occur easily, for example, with sliding message panels. However, in order to avoid damage or vandalism, it should not be *too* easy for sign changes to be made.

In order to ensure that the sign system continues to be functional, periodic evaluation is needed, similar to a 12,000-mile car tune-up. Each sign in the system needs to be inspected for accuracy, legibility, and condition. In addition, information about sign-related wayfinding problems may be identified by various departments.

Spacing and Location

Individuals attempting to make their way around an unfamiliar building require a great deal of information. They must "read" the environment, not only in the literal sense of reading signs or directories but also in terms of gathering information from other cues; corridors, windows, stairways, doors, and the type and configuration of furniture. They must use these visual cues to decide if a particular pathway is likely to lead to their destination.

To the person trying to find a particular destination, what is printed on signs is critical—including the typeface, color, letter size, and terminology. But no matter how good the sign is, no matter how legible or clearly worded, if the information is not available where it is needed, the sign's usefulness is drastically diminished. Paying particular attention to the placement and spacing of signs is essential to reduce the maze-like impression of the health care environment. The problem is to determine how many signs are enough or how many are too many, as well as where to locate a sign. There are obvious trade-offs between spacing signs so closely that they become overwhelming and spacing them so infrequently that first-time users become lost.

In determining where signs should be placed, a commonly advocated rule of thumb is to place signs at major decision points, that is, points along the path or corridor where the individual must decide whether to continue in the same direction or to turn.[23,27,30] It has also been suggested that signs be placed some distance beyond these major decision points in order to reassure people that they are on the right track.[17] Although using decision points as a placement criterion is intuitively satisfying, there has been no functional definition of the term *decision point* up until now. The purpose of the study reported in Research Box #3 was to determine where signs should be placed along hospital corridors and to develop a design-relevant definition of the concept of decision point.

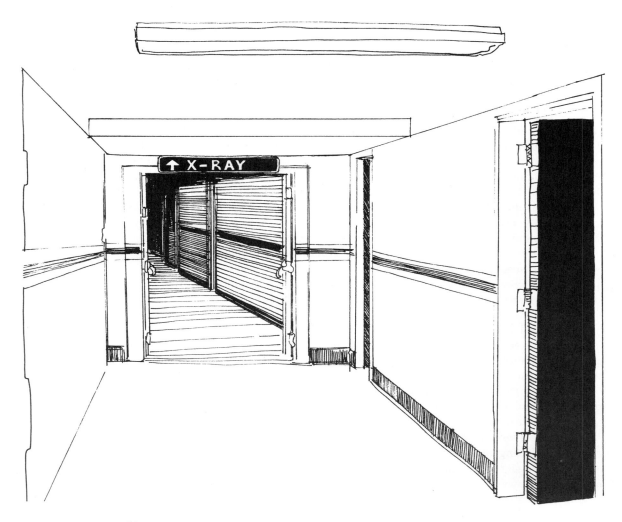

Signs reassuring users that they are on the right route are needed in corridors where an environmental feature indicates entrance to a new area.

Research Box #3: Spacing Signs

To simulate a typical wayfinding experience that patients and visitors would encounter in a hospital, participants in a study at the University of Michigan Hospitals were asked to locate a predetermined destination: the cyclotron.[1] A 660-foot-long corridor in the existing hospital was selected. The length of this corridor closely approximated the longest possible horizontal distance from entrance to destination that patients and visitors could traverse in the new hospital being designed for the university.

Although distance traveled was an important criterion in selecting the experimental setting, its complexity and the existence of various alternative destinations were also important. The portion of the corridor used in the study started at the Physical Medicine and Rehabilitation Department, passed by a major intersection, continued through the Pharmacy and Radiation Therapy departments, passed the Pain Clinic, and ended at a right turn that would take the individual to the cyclotron, the participants' destination. Randomly selected hospital visitors were escorted to the Physical Medicine and Rehabilitation Department and told that their task was to find the cyclotron.

Because the interest was in determining the ideal spacing and placement of signs, the number of signs strategically mounted along the corridor was systematically varied to see if people experiencing different conditions responded differently. As the participant walked along the corridor, the interviewer recorded the number of times the participant asked for directions, the number of times the participant made a wrong turn, the number of times the participant noticeably hesitated, and the amount of time it took the participant to find the cyclotron. After finding the destination, participants were asked to suggest locations for new signs as well as to report any feelings of stress brought about by trying to find the cyclotron.

When the participants' behavior and attitudes were compared across the conditions, it became obvious that the number of signs available at key decision points had a significant effect. Overall, the greater the number of signs available, the more likely the participant was to find the destination faster, to make fewer requests for signs, to hesitate or to ask directions less frequently, and to report a lower level of stress.

The results of this study make it clear that the basis for decisions about the location of signs should be the identification of key decision points rather than an arbitrary distance figure. However, the significance of the study is in defining what those key decision points are. The results of the study point to the placement of directional signs at every major intersection, at major destinations, and where a single environmental cue or a series of such cues (such as change in flooring material, change in color scheme, or a noticeable architectural feature such as a constriction in the hallway) conveys a message that the individual is moving from one area into another. If there are no key decision points along a given route, the results indicate that signs should be placed every 150 to 250 feet.

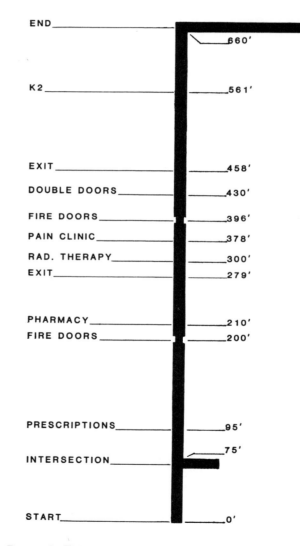

See Research Box #3: This graphic shows the research route for a sign-spacing study along a hospital corridor.

The following are suggested guidelines for locating signs in health care facilities:

● Determine sign locations in conjunction with mechanical and electrical fixtures (such as lights, sprinkler nozzles, and air vents) so that prime sign locations are not blocked.[1]

● Place signs at major decision points along the path. Decision points are places along the corridor where the individual must decide whether to continue in the same direction or to turn (such as at major intersections, at major destinations, and where a single environmental cue or a series of such cues indicates that the individual is moving into a new area).[1]

● Consider placing reassurance signs between 150 and 250 feet (45 and 75 meters) after major decision points, if another decision point has not been reached in the interim.[1,17]

● Place directory panels in central locations.[16,24]

● Locate information consistently so people learn to look for it in a certain place, for example, next to the elevators.[3,26,29,31]

Research Route Scenarios

(Circles represent sign placement)

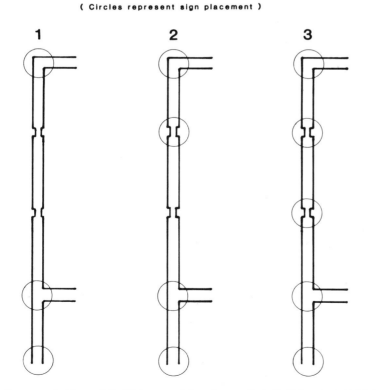

See Research Box #3: This graphic shows the three ways signs were located for a sign-spacing study along a hospital corridor.

Color Coding

Successful wayfinding depends upon reading the physical environment as well as upon reading signs. As individuals make their way through the environment, they will be helped or hindered by available cues. By designing particular cues, such as establishing color coding for departments or floors and using colored lines, banners, or lights, an integrated orientation system can be developed (see Research Box #4).

Colored lines on the floor have long been used in hospitals as easy ways to guide patients and visitors to their destinations. Although this component of a wayfinding system seems to be highly preferred and used by patients and visitors, colored lines on floors or walls are not an intrinsic solution to the wayfinding problem.[1] In large health care facilities with many destinations, it is impossible to have colored lines leading to each destination without creating a multicolored spaghetti of lines on the floor or wall. In a large hospital with many public destinations, a system of floor

---

Research Box #4: Using Banners and Colored Lights to Aid Wayfinding

In conjunction with the construction of a new entry, designers at Bellevue Hospital in New York City developed a new orientation system.[33] The design included carpeting, maps, color coded neon lights and banners, and a numbering system to identify patient destinations.

Several months after the renovation, researchers evaluated the success of the new design. Overall, patients and visitors responded positively. They felt that the appearance of the entry and corridor was much improved and that it showed that Bellevue "was doing something nice for them." Likewise, they noted that the attention paid to the orientation system showed that Bellevue cared about their comfort.

The orientation system itself received mixed reviews. The color cod-ing system of lights and banners seemed to be well understood: 81.7 percent of those interviewed knew what destinations were represented by the various colors. Some respondents felt that the increased interest provided by the lights and banners along the corridor made the journey seem shorter than it actually was. However, patients and visitors found the use of numbered banners (indicating various service areas) and numbered windows (indicating specific locations, such as the screening nurse and the clinic registration area) confusing as destination markers. As a result of this evaluation, the researchers recommended that windows be renamed, using words such as *nurse* or *registration* instead of numbers.

---

lines might work if they led only to major destinations. However, lines on the floor can be covered by carpeting in spots or lost to renovations, and lines on the wall may conflict with signs, artwork, doorways, or other design features.[2]

Small health care facilities with uncarpeted corridors may be best suited to using colored lines as a component of their wayfinding system. In order to be effective, however, only a small number of colors should be used, and these should be highly contrasting to make them easily distinguishable to patients and visitors.

Unfortunately, color coding is often wrongly thought to be an easy solution to wayfinding problems.[32] For example, in very large, complex buildings there are more floors and more potential destinations than any simple color scheme can accommodate. Because most people (let alone those under stress) cannot remember a single shade within a large number of different colors, this approach does not help, but instead adds to the visual confusion.

Another problem with color coding, even in relatively simple, small-scale facilities, is that it is not used strictly for wayfinding purposes. That is, color will be used for decoration in the same area where it is supposed to have meaning for wayfinding. If people cannot tell when color is supposed to mean something and when it is not, color can become ineffective as a wayfinding cue.

If color coding of spaces or color coded lines are to be used, the following recommendations may be helpful in making design decisions:

- Use colored floor lines along with other wayfinding aids as part of an overall system.[1]

- If a facility chooses to use a system of colored lines on the floor, use a small number of highly contrasting colors leading only to major destinations.

- If a color coding scheme has been determined necessary, use it logically and consistently throughout the health care facility. Avoid using colored bands or lines for decoration in facilities where bands or lines are used as wayfinding cues.[22]

Interior You-Are-Here Maps

In chapter 2, we described ways in which You-Are-Here (YAH) maps can help people orient themselves outside the building and find their way from one building to another. Similarly, interior YAH maps can help patients and visitors gain an overall understanding of the building layout. However, the map must be well designed if it is to be a useful addition to the overall wayfinding system (see Research Box #5 and Research Box #6). Individuals using a YAH map must be able to locate themselves accurately in relation to their destination, and to gain enough information from the map to select an appropriate route. Based on available research, the following principles of You-Are-Here map design are worth considering:

- Provide labels on the map that correspond to signs on the walls.[26]

- Place the map near an asymmetrical part of the building so that people have some feature to key on.[26]

Research Box #5: Determining Alignment in You-Are-Here Maps

Until recently, little research-based information has been available concerning the design of You-Are-Here maps. To begin to fill this void, researchers at State University of New York at Stony Brook conducted two experiments examining the effectiveness of alternative designs for You-Are-Here maps.[35] Both experiments looked at the use of You-Are-Here maps in terms of a spatial problem-solving process.

Experiment 1: In a laboratory experiment, students examined a series of 16 slides depicting various YAH maps. The slides differed in where the YAH arrow pointed (that is, whether the YAH map was aligned so that "forward is up") and in the simulated destination that participants were asked to find. After being shown each slide, participants were asked to indicate on a response sheet which direction they would go in order to find their destination. In the second part of this experiment, participants were again shown slides, but this time they were first given a detailed explanation of how to "read" YAH maps and how to orient themselves using the YAH arrow.

Results from both phases of the experiment were quite similar. When the YAH arrow was aligned so that "forward is up," participants gave correct direction-finding responses far more often than when the YAH arrow was not so aligned. Even when given explicit and detailed instructions on how to use the YAH map and arrow, participants consistently misread misaligned maps.

Experiment 2: In the second experiment, participants were asked to find a particular location within the university library. After being escorted to the starting point, participants were shown one of four different maps of the library floor plan (two of the maps were properly aligned and two were misaligned) and asked to find a particular destination. Time spent examining the map and time spent searching for the destination were recorded. Each participant completed the procedure twice, once after viewing an aligned map and once after viewing a misaligned map. Different destinations were assigned for the two trials.

Results were consistent with those of the first experiment. People viewing the aligned maps found their destination significantly more often than those viewing misaligned maps. In addition, those given misaligned maps spent significantly more time viewing the map as well as significantly more time searching for the destination than did those given aligned maps.

- Align the map so that forward is up, (the direction the person is facing while looking at the map should be at the top of the map) and make sure the map is aligned with the building layout.[26]

- Incorporate memorable architectural elements, such as landmarks, into the map design.[26]

- Simplify the map area and highlight public corridors and destinations. Staff areas are not relevant for visitors and need not be emphasized.

- Provide insets on the map showing the relation of the mapped portion of the building to the rest of the health care facility.[34]

- Draw the You-Are-Here arrow pointing in the direction and at the spot the viewer is facing while looking at the map.[26]

Research Box #6: Perspective vs. Plan View in You-Are-Here Maps

As part of a series of ongoing studies of wayfinding, the Patient and Visitor Participation Project at the University of Michigan Hospitals undertook an examination of the design of interior YAH maps.[34] The purpose of this study was to examine two questions not previously addressed in the literature. The first question concerned whether or not hospital patients and visitors would find *a plan view* graphic or *a perspective bird's-eye view* graphic a preferred way of representing the space they were in. The second question concerned whether or not hospital patients and visitors would find it easier to understand a YAH map *with an inset* depicting the location of the focal area in the context of the Medical Center Campus or a map *without such an inset.*

Seventy randomly selected patients and visitors were shown a series of YAH graphics (see below) and asked to voice their preferences. Respondents were asked to choose between:

1. Perspective view (no inset) vs. Plan view (no inset)

2. Plan view (no inset) vs. Plan view (with inset)

3. Perspective view (no inset) vs. Perspective view (with inset)

4. Perspective view (with inset) vs. Plan view (with inset)

Although this research did not examine which map type was superior in helping people find their way, it did show which map type people preferred to look at. The results of this study clearly showed that the perspective view was preferred over the plan view, whether presented with or without the inset. Maps with insets were preferred over those without, whether dealing with plan views or perspective views.

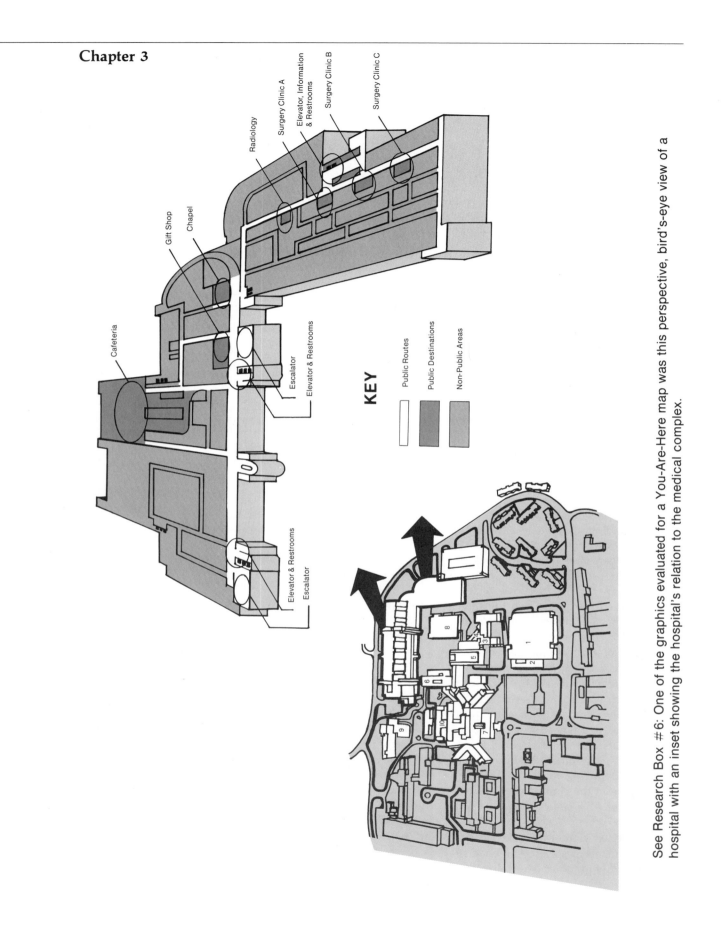

KEY

Public Routes

Public Destinations

Non-Public Areas

See Research Box #6: One of the graphics evaluated for a You-Are-Here map was this perspective, bird's-eye view of a hospital with an inset showing the hospital's relation to the medical complex.

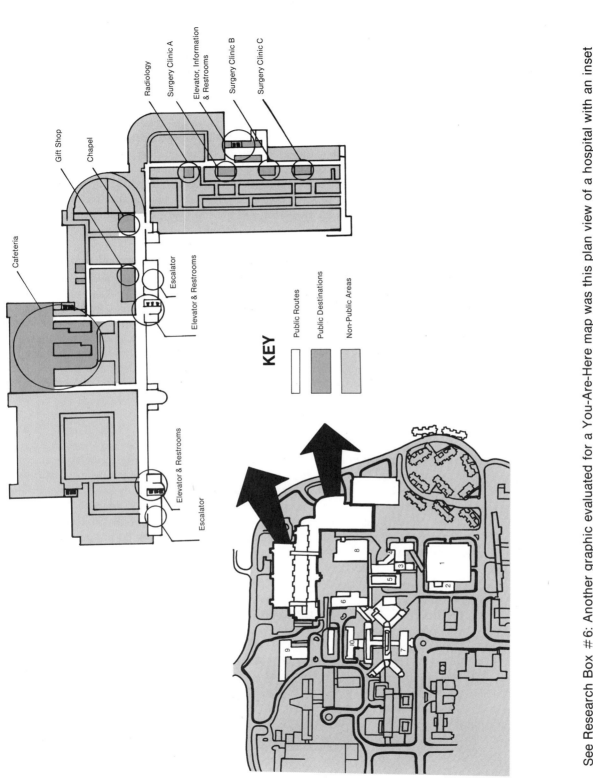

Cafeteria

Gift Shop

Chapel

Radiology

Surgery Clinic A

Elevator, Information & Restrooms

Surgery Clinic B

Surgery Clinic C

Escalator

Elevator & Restrooms

Elevator & Restrooms

Elevator & Restrooms

Escalator

KEY

Public Routes

Public Destinations

Non-Public Areas

See Research Box #6: Another graphic evaluated for a You-Are-Here map was this plan view of a hospital with an inset showing the hospital's relation to the medical complex.

Directions Given by Staff

Some people will need the reassurance that can be obtained only from another human being, regardless of the extent and quality of the overall wayfinding system, including signs, landmarks, the architecture, color coding, or lines on the floor. Although information desks specifically designed to handle this service may be available, other staff and volunteers will still be asked for directions from time to time.[6] Unfortunately, many staff members may not have skills necessary to give directions well. Large health care facilities should therefore consider instituting an ongoing staff training program in giving directions as consistently and accurately as possible.

For example, in light of the imminent occupancy of more than 1 million square feet of new facilities, the University of Michigan Hospitals recognized the need to train more than 800 staff members about details of the new wayfinding system, with special emphasis on giving directions. Training sessions were designed for the different needs of three groups: persons whose major duties involve giving directions, such as information desk attendants, diagnostic and treatment department receptionists, and inpatient unit clerks; persons whose major duties involve traversing the facilities, including messengers, transporters, and phlebotomists; and persons, such as maintenance and security personnel, whose major duties involve quickly locating specific rooms in the facilities.[36,37]

Future Wayfinding Systems

The high tech revolution has reached the realm of wayfinding. New computerized systems are being developed to help individuals select the appropriate destination, personalize their route choice and even generate a map that they can take with them. Computerized systems may not be appropriate for all or even most health care facilities. Nevertheless, the availability of such systems highlights the need to consider a variety of methods and the importance of developing an integrated wayfinding system that serves users' specific needs.

Corridor Function and Amenities

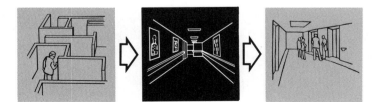

Corridors in health care facilities are often quite long, sometimes running several hundred feet in length. A long corridor of blank walls and undifferentiated doors may be not only uninviting but also a source of visual distortion.[38] Inpatients often need to get up and walk around for therapeutic reasons, and corridors that are perceived to be long and uninteresting will not encourage this activity. Corridors that have windows or other interesting things to look at are likely to be more inviting. However, the simple layout of the corridor should not be sacrificed in order to add to the visual complexity and richness (see also chapter 8).[3] Corridor interest may be increased in a number of ways:

- Use special graphics—including murals, photographic enlargements, wall hangings, paintings, reproductions, and pictorial symbols—to create mood and color. These can also signal changes in direction or use.[3]

- Consider putting some art on the ceiling at particular destinations to provide a focus for those patients on gurneys.[39]

- Route corridors to have views of landscaped areas to provide a focus for attention and wayfinding.[40,41]

- Provide windows along corridors, rather than at the end of corridors.

Carpeting

Carpeted corridors are often suggested as a way to humanize the health care environment. In general, carpeting is considered more comfortable, warmer, and more home-like than most hard-surface flooring.[42,43] Carpeting has also been found to reduce ambient noise levels and injurious falls.[43-46] With proper care, carpeting should pose no microbiological hazard to the typical patient.[47]

Along with the benefits, carpeting in corridors does have its drawbacks. Dietary carts, beds, gurneys, diagnostic machinery, and wheelchairs are more difficult to move on carpeted surfaces, although special casters and a low-pile unpadded carpet may alleviate the problem.[42,46,48] The type of carpeting selected is crucial. Specifications that need to be carefully considered include fire safety, degree of stain resistance, ability to lessen static electricity, ability to minimize friction of wheeled equipment, and the presence of a permanent antimicrobial finish.

Lighting

A corridor's lighting can significantly influence its ambience. The use of task and mood lighting is hardly new, but lighting can serve a number of other functions, especially in an area where the accurate rendition of patient skin tones is less important. Corridors must be lit in a way that facilitates safe and comfortable movement. For example, lighting can be used to signal changes like the beginning of a ramp or a different floor surface. Subtle variations in how the corridor is lit can also become an element of the wayfinding system by indicating turns, distinguishing the circulation path from other spaces, and highlighting meaningful spaces or information along the way. Lighting can also define areas along the hallway and visually break it up into segments, avoiding a tunnel effect. To improve corridor lighting consider these steps:[49]

- Avoid overlighting the corridor. One approach is to use a continuous band of low intensity light, rather than periodic bright lights that can appear glaring.

- Avoid corridor lighting that shines in patients' eyes as they are wheeled along in gurneys. This can be accomplished by using linear fluorescents mounted on one side of the ceiling or wall.

- Avoid a tunnel effect by mounting linear fluorescents on the sides of the corridor. Switch sides at corridor intersections, but no more frequently than every 75 to 100 feet (22.5 to 30 meters).

- Use special lighting color or intensity to highlight information, such as a sign, or meaningful spaces, such as a reception area.

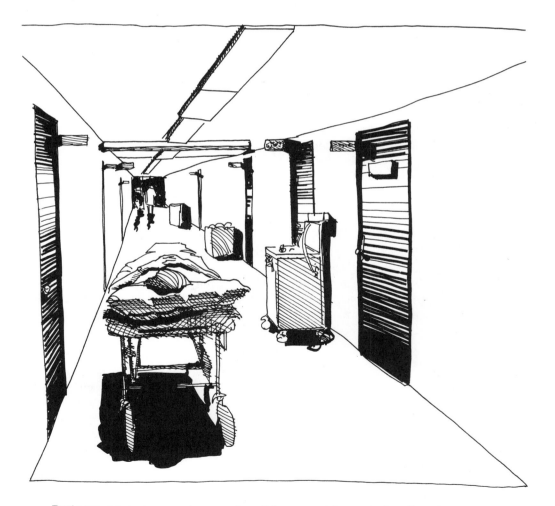

Patients on gurneys who must wait in a corridor may be disturbed by glaring ceiling light, noise, or lack of privacy.

Handrails and Seating

For many patients, just walking down the hall seems like a major expedition. Frail from illness or age, they may need physical support while walking or places to sit and rest along the way. Handrails positioned along the corridor can give these patients both the psychological and physical support they need to get up and around. Patients unsure of their strength may be encouraged to venture down a hallway where handrails are plainly available. Strategically placed seating alcoves will provide needed rest for the postsurgery patient who is out for a walk or the cardiology outpatient who must walk long distances to the clinic while suffering with angina.

In some facilities, handrails are incorporated into the design of wall bumper guards. Although this allows one design feature to serve two purposes, some precautions should be taken to make sure that these bumper guards are still usable as handrails. To insure that patients and visitors can firmly grasp the handrails, the handrail portion of the bumper guard should be rounded to fit a person's hand with a sizeable indentation on the back to allow the fingers to grip. It should be between 1 ¼ and 1 ½ inches (32 to 38 mm) in diameter. In addition, the handrail should be mounted 1 ½ inches (38 mm) from the wall, and between 32 and 34 inches (81.2 to 86.3 cm) from the floor. This clearance allows gripping without the chance of a person's arm becoming lodged between the wall and the handrail in the event of a fall.[50-52]

Traveling from Floor to Floor

Corridors are used to get from one part of the same floor to another and from one building to another; elevators and stairways are used to get from floor to floor. In many ways, the design and behavioral issues are similar. In both cases, patients and visitors need to travel comfortably and safely, and they need to find their way easily.

Elevators

For elevators, the primary concern is that patients and visitors be able to enter the elevator easily, reach the control panel, and understand how to use it:

- Install elevators with doors that are wide enough to accommodate a stretcher and the associated personnel and equipment—approximately 4 feet (1.2 meters).

- Because elevators will be used by inpatients who are likely to move and respond slowly, adjust doors to close slowly.

- Indicate elevator floor designations using raised numerals and braille.[50]

- On the control panel, consider using "redundant" cues for certain buttons, such as:

1 Main

- If control buttons use letters to identify floors, display easily understood explanations next to the buttons. For example:

> MZ Mezzanine
> PL Plaza Level—Street
> G Garage

- Use clear symbols and words to indicate buttons to be used for door opening, door closing, and emergency.

- Configure control buttons on the panel in a way that reduces confusion. For example, use 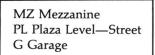 rather than

- Install elevator controls within the easy reach of someone in a wheelchair.[50]

- Provide an understandable and easy-to-read display indicating which floor the elevator is on.

- Design elevator lighting so it does not cause reflective glare on the floor number display.

- Use damage-resistant materials in the elevator cab.

- Provide a sign in the elevator lobby, opposite the elevator and in clear view of those riding the elevator, indicating which floor the elevator is on.

- Provide metal tactile numbers for floor designation on each floor, 60 inches (1.5 meters) above the floor on the fixed point at the open side of the elevator door or, when center-opening doors are used, on both sides.[53]

- Outside the elevator, provide call buttons with clear symbols for indicating up or down.

- Provide easily understood lighted symbols indicating if a particular elevator is going up or down.

- In elevator lobbies, provide a place for patients and visitors to sit while waiting for the elevator.

- In large hospitals, consider designating certain elevators for the public and outpatients, and others for staff and inpatients.

Stairways

If stairways were cheerful, clean, safe, and well-identified, more patients, visitors, and staff might use them. Not only would the often crowded conditions in elevators be alleviated, but those using the stairways would get beneficial exercise. Encouraging more frequent and safe use of stairways can be accomplished in these ways:

- Avoid stairs with protruding treads or open risers, because they are difficult for vision-impaired and mobility-impaired individuals to navigate.[50]

- Provide round handrails (1 ¼ to 1 ½ inches in diameter) with sufficient clearance between the handrail and the wall (1 ½ inches). In this way, the handrail can be easily gripped without the chance that a person's arm will become lodged in the gap in the event of a fall.[50]

- Provide handrails on both sides of the staircases.[50]

- Extend handrails beyond the first and last steps of the staircase.[50]

- Avoid constructing stairways out of slippery materials.[50]

- Avoid the simultaneous change of several environmental factors (such as lighting, view, floor surface) on the stairway.[54]

- Minimize the distance an accident victim might fall by providing landings at frequent intervals.[54]

- Provide sufficient illumination in the stairway without glare or shadows, so that patients and visitors with vision problems are not hindered.[54]

- Provide visual cues that distinguish stairway treads from risers.[54]

- Consider providing artwork in stairwells to make them visually interesting.

Unplanned Uses of Corridors, Elevators, and Stairways

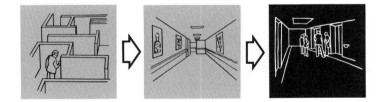

Corridors, elevators and stairways are the no-man's-land of the health care facility. They are rarely within the jurisdiction of any particular department or person. Consequently, they are given less day-to-day attention than may be needed. Circulation areas often become ad hoc storage areas for wheelchairs, linen, and gurneys; impromptu conference rooms for doctors and other medical personnel; and informal waiting areas for patients and visitors. With all of the unscheduled and often unplanned uses, corridors can become cluttered and noisy.

These unplanned uses affect patients and visitors in at least two ways, by reducing privacy and creating a poor image of the facility. When medical staff confer in hallways or elevators, information about a patient's condition may be overheard. This may not only breach the standard of confidentiality, it may also cause unnecessary alarm in those overhearing it. Furthermore, families forced to hear private and distressing information about the patient in a public corridor often feel angry and upset about the setting as well as the content of the news. As a result, they may be less likely to ask important questions of the staff. Cluttered corridors also create a poor public image of the health care facility. Consumers may wonder if the apparent lack of organization and order carries over to patient care.

Although it is probably unrealistic to assume that all unplanned use can be eliminated, much of the clutter and noise can be reduced by constructing alcoves and other storage areas, providing sufficient conference room space, and designing comfortable waiting rooms and lounges.

Conclusion

This chapter has described the nature and importance of the wayfinding system of a health care facility. Consisting of a series of mutually reinforcing cues and design elements, such a system can make it possible for first-time users to find their way correctly and confidently.

The chapter also looked at design features for circulation areas in health care facilities, including corridors, elevators, and stairways. Attention to lighting, handrails, artwork, carpeting, and other design details can make these circulation areas more pleasant, in addition to facilitating their use as passageways.

Design Review Questions

Making One's Way through the Facility

Landmarks and Building Layout

☐ Has the wayfinding system been designed to satisfy the orientation needs of the first time health care facility user?[1]

☐ Has the development of a wayfinding *system* been planned, rather than relying on a single element? Does this system include such components as the basic layout of the building and site, interior and exterior landmarks, views to the outside, signs, terminology, color coding, floor and room numbering systems, verbal directions, You-Are-Here maps, handout maps, and directories?[3]

☐ When possible, have related health care facility functions been located close to one another?[1]

☐ If a new health care facility is being designed, has the impact of the building's form on wayfinding been considered?[15]

☐ Have interior landmarks been developed using the architecture, lighting, color, texture, artwork, and plants?[1]

Floor and Room Numbering Schemes

☐ Do floor number designations logically relate to the main entry floor and indicate whether floors are above or below ground level?

☐ Have the relationships been considered among floor numbers of buildings that are linked together, so that, for example, floor 2 of one building does not link to floor 4 of another?[1]

☐ Have the floors been designated so that floor numbers can be easily used in the room numbering system for each level (for example, rooms on floor 5 would all begin with the number 5)?[6]

☐ Do rooms on the floors below the entrance level begin with a prefix likely to be widely understood by first-time users?[6]

☐ Is the room numbering system flexible enough to allow for future expansion and renovation without disruption of the sequence?[1]

☐ Is the numbering system used consistently on floors having similar use and layout?[1]

☐ Has a differentiation been made between those numbers needed by patients and visitors and those used only by staff?[1]

Notes

Design that Cares: Planning Health Facilities for Patients and Visitors, by Janet R. Carpman, Myron A. Grant, and Deborah A. Simmons. ©1986 by American Hospital Publishing, Inc.

☐ Are major patient and visitor destinations identified primarily by name?

☐ If the number of a room is its primary means of identification by patients and visitors, have the numbers been made large enough to be easily seen?[1]

☐ Are patient room numbers placed so that they are visible when the door is open?

☐ Has the use of a combination of letters and numbers to identify a space been avoided?[1]

☐ If letters and numbers must be used in the same sign, have those letters that may be interpreted as numbers (such as I, O, and Q) been avoided?[1]

☐ Does the numbering system start as close as possible to the main entry point for that floor?[22]

☐ Has a simple numbering system been used?[22]

☐ Have signs been constructed out of materials that will resist damage and that are easily stocked and replaced?[1]

☐ Has the coordination of room and telephone numbers been considered?[1]

Terminology

☐ Have the names for each department been tested for patients' and visitors' comprehension?[1]

☐ Has consistent terminology been used on signs throughout the facility?[22,24]

☐ Does each department use consistent terminology on its signs and in both written and verbal communications with patients and visitors?[22,24]

☐ Has the use of ambiguous terms been avoided?[24,25]

☐ Have messages been stated in positive terms whenever possible?[1,22]

☐ Has sign copy been written so that it is well within a sixth-grade reading level?[22]

Symbols and Pictographs

☐ Have the symbols that might be used been tested for comprehension by patients and visitors?[1]

☐ Has the entire symbol system been coordinated so that the styles, colors, shapes, and backgrounds remain consistent?[25]

☐ Has the number of symbols used been limited?[25]

☐ Is there only one symbol per message?[25]

Notes

☐ Are pictographs almost always used only as a supplement to verbal information?[25]

☐ Are arrows used only as direction indicators?[23]

Signs

Mounting and Typeface

☐ Have signs that project from the plane of the wall or those that are hung from the ceiling been mounted so that their bottom edge is at least 7 feet (2.1 meters) above the floor?[22]

☐ Have sharp edges or exposed fasteners been avoided in the design of signs?[27]

☐ Has the lighting been carefully planned to avoid producing glare on the signs?

☐ Are signs placed to provide maximum visual exposure, particularly along routes of travel?[28]

☐ Are both upper-case and lower-case letters used?[22,28]

☐ Have sans serif typefaces been used?[22]

☐ Have words been aligned at the left margin?[22]

☐ Are letters two to three times larger than the minimal size necessary for reading by a person with normal vision?[29]

☐ Is the minimum letter size based on a ratio of 1 inch (2.5 cm) of letter height for each 25 feet (7.5 meters) of distance?[28]

System Maintenance

☐ Is one person in charge of managing and maintaining the sign system?

☐ If possible, has an easily accessed and manipulated computer-assisted data base been developed to catalog all signs, their locations, and messages?

☐ Does sign design allow easy message changes without inviting vandalism?

☐ Is the sign system regularly reviewed for message validity and for damage?

Spacing and Location

☐ Has sign location been determined in conjunction with mechanical and electrical fixtures so that prime sign locations are not blocked?[1]

☐ Are signs placed at major decision points along the path?[1]

Notes _____

Design that Cares: Planning Health Facilities for Patients and Visitors, by Janet R. Carpman, Myron A. Grant, and Deborah A. Simmons. ©1986 by American Hospital Publishing, Inc.

☐ Have reassurance signs been placed between 150 and 250 feet (45 and 75 meters) after major decision points, if another decision point has not already occurred?[1,17]

☐ Have directory panels been placed in central locations?[16,24]

☐ Is information located consistently so people can learn to look for it in a certain place?[3,26,29,31]

Color Coding

☐ Are colored floor lines used along with other orientation aids as part of an overall system?[1]

☐ If a system of colored floor lines is used, does it consist of a small number of highly contrasting colors leading only to major destinations?

☐ If a color coding scheme is necessary, has it been used logically and consistently throughout the hospital?[22]

☐ Have colored bands or lines been avoided as decoration in facilities where these features are used as wayfinding cues?[22]

Interior You-Are-Here Maps

☐ Have labels been provided on the map that correspond to identification signs on the walls?[26]

☐ Has the map been placed near an asymmetrical part of the building so that people have some feature to key on?[26]

☐ Has the map been oriented so that forward is up, (that is, the direction the person is facing while viewing the map is at the top of the map)?[26]

☐ Is the map aligned with the building layout?[26]

☐ Have a number of dominant architectural elements, such as landmarks, been incorporated into the map?[26]

☐ Has the map been simplified by highlighting public corridors and destinations, and deemphasizing staff areas?

☐ Has an inset been provided on the map showing the relation of the mapped portion of the building to the rest of the health care facility?[34]

☐ Has the You-Are-Here arrow been drawn so that it points in the direction and at the spot the viewer is facing while looking at the map?[26]

Notes

Design that Cares: Planning Health Facilities for Patients and Visitors, by Janet R. Carpman, Myron A. Grant, and Deborah A. Simmons. ©1986 by American Hospital Publishing, Inc.

Giving Directions
☐ Has the facility considered instituting an ongoing staff training program in giving directions so that directions can be given as consistently and accurately as possible?

Corridor Function and Amenities
☐ Have special graphics including murals, photographic enlargements, wall hangings, paintings, reproductions, and pictorial symbols been used to create mood and color?[3]

☐ Has the facility considered locating some art on the ceiling at particular destinations to provide a focus for those patients on gurneys?[39]

☐ Where possible, are corridors routed with views to landscaped areas to provide a focus for attention and wayfinding?[40,41]

☐ Have windows been provided along corridors, rather than at the end of corridors?

Carpeting
☐ In selecting a carpet, have such specifications been considered as fire safety, degree of stain resistance, ability to lessen static electricity, ability to minimize friction on wheeled equipment, and presence of a permanent antimicrobial finish?[47]

Lighting[49]
☐ Has overlighting been avoided?

☐ Has corridor lighting been arranged so that it does not shine in the eyes of patients being wheeled along in gurneys?

☐ Has a tunnel effect been avoided?

☐ Has special lighting color or intensity been used to highlight information or meaningful spaces?

Handrails and Seating[50-52]
☐ Is the handrail or the handrail portion of a bumper guard rounded on top and behind to fit a person's hand and designed to be between 1 1/4 and 1 1/2 inches (32 to 38 mm) in diameter?

☐ Has the handrail been mounted 1 1/2 inches (38 mm) from the wall?

Notes

Design that Cares: Planning Health Facilities for Patients and Visitors, by Janet R. Carpman, Myron A. Grant, and Deborah A. Simmons. ©1986 by American Hospital Publishing, Inc.

☐ Has the handrail been mounted between 32 and 34 inches (813 to 864 mm) from the floor?

☐ Are seating alcoves provided where inpatients and outpatients might need them?

Traveling from Floor to Floor

Elevators

☐ Have elevator doors been installed that are wide enough to accommodate a stretcher and the associated personnel and equipment?

☐ Have elevator doors been adjusted to close slowly?

☐ Have floor designations been indicated with raised numerals and braille?[50]

☐ On the control panel, has redundant cueing like "1 Main" been used for certain buttons?

☐ If control buttons use letters to identify floors, have easily understood explanations been displayed next to the buttons?

☐ Have clear symbols and words been used on buttons for door opening, door closing, and emergency?

☐ Have the control buttons been configured in a way that reduces confusion?

☐ Have the elevator controls been installed within easy reach of someone in a wheelchair?[50]

☐ Is the floor display understandable and easy to read?

☐ Has elevator lighting been designed so that it does not cause reflective glare on the floor number display?

☐ Has the elevator cab been constructed of damage-resistant materials?

☐ Have signs indicating which floor the elevator is on been placed in the elevator lobby directly opposite the elevator and in clear view of those riding the elevator?

☐ Have metal tactile numbers for floor designation been installed on each floor, 60 inches (1.5 meters) above the floor on the fixed point at the open side of the elevator door or, when center-opening doors are used, on both sides?[53]

☐ Outside the elevator, are there call buttons with clear symbols for indicating up or down?

Notes _____

Design that Cares: Planning Health Facilities for Patients and Visitors, by Janet R. Carpman, Myron A. Grant, and Deborah A. Simmons. ©1986 by American Hospital Publishing, Inc.

☐ Are easily understood, lighted symbols provided, indicating if a particular elevator is going up or down?

☐ Has a place been provided for patients and visitors to sit while waiting for the elevator?

☐ Has the facility considered designating separate elevators for the public and outpatients, and for staff and inpatients?

Stairways

☐ Have stairs with protruding treads or open risers been avoided?[50]

☐ Are handrails 1 ¼ to 1 ½ inches round and mounted 1 ½ inches from the wall?[50]

☐ Have handrails been provided on both sides of the staircases?[50]

☐ Do handrails extend beyond the first and last steps of the staircase?[50]

☐ Are stairways constructed of nonslippery materials?[50]

☐ Has the situation been avoided in which several environmental factors (such as illumination, view, or floor covering) change simultaneously on the stairway?[54]

☐ Are landings provided at frequent intervals?[54]

☐ Has sufficient illumination (without glare or shadows) been provided?[54]

☐ Have visual cues been provided that distinguish stairway treads from risers?[54]

☐ Has the facility considered providing artwork in stairwells to make them visually interesting?

Unplanned Uses of Corridors, Elevators, and Stairways

☐ Have adequate storage areas been planned so that equipment can be easily placed out of sight?

☐ Is there sufficient conference room space where doctors and other medical personnel can hold impromptu meetings?

☐ Are a sufficient number of consultation rooms planned where medical staff can meet privately with a family?

Notes_____

Design that Cares: Planning Health Facilities for Patients and Visitors, by Janet R. Carpman, Myron A. Grant, and Deborah A. Simmons. ©1986 by American Hospital Publishing, Inc.

References _____

1. Carpman, J. R., Grant, M. A., and Simmons, D. A. *No More Mazes: Research About Design for Wayfinding in Hospitals.* Patient and Visitor Participation Project, Office of the Replacement Hospital Program, University of Michigan, Ann Arbor, 1984.

2. Shumaker, S., and Reizenstein, J. E. Environmental factors affecting inpatient stress in acute care hospitals. In: Evans, G. W., editor. *Environmental Stress.* New York: Cambridge University Press, 1982.

3. Weisman, G. D. Wayfinding and architectural legibility: design considerations in housing environments for the elderly. In: Regnier, V., and Pynoos, J., editors. *Housing for the Elderly: Satisfaction and Preferences.* New York: Garland Publishing, Inc., 1982.

4. Winkel, G., Olsen, R., and others. The museum visitor and orientational media: an experimental comparison of different approaches in the Smithsonian Institution, National Museum of History and Technology. Environmental Psychology Program, City University of New York, no date.

5. Christensen, K. An impact analysis framework for calculating the costs of staff disorientation in hospitals. Unpublished report, University of California at Los Angeles, Los Angeles, no date.

6. Carpman, J. R., Grant, M. A., and Simmons, D. A. Wayfinding in the hospital environment: the impact of various floor numbering alternatives. *Journal of Environmental Systems.* 1984 May. 13(4):353-64.

7. Zimring, C. M. The built environment as a source of psychological stress: impacts of buildings and cities on satisfaction and behavior. In: Evans, G. W., editor. *Environmental Stress.* New York: Cambridge University Press, 1982.

8. Corlett, E. N., Manenica, I., and Bishop, R. P. The design of direction-finding systems in buildings. *Applied Ergonomics.* 1972 June. 3(2):66-69.

9. Weisman, G. D. Way-finding in the built environment. *Environment and Behavior.* 1981 Mar. 13(2):189-204.

10. Best, G. Direction-finding in large buildings. Master's thesis, University of Manchester, Manchester, England, 1967.

11. Wener, R. E., and Kaminoff, R. D. Improving environmental information: effects of signs on perceived crowding and behavior. *Environment and Behavior.* 1983 Jan. 15(1):2-20.

12. Reizenstein, J. E., and Vaitkus, M. A. Hospital visitors and environmental stress. Patient and Visitor Participation Project, Office of the Replacement Hospital Program, University of Michigan, Ann Arbor, in progress.

13. Berkeley, E. P. More than you want to know about the Boston City Hall. *Architecture Plus.* 1973 Feb. 1(1):72-77, 98.

14. Hunt, M. Environmental learning without being there. *Environment and Behavior.* 1984 May. 16(3):307-34.

15. Weisman, G. D. Way-finding in the built environment: a study in architectural legibility. Ph.D. dissertation, University of Michigan, Ann Arbor, 1979. Available from UMI, 300 N. Zeeb Road, Ann Arbor, MI 48106.

16. Passini, R. Wayfinding: a study of spatial problem-solving with implications for physical design. Ph.D. dissertation, Pennsylvania State University, University Park, 1977. Available from UMI, 300 N. Zeeb Road, Ann Arbor, MI 48106.

17. Downs, R. Mazes, minds, and maps. In: Pollet, D. and Haskell, P., editors. *Sign Systems for Libraries.* New York: R. R. Bowker Co., 1979.

18. Kaplan, S. Adaptation, structure, and knowledge. In: Moore, G., and Golledge, R., editors. *Environmental Knowing: Theories, Research and Methods.* Stroudsburg, PA: Dowden, Hutchinson and Ross, Inc., 1976.

19. Appleyard, D. Why buildings are known: a perspective tool for architects and planners. *Environment and Behavior.* 1969 Dec. 1(2):131-56.

20. Devlin, A. Housing for the elderly: cognitive considerations. *Environment and Behavior.* 1980 Dec. 12(4):451-66.

21. McLaughlin, H. The monumental headache: overtly monumental and systematic hospitals are usually functional disasters. *Architectural Record.* 1976 July. 160(1):118.

22. American Hospital Association. *Signs and Graphics for Health Care Facilities.* Chicago: AHA, 1979.

23. Selfridge, K. M. Planning library signage systems. In: Pollet, D., and Haskell, P., editors. *Sign Systems for Libraries.* New York: R. R. Bowker Co., 1979.

24. Marks, B. The language of signs. In: Pollet, D., and Haskell, P., editors. *Sign Systems for Libraries.* New York: R. R. Bowker Co., 1979.

25. Follis, J., and Hammer, D. *Architectural Signing and Graphics.* New York: Watson Guptill, 1979.

26. Levine, M. You-are-here maps: psychological considerations. *Environment and Behavior.* 1982 Mar. 14(2):221-37.

27. Kamisar, H. Signs for the handicapped patron. In: Pollet, D., and Haskell, P., editors. *Sign Systems for Libraries.* New York: R. R. Bowker, Co., 1979.

28. Institute of Signage Research. Technical and psychological considerations for sign systems in libraries. In: Pollet, D. and Haskell, P., editors. *Sign Systems for Libraries.* New York: R. R. Bowker, Co., 1979.

29. Wechsler, S. Perceiving the visual message. In: Pollet, D., and Haskell, P., editors. *Sign Systems for Libraries.* New York: R. R. Bowker Co., 1979.

30. Daniel, E. H. Signs and the school media center. In: Pollet, D., and Haskell, P., editors. *Sign Systems for Libraries.* New York: R. R. Bowker Co., 1979.

31. Wilt, L., and Maienschien, J. Symbol signs for libraries. In: Pollet, D., and Haskell, P., editors. *Sign Systems for Libraries.* New York: R. R. Bowker Co., 1979.

32. Fusillo, A. E., Kaplan, S., and Whitehead, B. Human environmental considerations in health facility design. Unpublished report, Systems Science Institute, University of Louisville, Louisville, no date.

33. Olsen, R. V., and Pershing, A. Environmental evaluation of the interim entry to Bellevue Hospital. Unpublished report, Environmental Psychology Department, Bellevue Hospital, New York, 1981.

34. Carpman, J. R., and Grant, M. A. Executive summary: design of interior "you-are-here" maps. Unpublished research report #29, Patient and Visitor Participation Project, Office of the Replacement Hospital Program, University of Michigan, Ann Arbor, 1984.

35. Levine, M., Marchon, I., and Hanley, G. The placement and misplacement of you-are-here maps. *Environment and Behavior.* 1984 Mar. 16(2):139-57.

36. Carpman, J. R. Description of the wayfinding training program for the new University of Michigan Hospital and Health Care Center. Unpublished report, Ann Arbor, 1985 Oct.

37. Carpman, J. R. *You Can Get There from Here: Wayfinding System for the New University Hospital and Health Care Center.* Booklet, Office of Planning and Marketing, Office of Human Resource Development, University of Michigan Hospitals, Ann Arbor, 1985 Nov.

38. Spivak, M. Sensory distortions in tunnels and corridors. *Hospital and Community Psychiatry.* 1967 Jan. 18(1):12-18.

39. Shaw, H. Anti-stress art. *Nursing Times.* 1976 June 24. 72(25):960-61.

40. Bobrow, M. L., and Thomas, J. Achieving quality in hospital design. *Hospital Forum.* 1976 Sept. 19(4):4-6.

41. Calderhead, J., editor. *Hospitals for People.* London: King Edwards's Hospital Fund for London, 1975.

42. Greco, J. T. Carpeting vs. resilient flooring. *Hospitals.* 1965 June 16. 39(2):55-58, 102-10.

43. Cheek, F. E., Maxwell, R., and Weisman, R. Carpeting the ward: an exploratory study in environmental psychology. *Mental Hygiene.* 1971 Jan. 55(1):109-18.

44. Pierce, G. Carpeting cuts maintenance costs. *Canadian Hospital.* 1973 Apr. 50(4):55-60.

45. Snyder, J. Carpeting in the modern hospital. *Canadian Hospital.* 1966 Apr. 43(4):56-68.

46. Vestal, A. J. Analysts discuss pros and cons of carpeting in hospitals. *Hospital Topics.* 1972 Feb. 50(2):45-48.

47. Simmons, D. A., Reizenstein, J. E., and Grant, M. A. Considering carpets in hospital use. *Dimensions in Health Service.* 1982 June. 59(6):18-21.

48. Deschambeau, G. L. More effort needed to move cart on carpet than tile, study finds. *Modern Hospital.* 1965 July. 105(1):30.

49. Hayward, D. G. Working notes, Office of Hospital Planning, Research and Development, University of Michigan, Ann Arbor, 1982.

50. Harkness, S. P., and Groom, J. N. *Building Without Barriers for the Disabled.* New York: Watson Guptill, 1976.

51. American National Standards Institute. *American National Standards Specifications for Making Buildings and Facilities Accessible to and Usable by Physically Handicapped People.* (A117.1-1980) New York: ANSI, 1980.

52. Carpman, J. R., and Grant, M. A. Executive summary: Color, cubicle curtains, handrails. Unpublished research report #23, Patient and Visitor Participation Project, Office of Hospital Planning, Research and Development, University of Michigan, Ann Arbor, 1983.

53. Michigan Department of Labor. *Barrier-Free Design Codes.* Lansing: Michigan Department of Labor, 1985.

54. Templer, J. A., Mullet, G. M., and Archea, J. *An Analysis of the Behavior of Stair Users.* Springfield, VA: National Technical Information Service, 1978.

Chapter 4
Waiting and Reception Areas

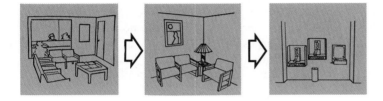

Reception   Waiting   Related Needs

Regardless of their medical condition, familiarity with the building, or personal status, patients and visitors are likely to spend some of their time waiting while in the health care facility. Patients wait to be admitted, to see the doctor, and to receive test results. Visitors wait for progress reports and a chance to see the patient. Waiting takes place in many different types of spaces throughout the facility—in clinics, the main lobby, on the patient floor, and in hallways. Some of these spaces are little more than a room with some seating, others will be associated with a reception area, and still others, such as the main lobby, serve a number of functions.

Long, tedious hours of waiting are an unfortunate fact of life in most health care facilities, but good design can help lessen some of the negative aspects of this experience. This chapter looks at design and behavior issues related to waiting and reception areas. While waiting, patients and visitors need to know they have not been forgotten by those in charge; they need to be physically comfortable; they need to be close to amenities such as phones, rest rooms, drinking fountains; they need to have things to do, watch, or read; and they need to be able to choose whether to interact with others or keep to themselves.

Entering a Reception and Waiting Area————

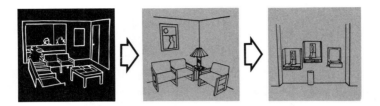

When they arrive at a reception and waiting area, patients and visitors need information; they need to know where to go, what they should do, how they should act and what will happen next. A major purpose of the entrance to the reception and waiting area is to provide this information. It should let people know that they have found their destination and provide them with information about what to do next.

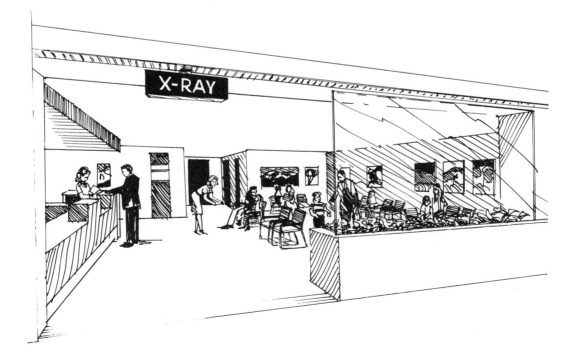

It is helpful to patients and visitors to be able to look in and identify a waiting and reception area from a distance. Once inside, good visual connection is important between the clerk and the persons waiting.

One study of waiting behavior in an admitting department found that without appropriate wayfinding information, patients often had difficulty finding their destination.[1] Once inside the admitting department, the lack of available information caused chaos and congestion. Not knowing that they should register so that paperwork could be started, patients simply stood around waiting to be called. Patients' waiting experiences were eased by providing information (such as signs directing patients and visitors to nearby services like rest rooms, telephones, and the cafeteria), a brochure explaining admitting department procedures, and a welcome sign with directions for registering (see Research Box #1).

Research Box #1: Providing Information in Waiting Areas

Waiting can be stressful for patients, and a lack of information can aggravate the situation. To test the effect of providing information, a study was conducted in the admitting department of a major urban hospital.[1]

The study compared two groups of patients: those who were given the traditional amount of information and those who were provided a number of information aids—orientation signs, a brochure explaining hospital policies, a letter answering frequently asked questions and a welcome sign describing registration procedures. While they waited in the admitting department, participants in the study were observed for five-minute intervals. At the end of the admitting process, before being escorted to their rooms, patients were interviewed. The interview concerned such topics as attitudes toward the hospital, perceived waiting time, and knowledge about the admitting process.

Those patients who were given increased information expressed significantly greater knowledge and familiarity with the admitting process, relied significantly more on signs rather than asking hospital staff for assistance, initiated approximately half as many contacts with registration desk staff, and were more likely to believe that something had been done by the hospital to ease their wait, than did the group that had not received such information. Although the study did not examine the effectiveness of different types of information or different ways of presenting information, it did show that providing information could significantly ease the stress of the waiting experience.

The following suggestions will help in designing a comfortable transition from the entrance area to the reception and waiting area:

- Make the entrance distinct from the corridor.[2]

- Use signage and other wayfinding aids to direct patients and visitors to the waiting area.

- Provide an identification sign easily seen from the corridor to let patients and visitors know they have arrived at their destination.

- At the entrance to the waiting and reception area, place signs directing patients and visitors to nearby services.[1]

- Provide patients with information about policies and procedures before they are seen in outpatient clinics and admitting departments.

Design for Reception and Registration

Health care facilities are often thought of as somewhat inhumane places where patients are processed like things rather than treated with special care. An assembly line atmosphere is not necessary or desirable, and the reception area can play an important role in projecting a more caring image. The circulation pattern created by the reception desk, its proximity to other spaces, and its design will influence the image that is projected.

In diagnostic and treatment areas, the reception desk will often provide the strongest cue to patients or visitors that they have arrived at the appropriate destination. How the reception desk is oriented will help individuals determine where they should go next by helping to define the circulation path and creating a natural queuing pattern that does not interfere with circulation in the waiting area.

In placing a reception desk, consider the following:[2]

- Position the desk so that it faces the majority of incoming patients and companions.

- Place the desk so that a queuing line does not infringe on the waiting or circulation areas.

- To ensure the patient's auditory privacy, make sure the queuing line forms approximately 4 feet (1.2 meters) away from the counter.

The reception area is a major focal point in the waiting area. In addition to functioning as a greeting, information exchange, and registration area, it provides a sense of security for those waiting. Being able to see, and be seen by, staff at the reception desk reassures patients and companions that they have not been forgotten. Those who are ill are reassured that help is available if needed.

A sense of security can be provided in the following ways:[2]

- Position the reception desk so that staff members have a clear view of people coming into the reception and waiting area.

- Position the reception desk so that staff members have a clear view of the entire waiting room.

How the reception and registration desks are designed can affect the patient's comfort and perceived privacy. For example, when registering, patients will often be carrying purses, briefcases, and other personal belongings. They will appreciate having a place to put these items while they talk with the clerk and fill out papers. Patients with poor vision, many of whom are older people with failing eyesight, would benefit from completing their paperwork on a counter surface colored to contrast with the clinic's forms. Some people have a hard time seeing where the form ends and the counter begins. Surfaces and lighting that prevent glare will be appreciated, too. In addition, patients may need to discuss personal matters with the staff while registering. The design can create an atmosphere of privacy.

The desk itself also influences the patient's image of a health care facility. A desk that is sterile and uninteresting, bare of anything but signs and registration forms, may seem institutional; and a cluttered desk, stacked high with noisy equipment and paperwork, may seem unapproachable. A desk where staff members have room to display a few personal items and where unnecessary equipment is out of sight may seem more friendly.

A number of factors can help make the registration desk and reception area more appealing to patients and visitors:[2]

- Screen from public view all work surfaces and equipment that are not reception related.

- Construct registration desks and counters of nonglare material. Avoid creating sharp edges.

- Provide nonglare task lighting.

- Allow reception and registration staff to personalize their spaces by displaying personal photographs and other knick-knacks.

- Provide wide counters or shelf space for patients' purses, briefcases, and other personal items.

- Screen patients visually and acoustically between registration stations by providing partitions or booths.

- Make sure the registration desk or reception area accommodates wheelchair users and others who may need to sit, including counter space at an appropriate height.

- Provide a chair for those who may need to sit down.

- Provide a place to store coats.

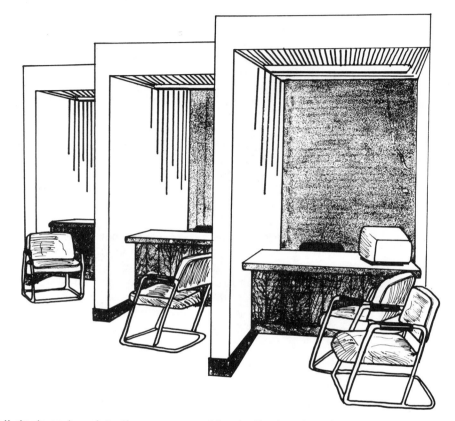

This well-designed registration area provides both visual and acoustical privacy for patients and a degree of separation for staff.

Waiting Areas

Health care facilities contain waiting areas for a variety of functions and areas: the main lobby, treatment waiting, diagnostic test waiting, surgery waiting, emergency room waiting, intensive care unit waiting, inpatient unit waiting, and others. Although family members and friends who find themselves in these waiting areas will have different design-related needs, some issues are common to all of them. We will discuss these first, and return to some special waiting areas at the end of the chapter.

Size and Location

A waiting area that is constantly crowded, forcing some patients and visitors to stand or move into the hallway, is likely to aggravate individual levels of stress and discomfort. On the other hand, a waiting room that is oversized or underused wastes space and resources. It is important to gauge properly the size of waiting rooms to their use, carefully balancing the need to accommodate peak loads with the need to conserve space (see Research Box #2). Although space allocation estimates are often imprecise, a rule of thumb is to provide approximately 15 net square feet (1.3 square meters) per person during peak load periods.[2]

The waiting room's location is also important. A waiting room hidden down a remote hallway, away from amenities like rest rooms and telephones, may seem too isolated. A waiting area in a hallway, or one that isn't much more than an alcove off a busy corridor, will not be very comforting and may indicate to patients and visitors that the facility does not care enough to provide adequate space.

When locating waiting areas, consider the following:[2]

- Place waiting rooms so that they are protected from the corridor but are near a major circulation path.

- Make sure that patients and visitors in a diagnostic or treatment waiting area can see and be seen by the receptionist.

- Locate waiting areas adjacent to rest rooms, drinking fountains, vending machines, phones, and other amenities.

Related Activities

People using a waiting area differ in age, sex, infirmity, and in how they would like to spend their time while waiting. Some like to people-watch; others want to read quietly or talk with friends or relatives; still others prefer to watch television, work on crafts, or play with their children. Even though the stress created by waiting can be reduced if people are given choices about what to do with their time, many waiting areas do not accommodate this wide range of activities.[4] The key is to provide environmental supports for as many different activities as possible—quiet activities such as reading, moderately active pursuits such as watching television, and more active ones such as playing with children.

Separate activity areas can be created by incorporating features into the design that draw people to an appropriate area. Those who are interested in an activity will be drawn to the area that provides it (see Research Box #2), whereas those who would like solitude will be drawn to quieter areas. A number of design features, such as an aquarium, mobiles, paintings, posters, plants, television, and reading material, can create such an area.[2]

Interior and exterior windows provide important focal points for activity, because many people enjoy looking out onto a pleasant scene. Windows also help patients and visitors feel less isolated. Visitors who must wait for what seems like inordinate lengths of time with little information about a patient's status can benefit from being at least visually connected to the unit's peripheral activity. They do not wish to feel removed from what is going on by being in a secluded waiting area with no way to see out. In one study, when visitors were shown a three-dimensional model of a typical waiting area and asked to choose between a solid wall and a glass wall for the separation between the waiting area and the hallway, the vast majority preferred the glass wall.[5] The glass wall made the visitors feel a part of what was going on while also providing something interesting to watch.

Many people find it preferable to catch a glimpse of activity in a waiting area or to be able to see into it before entering. For the patient or visitor, previewing waiting

Research Box #2: Observing Waiting Room Use and Behavior

By observing patients and visitors using hospital waiting areas, researchers at the University of Utah described typical waiting behavior as well as the behavioral effects of certain design features.[3] The study focused on waiting area size, activities, and the environmental features necessary to support these activities.

Observers recorded patients' and visitors' spatial behavior in 12 different lobbies (four main lobbies, four outpatient lobbies, and four medical or surgical floor lobbies) in four different hospitals. Researchers recorded the number of people using the waiting area at any one time, their behavior (conversing, standing, reading), where the behaviors took place, and general demographic information.

The data gathered enabled the researchers to describe the most frequent activities (people-watching, conversation), where particular activities usually took place, and the relationship between these activities and environmental features. For example, reading typically took place in areas removed from distractions and was more likely to occur if a magazine rack was available. Such information can be valuable in determining the kinds of amenities that are appropriate in various types of areas.

Design-related recommendations included providing parts of waiting areas specially designed for children, designating sections farthest away from circulation as reading areas, locating information desks so they are easy to see and approach, and setting aside areas where people can wait for transportation.

area activity eases the transition from a corridor where they are relatively anonymous to the seemingly intimate group setting of a waiting room. Previewing enables the person to decide whether or not to go in at all, making unnecessary what otherwise might be an awkward exit. It also gives the user an opportunity to decide in advance about where to sit and place belongings.

It is important to make sure that waiting area activities do not conflict. For example, television may provide the primary and most popular source of diversion for both patients and visitors, but the key to designing a television space effectively is to make sure the television doesn't interfere with nonwatchers. If television is installed, its sound and view should be screened from other activity areas in the waiting room.[6] Dividers and alcoves can break up a waiting area into smaller activity areas. Plants also help divide the space into smaller areas, and they provide a degree of visual privacy and something pleasant to look at. If a waiting area is too small to allow separate activity areas, it may be better not to provide television.

Seating Arrangements

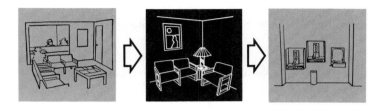

People in waiting areas tend to congregate in groups of different sizes. Some people prefer to be alone, others want to be with one or two people, and some come in larger groups. If movable furniture cannot be supplied, it is important to provide seating that accommodates individuals, groups of two or three, and larger groups.

Seating arrangements also affect patients' and visitors' abilities to converse comfortably. People like to sit at angles to one another or face to face.[7-9] The typical fixed-seating arrangement—with people sitting side by side as in airports or bus stations—is not conducive to conversation. An inward-facing seating arrangement is more likely to facilitate conversation.

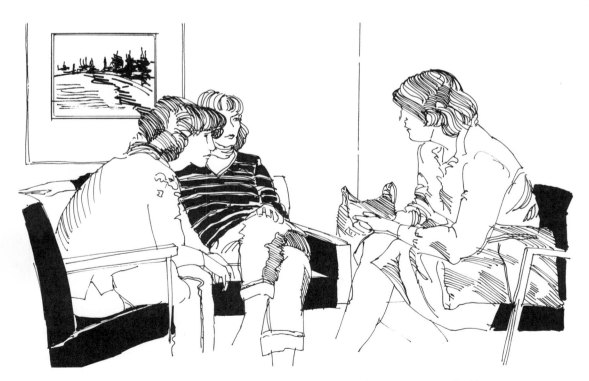

Persons in waiting areas will be able to hold conversations more easily if some seating is arranged in small, inward-facing groups.

Waiting areas also need to accommodate people in wheelchairs. By providing movable seating, the area can make room for a person in a wheelchair *within* the seating arrangement as opposed to isolating the person in a special area.

The following recommendations may be helpful in making seating design decisions:

- Provide seating that enables people to arrange themselves in different-size groups.[6]

- Provide seating that enables people to position their bodies comfortably for conversation, with regard to both the distance from one seat to another and the angle at which one person can face another.[7-9]

- If the waiting area is likely to be used by those in wheelchairs, provide wheelchair space among the seats.

Seating Comfort

Providing comfortable seating is particularly important because patients and visitors may spend hours in waiting rooms. For visitors of inpatients, the hours may turn into days. Seating must accommodate a wide variety of people, including those who are elderly or weak and who cannot easily get up from low, conventional seating or who cannot sit for long periods of time on backless chairs. Comfortable seating gives good back and arm support and does not cut off leg circulation (see Research Box #3). Firm cushion support, padded arms, and a space to place the feet under the body's center of gravity are other ways seating design can accommodate users' needs. Armrests help give patients and visitors a sense of separation from others in a crowded waiting room (see chapter 8).

The following are suggested guidelines for providing comfortable seating:

- Provide seating that will accommodate a wide range of users, including children, pregnant women, heavy or tall people, elderly people, and the physically weak.[2]

- Whenever possible, provide seating that has backs and arms, and supports thighs, lower back, upper back, and neck.[10-12]

- Avoid seating that has sharp edges.[10-12]

- Select seating material that will be comfortable, neither scratching users nor causing them to perspire.[10-12]

- As an aid in rising and in sitting down, provide seating with firm support at the front edge, room for the sitter's feet to tuck under the front of the chair, and arms that extend out to or slightly past the front edge of the seat.

- When seats are placed next to each other, use armrests on some to give people a sense of separation from their neighbors.[12]

Research Box #3: Evaluating Waiting Room Seating

Perhaps one of the best ways to evaluate waiting room seating is to install different types of chairs in actual waiting areas. To this end, a study was conducted to evaluate patients' and visitors' detailed impressions about the comfort of 18 different seats currently being used at the University of Michigan Hospitals.[12] The information collected in this study—combined with cost, availability, and departmental wishes—was used in selecting the seating that would be purchased in the future.

Patient and visitor interviewees sat in test chairs for varying periods of time (10 minutes or less, 11-20 minutes, 21-30 minutes, and 30 minutes or more). Some questions focused on specifics of chair comfort, including ease of getting into and out of the chair and provision of thigh, lower back, upper back, and arm support. Other questions asked about chair size, stability, and appearance.

Finally, two questions focused on sitting in close proximity to others, a common situation in waiting areas.

An important finding of this study was that when waiting area seats need to be placed next to each other, as is often necessary to maximize the number of people who can be seated, it is important to use a seat with an armrest in order to give people some sense of their own territory and some sense of separation (if only symbolic) from their immediate neighbor. The difference in comfort was statistically related to the presence or absence of armrests. Armrests also provide assistance to people in sitting down and rising. In addition, the study suggests that special attention be given to the older patient and visitor, for whom the issues of back, thigh, and arm support and ease of sitting down and rising are especially important.

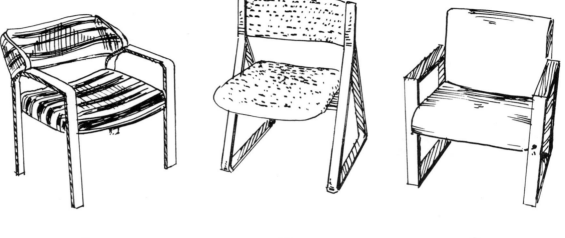

A   B   C

Waiting room seating should provide as much comfort and support as possible. Seat A's low back makes it uncomfortable over a period of time. Seat B has no armrests and is therefore difficult to get in and out of for many patients and visitors. Also, without armrests to provide some separation, people often feel uncomfortable sitting right next to others they don't know. Seat C is comfortable and has a high back and armrests.

Flooring, Wall Covering, and Lighting

People like to have interesting things to look at while waiting. Interior design details like floor covering, artwork, and lighting can make a big difference, especially to people waiting for long periods of time. Attention to the design of floors, walls, and ceilings can help create a comfortable and safe waiting environment.

Patients and visitors should not have to worry about their safety inside the facility, and nonskid floor surfaces help alleviate this problem. Flooring for a waiting area must also suit physically disabled people, dampen noise, and be visually appealing. The consensus of researchers seems to be that very low-pile carpeting without a pad is functional, if it can be negotiated by handicapped users.[13] Other types of surfaces are also appropriate.

People with failing eyesight, particularly older people, have trouble distinguishing between floors and walls, especially at edges. Contrasting colors or intensities will help them negotiate the environment. The volume of traffic coming into a health care facility, added to the number of people likely to be in the waiting area, can result in a noise problem. Flooring material, in addition to such other design features as acoustical ceiling material, can help reduce noise.

Lighting also affects the ambience and comfort of the waiting area. Generally, bright, cool fluorescent lighting is considered institutional, while indirect, warm fluorescent or incandescent lighting is considered friendlier. Table lamps create a more home-like atmosphere and provide adequate lighting for reading or doing handi-crafts. Lighting design is particularly critical for older people, who may need higher intensities of light than younger people, but whose eyes cannot tolerate glare. Consequently, the illumination level, distribution, color, and manner in which the light interacts with other design features are all important considerations:[14]

- Design lighting so that it is intense enough for reading, yet not overly bright or glaring.

- Consider indirect lighting and other "noninstitutional" lighting such as table lamps and recessed spotlights for waiting areas.

- Consider the interaction between lighting, flooring, and other surfaces in order to avoid glare.

- Avoid lighting that produces excessive heat.

Related Amenities

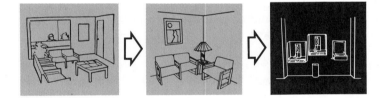

Waiting is not a unidimensional activity; patients' and visitors' lives do not stop once they enter the waiting area. They still may need to use a rest room, look after their children, contact someone by phone, learn more about their illness, or get something to eat. The availability of these amenities will help ease the stress of the waiting experience.

Places for Patient and Family Education

One way of reducing stress for patients and visitors is to provide specific information about the patient's illness or about the medical procedures they will undergo. Medical equipment can be frightening and stress-inducing, particularly in such departments as cardiology, nuclear medicine, radiation therapy, or magnetic resonance imaging. An area devoted to education should be provided within these departments and others where pretreatment orientation would be helpful. An education area should enable a health care professional to talk with the patient and companion in a comfortable setting. Audiovisual materials that show the equipment and settings for the medical procedures should be available and easily presented. Programs that recognize and accommodate patients' and family members' fears and their need to understand more about the medical situation facing them—and well-designed, dedicated space to house these programs—can go a long way toward conveying a sense of caring.

Places for Children

When people go to a physician's office for a brief examination, to the emergency department with an injured friend, or to the hospital for a diagnostic test, they may be accompanied by children, whether or not the facility officially welcomes them. The predictable presence of children in waiting rooms creates special design requirements. The environment needs to enable parents and children to wait comfortably, while not bothering other adults.[15]

Accommodating children in some waiting areas need not cause dramatic changes in facility design or policy. The first step is to decide which waiting spaces in adult-oriented facilities are most likely to be visited by children. Physician's offices, outpatient clinics, diagnostic areas, emergency departments, and main lobbies are top candidates.

Next comes the question of what environmental design features are desirable. One expert recommends providing children's play spaces that are physically identifiable and have an ambience of their own. These should be protected from major circulation paths and have materials that are visibly displayed and actively used. These play spaces can be small and should be easily seen from the reception desk and some of the waiting room seats, so they can be tacitly supervised by both parents and staff.[16]

Because children tend to be noisy when they are playing, provide adequate space and sound attenuation between a children's play area and the rest of the waiting room. Most waiting room seats should be oriented away from the play area and separated by a barrier of some sort, so adults who choose not to, do not have to become involved with children's play. The play space might also have a sunken or raised carpeted area where children and parents could play together. Another alternative is to provide special children's game tables, where board games can be played. These could also contain quiet electronic games appealing to both younger and older children.[16]

If you will be providing small play spaces for children within adult waiting areas, consider the following:[16]

- Create a play area in the most protected part of the room, out of the circulation flow.

- Place the play area within good visual and auditory range of the reception area, so the receptionist can act as a tacit supervisor.

- Use sound-attenuating materials in the waiting area.

- Place some adult seating clusters facing the play area and some directed away from the play area.

- Provide play materials that are sturdily constructed, have some inherent complexity, and, if possible, are usable by more than one child at a time.

- Avoid selecting toys with small pieces that are easily lost or swallowed.

- If only a very small space is available, consider filling it with a sunken area or raised platform. A low table, a book rack, and a storage unit with some craft materials, stuffed animals, construction toys, or games could be contained there.

- Consider using low, carpeted risers to form an enclosed play "pit."

- Provide some multiperson seating without arms, like couches, to enable a parent to comfort or hold a child.

- Provide some small tables containing board games or quiet electronic games.

Places for Personal Belongings

Most people walk around carrying something with them—purse, briefcase, bags, books, and assorted paraphernalia. During the winter months, hats, coats, gloves, and other cold weather gear add to the load. In addition, hospital visitors often bring flowers, gifts, and other items for the patient. In the absence of planned places for people to store their belongings, they will place these on seats, taking away potential seating space. Because personal belongings need to be accommodated, each waiting area should contain some coat hooks and tables or other places for people to place their things temporarily.[2]

Telephones

Telephones provide an important source of contact with the outside world. Patients and visitors need access to telephones for making arrangements or for keeping in touch with friends and family. Although inpatients may have a bedside phone available, outpatients and visitors rely on pay telephones. In using these phones, their greatest concerns are the proximity of the phones to the waiting room, privacy, and comfort while talking.

In years past, public telephones offered a number of environmental supports. There was often an enclosed booth to provide complete privacy, a seat to rest on, a shelf to put one's things on, a light to see the address book, and phone books to look up numbers. Most of these amenities have vanished. One reason for these changes relates to accessibility for handicapped persons. Handicapped access has necessitated a change in height of the phone and type of seating. An accessible, fully enclosed telephone booth is still obtainable, but at a high price. In general, the cost of space, special design features, and maintenance is the reason for fewer amenities in public telephones. Those who pay for these phones often want the most economical models.

Privacy on the telephone is so important that, in the absence of a convenient booth, some people will sometimes make sure no one uses the public telephone next to them by placing their belongings in the way. In light of this concern, some form of enclosure is advisable to provide acoustical privacy. In particularly busy areas such as the main lobby, total enclosure may be necessary (see Research Box #4).

Research Box #4: Choosing the Appropriate Telephone Enclosure

With the issue of providing access to pay telephones in mind, researchers at the University of Michigan Hospitals asked 206 patients and visitors about their choice of public phones for two different spaces: inpatient-floor waiting areas and the main lobby.[18] Participants were shown a series of drawings of public telephones having different types of enclosure. One was a telephone booth; one a semi-enclosed, wall-hung model; and the third was a wall-hung model with no enclosure.

Interestingly, patient and visitor responses indicated that they needed more telephone privacy in the main lobby than in the waiting areas. For the lobby, 54 percent of the patients and 42.5 percent of the visitors preferred the booth, whereas 39 percent of the patients and 50.9 percent of the visitors preferred the semi-enclosed model. Less than 7 percent of all those interviewed chose the open style phone. In contrast, for the patient-floor waiting areas, the majority of patients (64 percent) and visitors (67 percent) preferred the semi-enclosed, wall-hung telephone. Again, the nonenclosed, wall-hung phone was least preferred. Patients and visitors apparently felt that there would be fewer people on the inpatient unit floors and that they were less likely to need as much enclosure as they would in the main lobby. Consequently, the complete visual and acoustical privacy offered by the booth was not seen as necessary.

The telephone's location is also important. In one study, visitors were asked if telephones should be located inside the waiting areas or out in the hallway. More than two-thirds thought that phones should be located in the hallway.[5] Patients and visitors would rather conduct personal business outside the rather intimate group setting of the waiting room. Also, the hall location provides better access to the phone for all patients and visitors, in addition to those using the waiting rooms.

In brief, the use of public telephones can be facilitated in the following ways:

- Locate public telephones outside of, but very close to, public waiting areas.[2,5,17]

- For intensive care unit and surgery waiting areas, public phones may need to be located inside the waiting area to ensure that someone placing a call doesn't miss an incoming doctor's report on the patient's condition. These phone enclosures should provide acoustical privacy.[2,5,17]

- Use semi-enclosed public telephones in waiting areas and enclosed, handicapped-accessible booths in the main lobby.[5,18]

- Provide visual and acoustical barriers between semi-enclosed public phones.

- Provide a writing shelf near each phone.[2]

- Provide lights, seats, and telephone books whenever possible.

- Provide some public telephones with amplifiers for the hearing-impaired.

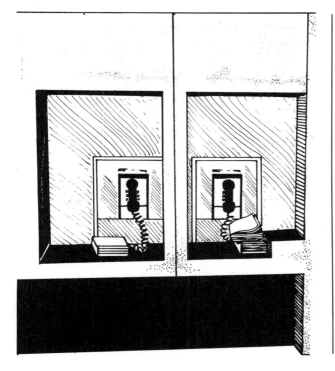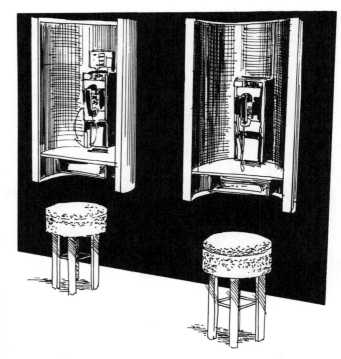

Patients and visitors often have to discuss personal information over the telephone and need some privacy. The telephones shown on the left provide no privacy at all, whereas the telephones shown on the right provide some spatial separation and acoustical buffering.

Refreshments

Eating is a popular way of passing time while waiting. For visitors or outpatients who must wait for several hours, snacks can tide them over until they have a chance to get a meal. Visitors of inpatients in particular have said that it would be nice to be able to "grab a cup of coffee" without having to leave the patient floor. Even though many people do not like the quality of food available in vending machines, they value the convenience of these machines and would like them available near waiting areas.[6] It is also important to provide readily accessible water fountains.

Of course, with food and drink there will be increased litter and spills. Providing wastebaskets may limit this problem, but realistically, increased housekeeping attention will probably be needed to keep the waiting areas clean.

Some considerations for making refreshments available to those waiting include the following:

- Provide vending machines close to waiting areas, perhaps in an out-of-the-way alcove.[2,6]

- Stock the vending machine with nutritious foods that have good eye appeal.[2]

- Consider accommodating those who would like something hot to drink by providing hot water, tea, cocoa, and coffee. This is particularly important in high stress waiting areas.[2]

- Provide appropriate trash receptacles.[2]

- Install water fountains that can be used by children and wheelchair users.[2]

Rest Rooms

Patients and visitors need convenient access to rest rooms. Because they often feel "tied" to the waiting room, afraid that if they leave they will miss an important message from the doctor, they need rest rooms close by.

Rest rooms should not be too close, however. Although waiting rooms are public areas, patients and visitors do not consider them thoroughfares for people who just need to use the rest room. In one study, three-fourths of the visitors interviewed preferred that rest rooms not be entered from inside the waiting room. Instead, they felt that rest rooms should be accessed from the hallway closest to the waiting room.[5] In addition to cutting down on traffic, visitors felt that they would have a higher level of acoustic and visual privacy by using rest rooms outside the waiting room.

The design of the rest room is also important. Even though rest rooms are one of the few places in a health care facility devoted to purely personal activities, many are not designed to handle activities like changing clothes, personal grooming, or diapering or nursing a baby. In waiting areas where visitors may spend the night, the need to accommodate personal grooming or clothes changing is even more acute. Many of these rather basic needs can be facilitated without much difficulty. In addition to satisfying handicapped-accessibility requirements:

- Make all public rest rooms accessible from hallways rather than through waiting areas.[5]

- Provide unobstructed counter space for diapering a baby in both men's and women's public rest rooms.

- Provide electrical outlets (for electric shavers and hairdryers) in both men's and women's public rest rooms.

- Provide several clothes hooks in each rest room.

- Make public rest rooms wheelchair-accessible whenever possible.

- If space permits, provide a comfortable chair.

Clocks

Time is a major concern in waiting rooms. Patients and visitors wonder how much longer they will have to wait, when they will be done, if they will have time to run errands on their way home, or if their parking meter has expired. Visible clocks will reassure some and free others from having to ask the reception desk attendants about the time. Clocks should have easily read numerals and be placed so that they can be seen from all or most seats in the waiting room. Providing at least one calendar in the waiting area will let patients and visitors plan future visits and take care of other personal business more easily.[2]

Smoking and Nonsmoking Areas

Smoking in public areas of health care facilities is an issue of great concern. Nonsmokers are bothered by the odor and potential health problems created by tobacco smoke. Although smokers represent a minority of health care facility users, their numbers (30 percent of the population in one sample) suggest that their needs are also important to consider, especially during a very stressful time in their lives.[5,18] Being told not to smoke may only add to their stress.

Given no spatial limitations, the ideal solution would be to build separate smoking and nonsmoking waiting areas.[5,18] Unfortunately, most facilities do not have this luxury and must deal with the problem in other ways, such as installing special ventilation devices and partitions or other screening so that waiting areas do not become "smoke-filled rooms."[2,6] Another alternative is to allow smoking in a few specially designated and controlled areas, such as a hallway. Still another possibility is to designate smoking and nonsmoking sections of the waiting area.

Another solution, of course, is to prohibit smoking in the facility altogether. As with many kinds of prohibition, however, this may not work. Evidence of the lack of effectiveness of this policy in one hospital has been reported.[18] Although the hospital prohibited smoking in the patient rooms, almost one-third of patients who smoked reported smoking in their room or bathroom.

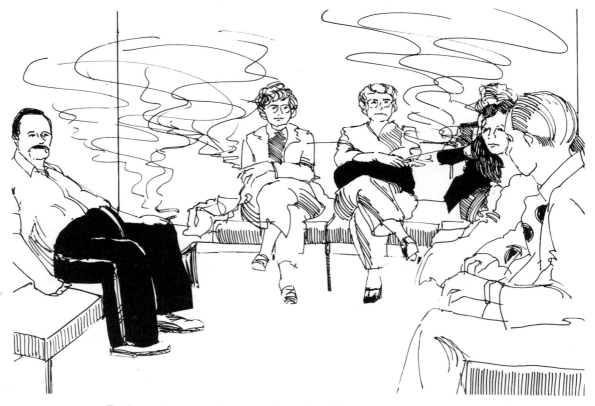

Both smokers and nonsmokers should be able to wait in comforting environments. When a waiting room is shared by both groups, the nonsmokers suffer, and when smoking is prohibited, the smokers suffer. Real solutions to this problem are expensive and hard to find.

Main Lobby

The main lobby is a special waiting area—the most visible and public space in the facility. It serves both real and symbolic functions. A number of activities take place within it, including talking, reading, people-watching, resting, and child-watching, as well as necessities like telephoning, using the rest rooms, and obtaining information. A variety of people use the main lobby, including inpatients well enough to walk a bit for a change of scene, visitors who are waiting for a patient or who want to get away from the waiting areas on the inpatient floors, children accompanying visitors, staff, and others who have business in the facility.

As with any diverse public group, there will be lobby users with special needs, such as the elderly and the physically handicapped. Symbolically, the lobby will make a statement in its visual image and especially in its functioning about what kind of place the health care facility is. Ideally, the lobby will project an image of a competent, professional health care facility that is sensitive to the needs of its users.

One of the major functions of the main entrance is to ease the process of picking up and dropping off companions. People should be able to stay warm and dry inside the lobby and still be able to see their ride approaching (see also chapter 2).

As a major public area and as the first part of the hospital people enter, the lobby will also be the logical place for interest groups to place written material. If this function is designed for, the material can be stored and displayed attractively. If it is not designed for, it is likely to occur anyway and in ways that will not be aesthetically pleasing.

Many people in the main lobby like to watch people going by, without putting themselves in the middle of the traffic. For this reason, the main corridor should be functionally separate from, but visually connected to, the lobby.

All guidelines for waiting areas apply to the main lobby as well. In addition, two important considerations are to:

- Arrange lobby seating so that those waiting inside the lobby can see cars driving up outside in the drop-off and pick-up area.

- Provide an attractive way of displaying newspapers, brochures, and other written material.

The general principle behind the design of a successful main lobby or any other waiting space is to give patients and visitors the maximum number of ways to reduce the stress associated with visiting a health care facility. Unfortunately, lobbies often do not meet this objective. For example, in a recent study, post-occupancy evaluation (POE) techniques were used to examine the adequacy of three hospital lobbies in Canada. Through interviews with visitors and staff and the use of a physical feature checklist, the researchers evaluated the overall design of the lobbies. Common problems included overcrowding, the need for furniture to be flexibly arranged into conversation groups, noise, conflicting circulation paths, lack of privacy in the admitting area, poor signage and lack of other wayfinding aids, and inadequate rest room services. Other problems included the presence of unattended children, poor illumination, inadequate security, annoying tobacco smoke, and excessive distance between the lobby and the parking lot.[19]

We recognize that patients' and visitors' needs cannot be the only considerations influencing main lobby design and that the needs of other groups (such as maintenance and housekeeping staff) are important and have a direct bearing on how the space will be perceived by patients and visitors. However, it is often possible for at least the most important requirements of all the various user groups to be accommodated.

High-Stress Waiting

Family and friends of patients in emergency, surgery, and intensive care units are likely to experience more stress than other visitors because they are concerned with patients in critical condition. In response to the emergency, they tend to behave differently from visitors in less stressful situations.

For example, these visitors tend to keep vigils in the waiting area, which may be as close as they can get to the patient's bedside. They spend long hours—sometimes days and weeks—in what is often a confined and isolated waiting space. Many times, the vigils are kept by a group of people. In order to accommodate large family groups, high-stress waiting areas need to be larger than others, with the flexibility to be split up into several different family areas. For family members who want to be physically close to each other, couches and other forms of comfortable multiple seating should be provided. For some people, the vigil goes on around the clock. Furnishings that are comfortable to sleep on, and staff who can provide pillows and blankets, can greatly add to the visitor's comfort.

Telephones that are located inside or immediately outside the waiting area and that offer acoustical privacy will help visitors avoid missing an important incoming call. An alcove where hot coffee and tea can be made will add to the facility's symbolic message of thoughtfulness.

When designing high-stress waiting areas:

- Locate family waiting areas close to relevant units.[20]

- Provide large waiting spaces that contain a sufficient number of separate family-size "territories."

- Provide couches, chairs, and other furnishings that can be arranged to enable family and friends to be comfortable for long periods of time.[20]

- Provide couches and other furnishings that can be slept upon comfortably.

- Locate telephones inside or immediately outside waiting areas and make sure that they are acoustically private.

- Provide an intercom or telephone connection between the nurses' station and the family waiting room.

- Provide a place where coffee and tea can be made.

- Provide lighting, finishes, artwork, and accessories that create a warm, intimate, noninstitutional image.

- Provide bathrooms adjacent to family waiting areas, with counters and electrical outlets that will help visitors freshen up, shave, or perform other daily hygiene functions.

- Provide pamphlets within the waiting area for family members to learn more about the patient's illness.[20]

- Provide a comfortable and private place for family members to grieve.[20]

Conclusion

This chapter has examined the behavioral issues involved in designing waiting and reception areas. The themes of physical comfort (such as the design of seating), social contact (such as acoustical privacy at a registration desk) and symbolic meaning (such as the proximity of rest rooms) are relevant here. With attention to these issues and their design implications, waiting areas can become comfortable and attractive settings rather than the afterthoughts they have often been in the past.

Design Review Questions ⎯⎯⎯⎯⎯⎯⎯⎯⎯⎯⎯

Entering a Reception and Waiting Area

☐ Is there an identification sign easily seen from the corridor, to let patients and visitors know they have arrived at their destination?

☐ Is the entrance to the waiting or reception area distinct from the corridor?[2]

☐ Have signage and other wayfinding aids been used to direct patients and visitors to the waiting area?

☐ Have signs been placed at the entrance to the waiting and reception area to direct patients and visitors to nearby services?[1]

☐ Have patients in outpatient clinics and admitting departments been given information about policies and procedures?[1]

Design for Reception and Registration

☐ Has the reception desk been positioned so that patients and companions can readily see where to go?[2]

☐ Has the reception desk been positioned so that a queuing line is formed that does not cause congestion in the circulation or waiting areas?[2]

☐ To ensure the patient's auditory privacy, does the queuing line form approximately 4 feet (1.2 meters) from the counter?[2]

☐ Has the reception desk been configured and positioned so that the staff has a clear view of people entering the reception or waiting area?[2]

☐ Has the reception desk been positioned so that the staff has a clear view of the waiting room?[2]

☐ Do the colors of the counters where patients will be writing contrast with forms they have to fill out?

☐ Have all work surfaces and equipment that are not reception-related been screened from public view?[2]

☐ Have the reception and registration desks and counters been constructed of nonglare material without sharp edges?[2]

☐ Has nonglare task lighting been provided?[2]

☐ Have reception and registration staff been allowed to personalize their space, putting up personal photographs and other knick-knacks?[2]

Notes ⎯⎯⎯⎯⎯⎯⎯⎯⎯⎯⎯⎯⎯⎯⎯⎯⎯⎯⎯⎯⎯

Design that Cares: Planning Health Facilities for Patients and Visitors, by Janet R. Carpman, Myron A. Grant, and Deborah A. Simmons. ©1986 by American Hospital Publishing, Inc.

☐ Have the reception and registration desks been designed with wide counters or shelf space and coat hooks for patients' personal items such as bags, purses, and briefcases?[2]

☐ Have partitions or booths been designed that screen patients visually and acoustically between registration stations?[2]

☐ Does the registration or reception desk accommodate wheelchair users and others who may need to sit and write?[2]

☐ Has a chair been provided for those who need to sit down?[2]

☐ Is there a place to store coats?[2]

Waiting Areas

Size and Location[2]

☐ Has the waiting room been sized to allow approximately 15 net square feet (1.3 square meters) per person during peak load periods?

☐ Have waiting rooms been placed so that they are separate from the corridor but near a major circulation path?

☐ Can patients and visitors in diagnostic and treatment waiting areas make visual contact with the receptionist?

☐ Are rest rooms, drinking fountains, vending machines, phones, and other necessary amenities adjacent to waiting areas?

Related Activities

☐ Where possible, have separate areas been created so that there is a quiet area for such activities as reading, a moderate-level activity area for television watching, and a high-level activity area for children?[4]

☐ Have interior and exterior windows been provided in waiting areas?[5]

☐ Can patients and visitors see into the waiting area before entering it?

☐ If television is available, has it been installed so that its sound and view are screened from other activity areas in the waiting room?[6]

☐ If a waiting room is too small to allow separate activity areas, has a television been omitted?

Notes

Design that Cares: Planning Health Facilities for Patients and Visitors, by Janet R. Carpman, Myron A. Grant, and Deborah A. Simmons. ©1986 by American Hospital Publishing, Inc.

Seating Arrangements

☐ Has seating been provided that enables people to arrange themselves in different-size social groups?[6]

☐ Does the seating enable people to position their bodies comfortably for conversation, with regard to both distance from one seat to another and the angle at which they face one another?[7-9]

☐ If the waiting area is likely to be visited by wheelchair users, have wheelchair spaces been provided among the seats?

Seating Comfort

☐ Does the seating accommodate a wide range of users, including children, pregnant women, heavy or tall people, elderly people, and the physically weak?[2]

☐ Has seating been provided that has backs and arms wherever possible, and that supports thighs, lower back, upper back, and neck?[10-12]

☐ Has seating with sharp edges been avoided?[10-12]

☐ Is seating material comfortable, neither scratching users nor causing them to perspire?[10-12]

☐ To aid people in rising and sitting, has seating been provided that has firm support at the front edge, room for the sitter's feet to tuck under the front of the chair, and arms that extend out to or slightly past the front edge of the seat?

☐ When seats are placed next to each other, have armrests been used in order to give people a sense of separation from their neighbors?[12]

Flooring, Wall Covering, and Lighting

☐ Has a nonskid floor surface been used?[13]

☐ Have flooring and ceiling materials been chosen that will help reduce noise?[13]

☐ Has lighting been installed that is intense enough for reading, yet not overly bright or glaring?[14]

☐ Has indirect and other "noninstitutional" lighting been considered, such as table lamps and recessed spotlights?[14]

☐ Has the interaction between lighting, flooring, and other surfaces been planned and arranged to avoid glare?[14]

Notes

Design that Cares: Planning Health Facilities for Patients and Visitors, by Janet R. Carpman, Myron A. Grant, and Deborah A. Simmons. ©1986 by American Hospital Publishing, Inc.

☐ Have floor and wall colors been selected to contrast, thus helping people with poor vision?[14]

☐ Has lighting that produces excessive heat been avoided?[14]

Related Amenities

Places for Patient and Family Education

☐ Is a patient education room adjacent to the waiting area in departments that do invasive or threatening procedures such as heart catheterization, CT scan, magnetic resonance imaging, and radiation therapy?

☐ Is the patient education room equipped with some programming, such as video cassettes, that explain the medical procedure in lay terms and show the space where it will occur?

Places for Children[16]

☐ Have adult waiting areas that are likely to be visited by children been identified and designed to accommodate children?

☐ Have play areas been located in the most protected part of each waiting space, out of the circulation flow?

☐ Have play areas been located within good visual and auditory range of the reception area?

☐ Have sound-attenuating materials been used in the waiting area?

☐ Do some adult seating clusters face the play area?

☐ Do some adult seating clusters face away from the play area?

☐ Have play materials been provided that are sturdily constructed, have some inherent complexity, and, if possible, are usable by more than one child at a time?

☐ Have toys been avoided that have small pieces that are easily lost or swallowed?

☐ If only a small space is available for children's waiting, has a sunken area or raised platform been considered?

☐ Have low, carpeted risers that form an enclosed play pit been considered?

☐ Has some multiperson seating without arms been provided?

☐ Have some small game tables been provided?

Notes _____

Design that Cares: Planning Health Facilities for Patients and Visitors, by Janet R. Carpman, Myron A. Grant, and Deborah A. Simmons. ©1986 by American Hospital Publishing, Inc.

Places for Personal Belongings

☐ Do waiting areas contain tables, coat hooks, or other means for people to store their coats, purses, and other belongings?[2]

Telephones

☐ Are public telephones located outside of public waiting areas but close to them?[2,5,17]

☐ For intensive care unit and surgery waiting areas, are acoustically private public phones available inside or immediately outside the waiting room?[2,5,17]

☐ Are semi-enclosed public telephones provided in visitor waiting areas?[5,18]

☐ Are enclosed, handicapped-accessible booths provided in the main lobby?[5,18]

☐ Are there visual and acoustical barriers between semi-enclosed public phones?

☐ Has a writing shelf been provided near each phone?[2]

☐ Have lights, seats, and telephone books been provided whenever possible?

☐ Have some public telephones been provided with amplifiers for the hearing-impaired?

Refreshments

☐ Are there vending machines close to waiting areas?[2,6]

☐ Have vending machines been stocked with nutritious foods that have good eye appeal?[2]

☐ Are hot drinks available nearby?[2]

☐ Have trash receptacles been provided?[2]

☐ Have water fountains been installed that can be used by children and wheelchair users?[2]

Rest Rooms

☐ Have entrances to rest rooms been placed so that they are entered from the hallway, not the waiting room?[5]

☐ Do both men's and women's rest rooms contain unobstructed counter space sufficient for diapering a baby?

☐ Have electrical outlets for electric shavers and hairdryers been provided?

☐ Have clothes hooks been provided in each rest room?

Notes

Design that Cares: Planning Health Facilities for Patients and Visitors, by Janet R. Carpman, Myron A. Grant, and Deborah A. Simmons. ©1986 by American Hospital Publishing, Inc.

☐ Have public rest rooms been made wheelchair-accessible whenever possible?

☐ If space permits, has a comfortable chair been provided?

Clocks

☐ Are there clocks with easily read numbers in all waiting areas?[2]

Smoking and Nonsmoking Areas

☐ If space is available, have separate smoking and nonsmoking waiting areas been provided?[5,18]

☐ If separate waiting areas are not possible, has the option of assigning one or two special smoking areas such as a hallway been considered?[2,6]

☐ If smoking occurs in general public areas, have special ventilation devices or partitions been installed?

☐ Have smoking and nonsmoking sections of public areas been designated?

Main Lobby (see also **Waiting Areas,** page 125)

☐ Has seating been arranged so that those waiting in the lobby can see cars arriving in the drop-off and pick-up area?

☐ Is the main corridor functionally separated from yet visually connected to the main lobby?

☐ Has an attractive display rack for magazines, brochures, and other written material been provided?

High-Stress Waiting

☐ Have family waiting areas been located close to relevant units?[20]

☐ Have large waiting spaces that contain a sufficient number of separate, family-size "territories" been provided?

☐ Have couches, chairs, and other furnishings been provided that enable family and friends to be physically close to one another?

☐ Has waiting room furniture been selected that is comfortable for long periods of time?[20]

☐ Have couches and other furnishings that can be slept on comfortably been provided?

Notes _____

Design that Cares: Planning Health Facilities for Patients and Visitors, by Janet R. Carpman, Myron A. Grant, and Deborah A. Simmons. ©1986 by American Hospital Publishing, Inc.

☐ Have acoustically private telephones been located inside or immediately outside these waiting areas?

☐ Has an intercom or telephone connection been provided between the ICU nurse station and the family waiting room?

☐ Is there a place in the waiting area where coffee and tea are available?

☐ Do the lighting, finishes, artwork, and accessories lend a warm, intimate, noninstitutional feeling to the waiting area?

☐ Have bathrooms been provided adjacent to family waiting areas, with counters and electrical outlets that will help visitors freshen up, shave, or perform other daily hygiene functions?

☐ Have pamphlets been provided within the waiting area for family members to learn more about the patient's illness?[20]

☐ Is there a comfortable and private place for family members to grieve?[20]

Notes

Design that Cares: Planning Health Facilities for Patients and Visitors, by Janet R. Carpman, Myron A. Grant, and Deborah A. Simmons. ©1986 by American Hospital Publishing, Inc.

References

1. Nelson-Shulman, Y. Information and environmental stress: report of a hospital intervention. *Journal of Environmental Systems.* 1983-1984. 13(4):303-16.

2. Petersen, R. W. Behavioral design criteria: patient and companion needs for reception and waiting areas. Unpublished report, R. W. Petersen and Associates, McMinnville, OR, 1981 July 31.

3. Pendell, S. D., Coray, K. E., and Veneklasen, W. D. Architectural/behavioral correlates of hospital lobbies. Architectural Psychology Symposium, Rocky Mountain Psychological Association, Salt Lake City, 1975 May.

4. Petersen, R. W. Behavioral design in OPD architecture: considerations for reception and waiting areas. In: *Proceedings of the Symposium on Pediatric Clinic and Emergency Architecture, 1981 June 26-28.* Chicago: American Academy of Pediatrics, Chicago, 1981.

5. Reizenstein, J. E., Grant, M. A., and Vaitkus, M. A. Visitor activities and schematic design preferences. Unpublished report #4, Patient and Visitor Participation Project, Office of Hospital Planning, Research and Development, University of Michigan, Ann Arbor, 1981.

6. Reizenstein, J. E., and Grant, M. A. Spontaneous design suggestions by patients and visitors. Unpublished report #6, Patient and Visitor Participation Project, Office of Hospital Planning, Research and Development; University of Michigan, Ann Arbor, 1981.

7. Sommer, R. The distance for comfortable conversation: a further study. *Sociometry.* 1962. 25:111-16.

8. Mehrabian, A., and Diamond, S. G. Seating arrangements and conversation. *Sociometry.* 1970. 34:281-89.

9. Mehrabian, A., and Diamond, S. G. Effects of furniture arrangement, props and personality on social interaction. *Journal of Personality and Social Psychology.* 1971 Oct. 20(1):18-30.

10. Carpman, J. R., and Grant, M. A. Outdoor seating evaluation. Unpublished research report #22, Patient and Visitor Participation Project, Office of Hospital Planning, Research and Development, University of Michigan, Ann Arbor, 1983.

11. Carpman, J. R., and Grant, M. A. Hospital patient room furnishings mock-ups. Unpublished research report #25, Patient and Visitor Participation Project, Office of Hospital Planning, Research and Development, University of Michigan, Ann Arbor, 1984.

12. Carpman, J. R., and Grant, M. A. Evaluation of waiting room seating. Unpublished research report #27, Patient and Visitor Participation Project, Office of Hospital Planning, Research and Development, University of Michigan, Ann Arbor, 1984.

13. Simmons, D. A., Reizenstein, J. E., and Grant, M. A. Considering carpets in hospital use. *Dimensions in Health Service.* 1982 June. 59(6):18-21.

14. Hayward, D. G. Working notes, Office of Hospital Planning, Research and Development, University of Michigan, Ann Arbor, 1982.

15. Alcock, A., Goodman, J., and others. Environment and waiting behaviors in emergency waiting areas. *Children's Health Care: Journal of the Association for the Care of Children's Health.* 1985 Spring. 13(4):174-80.

16. Olds, A. Psychological considerations in humanizing the physical environment of pediatric outpatient and hospital settings. In: Gellert, E., editor. *Psychosocial Aspects of Pediatric Care.* New York: Grove and Stratton, 1978.

17. Welch, P. Hospital emergency facilities: translating behavioral issues into design. Report, Department of Architecture, Harvard University, Cambridge, 1977.

18. Reizenstein, J. E., and Grant, M. A. Patient activities and schematic design preferences. Unpublished research report #2, Patient and Visitor Participation Project, Office of Hospital Planning, Research and Development, University of Michigan, Ann Arbor, 1981.

19. Hamilton, D. N. Lobby study. Unpublished report #2-A, Saskatoon Hospital Evaluation Project, University of Saskatchewan, Canada, no date.

20. Clipson, C. W., and Wehrer, J. J. *Planning for Cardiac Care: A Guide to the Planning and Design of Cardiac Care Facilities.* Ann Arbor, MI: Health Administration Press, 1973.

Chapter 5

Diagnostic and Treatment Areas

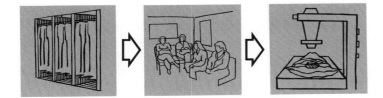

Undressing   Gowned Waiting   Diagnosis and Treatment

D iagnostic and treatment areas take on many different forms. In a private physician's office, the diagnostic, treatment, examination, and office spaces may all overlap, with one room serving multiple functions. Patients typically move from the waiting and reception area directly to the examination room, where they undress, wait, are seen by the physician, undergo the appropriate treatment, and dress again. The entire examination process takes place within one room. In an outpatient clinic or other large facility, a more complex variety of spaces may be found. Patients may move from an outer waiting and reception area to a dressing room, to a gowned waiting area, and finally to one of a number of diagnostic or treatment rooms.

No matter how many spaces are involved, patients' basic behavior remains the same: they must move from an initial waiting area, change clothes, find an appropriate place to store their clothes, maintain a sense of privacy while in the gown, undergo the treatment or examination, and then reverse the process. Many patients bring a companion to make the experience more pleasant.

This chapter explores the issues involved in a visit to a diagnostic or treatment area. We focus on the more complex of the possible scenarios, such as a visit to a hospital outpatient clinic, in order to look at the design and behavioral issues involved. (Specific needs and design issues relating to waiting and reception areas are discussed in chapter 4.) For design decision makers working with a less complex system, such as a physician's office, this chapter introduces the range of behavioral needs that must be accommodated within a limited amount of space.

The process and procedures that take place within diagnostic and treatment areas are not all the same. The needs of renal patients may vary significantly from the needs of those undergoing radiation therapy, for example. In each case, special equipment or the need for protective shielding may need to be factored into the design requirements of the facility. Unfortunately, space does not permit us to develop design criteria for each of the different treatment areas. Consequently, this chapter will focus on a generic diagnostic and treatment area, discussing those issues that pertain to the majority of patients and companions. Whenever possible, reference to special concerns will be integrated into the discussion.

Special Needs of the Patient

Patients visit examination, diagnostic, and treatment centers for a variety of reasons—they may be coming in for their annual physical, minor surgery, or prolonged treatment of a life-threatening disease. Depending on the circumstances, their mental and physical states differ dramatically. They may come to the facility alone or accompanied by family and friends. Depending on their past experience with the facility, they may be very familiar or totally unfamiliar with the examination or treatment process. Consequently, the facility must be flexible enough to accommodate a wide range of physical, emotional, and informational needs.

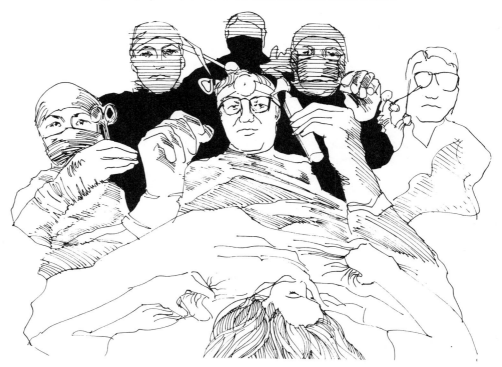

Patients are often fearful of the medical procedures that occur in diagnostic and treatment areas.

It is also important to remember that patients are unfamiliar with, and intimidated by, many medical procedures. Even the patient coming in for a simple procedure or examination may have fears: fear of disease, fear of machinery and procedures, fear of the unknown. The facility can do a great deal to ease these fears and lessen the trauma associated with medical technology. Good design can help "humanize" the experience. Policies as well as design can treat patients in a way that preserves their sense of order and limits unnecessary interaction with the more frightening aspects of medical procedures. For example, the facility might provide a videotape or slide-tape description of the procedure for patients who will be involved in complex or potentially intimidating protocols. This would allow patients to become familiar with various aspects of their examination or treatment in advance, in an unthreatening environment.

For many, the diagnostic and treatment area represents a foreign environment. Not only is the terminology often misunderstood, but patients may also find the physical layout of the clinic complex and confusing. (Wayfinding within the health care facility is discussed in chapter 3.) Getting from one point to another may be difficult. The patient may have a number of different destinations (the dressing room, gowned waiting, rest room, treatment room, physician's office, check-out area). If each of the possible destinations within the diagnostic area is located in sequence, patients can move easily from space to space. This arrangement eliminates backtracking, saves time, and reduces the chances of a patient's becoming lost.[1-4] It is important to provide clearly labeled examination or treatment rooms, so that patients who leave to use the bathroom can find their way back. Providing an understandable wayfinding system will not only help avoid confusion but also lessen the frequency of lost patients entering the staff's area.

Undressing and Dressing

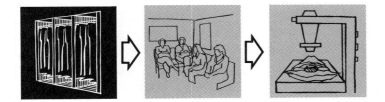

Many procedures and examinations require patients to wear a hospital gown. In some settings, such as a private physician's office, patients undress in the examination room. In many larger outpatient clinics, patients disrobe in a separate dressing room or cubicle before moving to the treatment area. In either case, patients will remove at least some street clothing and don a hospital gown. Although the process of dressing for treatment seems routine, for patients it is part of becoming psychologically as well as physically prepared for treatment or examination.

In giving up street clothes, the individual begins to take on the role of a patient. The design of the dressing room symbolically indicates to the patient how the facility views this role transformation. That is, the design of the dressing area may send the message that the patient is considered "just another body" to be treated. By paying attention to design details, however, the facility has an opportunity to show the patients that they are received as individuals who deserve to be treated with dignity.

In the process of gowning, the patient is usually forced into a less modest situation than when wearing ordinary street clothing. Thus, the facility must strive to ensure that the patient's privacy is respected:

- When planning separate changing rooms, provide a lockable door for the patient's security and privacy.[5]

- If a dressing room door cannot be locked because of safety concerns, install an indicator on the outside that shows the room is occupied.[2]

- When planning a group changing area with numerous dressing cubicles, provide curtains or doors that provide visual privacy.

- For gowned patients, provide bathroom facilities and water fountains out of the view of public space.[5,6]

- Locate the circulation path from dressing rooms to gowned waiting and examination or treatment rooms out of public view.

It is reasonable to expect patients, and in some instances their companions, to spend several minutes in the dressing room. The physical design of the dressing area will determine how comfortably this time is spent and whether or not a variety of activities (dressing and undressing, waiting, grooming, communicating with others) can be accommodated:

- Provide at least one dressing room or cubicle that is large enough to accommodate two people or someone in a wheelchair and a companion.[6]

- If dressing areas are also used as waiting spaces, provide an appropriate number of chairs and enough space to wait in comfortably.[7]

- Provide comfortable chairs and also a small stool or other piece of furniture that will help those who may have difficulty bending over to tie their shoes.[6,7]

- Keep dressing rooms slightly warmer than the rest of the facility, because patients are wearing only a hospital gown.[6,7]

- Provide a mirror that can be seen by short people, tall people, and wheelchair users.

- Carpet dressing room floors, because carpeting tends to be warmer for patients who have taken off their shoes.

- Install hooks and shelves in easily reached places for hanging clothes and storing personal items.

- Provide adequate lighting.

- Avoid isolating patients by providing some mechanism for the patient to communicate with staff.[6]

If patients leave the dressing room, or if the dressing room is to be used by another patient, some provision needs to be made for storing belongings. Unless the dressing room can be locked, unattended belongings create security and privacy problems. In the absence of secure, locked spaces, patients will have to carry valuables through diagnostic procedures and spaces where they may be misplaced.

One study showed that given a choice, most patients prefer leaving their belongings in a locker rather than taking them along.[8,9] With either system, there are management issues and design issues to consider. Lockers need to be operable by patients with varying physical abilities, and should be simple and extremely durable. They should be located in a place where they can be monitored directly by staff or by closed-circuit camera. If bags are used to store belongings, they need to be durable and easily stored out of the way in treatment rooms. Staff members need to help patients keep track of their bags.

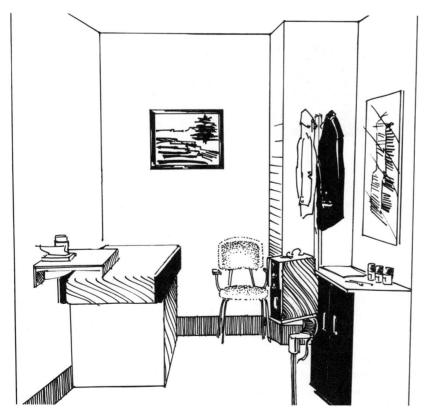

A well-designed examination room provides a chair to sit in while waiting, pleasant things to look at, distractions to help pass the time, a place to hang clothes, and a mirror for grooming after examination.

Typically, the patient will undress and don a hospital gown in the examination room, see the doctor, and then dress again before leaving. It is important to plan for the patient's comfort in the examination room by providing places for clothes and grooming aids. To maximize patient comfort:

- Where appropriate, install a privacy curtain to shield patients from exposure when the examination room door is opened. This is particularly important in rooms where patients need to undress completely.

- Provide hooks and shelves in easily reached places for hanging clothes and storing items.

- Provide a mirror that can be viewed by short people, tall people, and wheelchair users.

Gowned Waiting

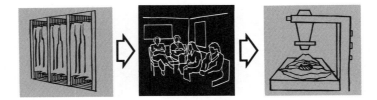

In many facilities, gowned patients are asked to wait in a common waiting area. (A detailed discussion of waiting areas can be found in chapter 4.) Jokes about the revealing nature of hospital gowns are legion, but the reality is that the gowns are considered embarrassing and humiliating by many patients.[10] What may seem adequate while waiting in an examination room with some privacy may seem too exposed in a group waiting area. As one study showed, if they must wear a typical hospital gown, many patients prefer to wait in rooms segregated by sex.[6] If a less revealing gown is provided, concerns over modesty are somewhat alleviated and patients feel more comfortable waiting with both sexes (see Research Box #1).[8,9]

Patients who must wear hospital gowns in public are obviously concerned about bodily privacy. By purchasing less revealing gowns or by providing a robe, the facility could show more respect for the patient's dignity and would not have to provide waiting areas segregated by sex. A more modest gown or a robe allows patients to feel more comfortable in a room where others are both dressed and gowned, so companions can more comfortably accompany patients throughout the process. Some manufacturers have responded to these concerns by offering hospital gowns that cover more of the patient's body than do traditional gowns.

Research Box #1:
Selecting Hospital Gowns

Recognizing that patients wearing gowns may be asked to spend time in a waiting room before going to the examination room, the University of Michigan Hospitals Patient and Visitor Participation Project staff interviewed both inpatients and visitors concerning their preferences.[8,9] Visitors were asked to imagine that they were coming to the hospital for a clinic appointment and going home again after the appointment. They were asked, if they had on a "typical" hospital gown, whether they would prefer waiting in a waiting area with both sexes, or with people of their own sex, or whether it would not make any difference. Most visitors said they preferred to wait with people of their own sex (72.6 percent), whereas inpatients were equally divided on the issue (50 percent said they would prefer to wait with members of their own sex, 7 percent said they would prefer both sexes, and 43 percent said it would make no difference).

The second question asked which type of waiting area they would prefer if they had on a "less revealing" hospital gown. Interestingly, when respondents were offered this more modest hospital gown, the proportion who said they would rather wait in an area with both sexes or that it would make no difference rose dramatically. Visitors were still more likely to prefer being with those of their own sex (40.6 percent) than were inpatients (18 percent). Even if they were wearing the less revealing gown, female visitors were more likely to prefer waiting with members of their own sex than were male visitors.

The responses to these questions point out the importance of bodily privacy to patients. This is also an example of the importance of seemingly small details like the design of a hospital gown. If less revealing gowns are provided, gowned-waiting areas could be combined and more respect shown for the patient's dignity.

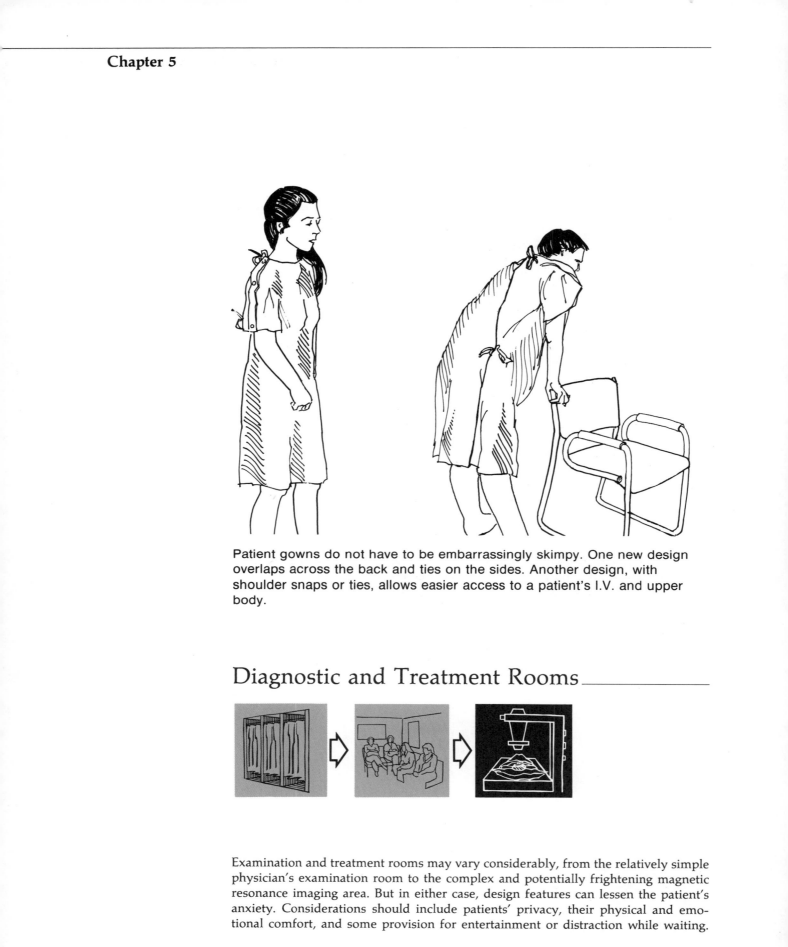

Patient gowns do not have to be embarrassingly skimpy. One new design overlaps across the back and ties on the sides. Another design, with shoulder snaps or ties, allows easier access to a patient's I.V. and upper body.

Diagnostic and Treatment Rooms

Examination and treatment rooms may vary considerably, from the relatively simple physician's examination room to the complex and potentially frightening magnetic resonance imaging area. But in either case, design features can lessen the patient's anxiety. Considerations should include patients' privacy, their physical and emotional comfort, and some provision for entertainment or distraction while waiting.

Maintaining Privacy

Because patients are partially or fully undressed during many procedures, it is important to maintain bodily privacy and reduce the chance of unintentional exposure. However, privacy involves being able to control what you can see or hear of others, as well as what others can see or hear about you. It may be as disturbing to overhear a discussion between a doctor and another patient as it is to know that your personal conversations can be overheard. A situation where one patient accidentally sees another patient disrobed may embarrass both persons. A general understanding of the issues, coupled with good planning, can limit the invasions of patients' visual, auditory, and bodily privacy:

- Position the examination or treatment room door and examination table so the patient is not exposed to people in the hallway when the door is opened.[7]

- Where appropriate, provide privacy curtains in examination and treatment rooms and encourage staff to use them.

- Where technicians follow the progress of the patient from an adjacent area, position the control monitor so it cannot be viewed by a passerby.[2]

- Provide auditory privacy in examination and treatment rooms. One approach is to construct walls from the floor to the underside of the structural slab, fully insulate with sound-attenuating material, cover both sides of the studs with drywall, then caulk all perimeter joints. In addition, install sound-attenuating material around pipes or duct work to reduce noise.[2]

- Provide a separate and private recovery or consultation room for patients who need time to recover physically and emotionally from some procedures.[11]

- Although many treatments (such as dialysis) may be best carried out in an open ward, also provide a private room for medical examination and consultation.[5]

Patient Comfort

Although planners of diagnostic and treatment facilities may wish it were different, the patient often spends a long time (on the average, 45 minutes) in the treatment room.[12,13] Much of this time is spent waiting for the physician or technician. It is important to consider the patient's comfort during the inevitable wait. The treatment room should be a psychologically comfortable place to wait, one that encourages peace of mind and provides a relaxed atmosphere. The need for an anxiety-reducing atmosphere is especially important for patients undergoing procedures with frightening or stress-inducing technology, such as a linear accelerator, heart catheter, or magnetic resonance imager.

When designing a comfortable room, consider the effects of each design feature. For instance, incandescent table lamps seem to be less stressful to those undergoing treatment than do overhead fluorescents.[14] Also, the ambience of the treatment room may affect the patient's psychological state. A setting that appears too cold and institutional may lessen the patient's willingness to talk about intimate details with the physician (see Research Box #2). These design features are likely to improve the comfort of the treatment room:

- When possible, provide two comfortable chairs in each examination or treatment room.

- If the protocol requires that patients are positioned for treatment while in the dark, provide a dim night-light so they do not become disoriented.[2]

- Minimize patient contact with medical equipment.[15,16]

- Use carpeting, wall coverings, wood paneling, and murals to soften the decor because a treatment area that creates a noninstitutional atmosphere may be comforting to the patient.[17]

- Select relaxing artwork (prints, kites, mobiles, etc.).

- Prepare patients psychologically for the treatment by describing and showing them what will be done.

Sitting on an examining table with nothing on but a paper gown is not a pleasant experience. Examination and treatment rooms often seem designed for the medical procedures that take place in them and not for the comfort of the patient. For example, many medical machines are sensitive to temperature fluctuations and must be kept within limited temperature ranges in order to function properly; others generate a great deal of heat as a by-product of their functioning. Crowding machinery in the treatment room may restrict patient movement unnecessarily and even pose a risk to the patient. Attention to these details can make a big difference:

- Attend to patients' thermal comfort in rooms that require unusual temperatures.[5,11]

- Because patients waiting in a hospital gown may become chilled at a temperature comfortable for fully clothed staff, keep examination rooms warmer than staff areas.[5,11]

- Where examination or treatment procedures are likely to be stressful, provide indirect, soft lighting. Also avoid situations where patients must stare into lights during treatment; if possible, provide a dimmer control.[16]

- Allow sufficient space in the treatment room to accommodate both the patient and the various pieces of medical equipment.

- Protect patients from being chilled by contact with metal medical instruments and equipment such as examination table stirrups. If possible, provide warmers for metal instruments.

Research Box #2:
Designing for Self-Disclosure

Staff who are delivering care often need detailed information from the patient in order to diagnose an illness or determine proper treatment. The degree to which the patients feel comfortable talking about personal issues may influence their ability to reveal this information.

Realizing that there may be environmental factors involved, researchers at Old Dominion University in Norfolk, Virginia, examined the effect of room environment on self-disclosure.[18] The study compared participant behavior within an architecturally "hard" room to that in an architecturally "soft" room. The "hard" room was relatively barren with cinderblock walls, a brown tile floor, and simple furniture. The "soft" room added a rug, pictures on the wall, indirect lighting, magazines, some upholstered furniture, and a variety of odds and ends.

Participants in the study (psychology students) were interviewed by a counselor and asked to talk about themselves. The researchers examined videotapes of the sessions to determine the amount of intimate self-disclosure occurring. Results showed that those interviewed in the "soft" room were significantly more willing to discuss intimate details than those interviewed in the "hard" room.

Providing Distraction

Among patients' greatest fears about medical diagnosis and treatment is that they will be diagnosed as having a serious disease or that treatment will be painful. Waiting with nothing to do only gives them time to dwell on these fears. Anxiety can be alleviated, however, if the examination and treatment area provides entertainment or distractions—ways for a patient and companion to amuse themselves while waiting, as well as things for patients to focus their attention on during treatment:[9]

- When patients undergo lengthy treatment procedures (such as dialysis or nuclear medicine scans) and visual privacy is not a concern, avoid separating patients and their companions. In addition, allowing patients to watch the activities going on around them may provide a source of interest and distraction.[4]

- Where examination or treatment procedures are apt to be lengthy, consider providing television, radio, musical tapes, and current magazines. Consider providing patients with choices about programming. Pillow speakers with accessible controls are one option.[5]

- Give patients something to focus their attention on. Where appropriate, provide windows into the hallway or the outdoors, or hang artwork on walls and ceilings.[15,17,20]

- Provide a patient-to-staff communication system in examination rooms.

- During particularly stressful procedures, such as radiation therapy or magnetic resonance imaging, it may be beneficial to provide the patient with means to commmunicate with the technician or a companion in the next room. A speaker and microphone system may be useful.

- During lengthy procedures, provide patients with the option of viewing monitors that show the progress of their treatment. This reassures some patients and helps them feel part of the overall process.[15]

- Consider providing other sorts of distractions, such as olfactory stimulus in record form (the smell of campfires, a cedar forest, and others are available from manufacturers). Although not necessarily appropriate for every patient, these may be welcomed by people who find "hospital smells" unpleasant.

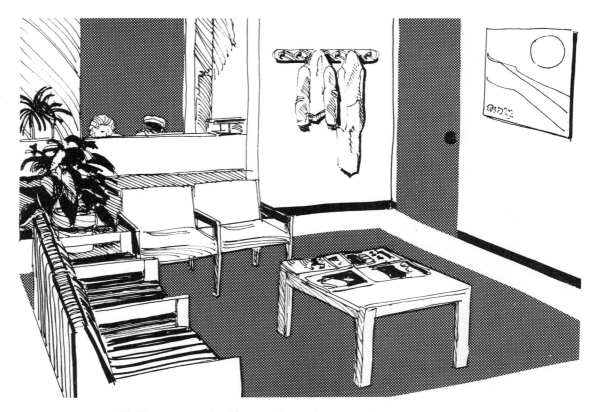

Waiting rooms in diagnostic and treatment areas do not have to be unpleasant spaces. Comfortable seating, distractions, and attention to aesthetics can contribute to a pleasant ambience.

Some General Considerations _____

The visit to a treatment area involves a number of discrete activities. The patient waits, undresses, waits again, consults with the medical staff, undergoes a treatment or examination, and dresses. At each point in this generalized sequence of events, we have tried to point out the needs of patients and their companions. Some of these needs are specific to a particular point in their progress through the examination procedure, such as the need for a mirror or other grooming aids in the dressing area. Other design and policy concerns relate to general needs—facilitating contact between patients and staff, satisfying bodily functions, and accommodating both inpatients and outpatients within the same facility.

Satisfying Bodily Functions

Patients and visitors spend time waiting, reading, and perhaps chatting quietly with each other. They move from one part of the facility to another and consult with the medical staff. They also use the bathroom, wash up, and get a drink of water or a cup of coffee. They need access to a public telephone, so they can make arrangements and keep in touch with activities outside the facility.

Public telephones, rest rooms, and water fountains that are accessible to wheelchair users need to be available to both patients and companions. Toilets and drinking fountains should be available near each stop in the journey (waiting, dressing, gowned waiting, and treatment). Gowned patients should not have to walk through public areas to get a drink of water, nor should a visitor have to travel into the treatment area to use a bathroom.[2,7,11]

Facilitating Contact between Patients and Staff

Patients visiting a particular facility vary dramatically in their physical capabilities. Some are very healthy, whereas others are seriously ill. However, the health care experience may leave them all feeling vulnerable and forgotten because they are often left alone to wait for what seems an interminable amount of time. To feel secure, patients need to know that if anything goes wrong, they will be able to get help. It is important for staff to have visual access to diagnostic and treatment waiting areas.[1] Visible and easily reachable call buttons or cords need to be available to patients who are left in bathrooms, examination rooms, dressing rooms, and other closed rooms.[16]

Accommodating Both Inpatients and Outpatients

In some health care facilities, inpatients and outpatients use the same treatment areas. Yet some people are uncomfortable around others who are sick; so for outpatients, being exposed to inpatients may be a disturbing or even frightening experience. And for inpatients, becoming the object of curiosity may be unpleasant. Therefore, inpatients and outpatients should be separated as much as possible.[1]

Inpatient waiting areas have certain unique requirements. First, they need to be spacious enough to accommodate patients on stretchers and in wheelchairs, as well as ambulatory patients.[2] Also, because stretcher patients will use waiting areas, special attention should be paid to the lighting and ceiling design. Some artwork on the ceiling would be appreciated by such patients. Finally, inpatient waiting areas need to be visually monitored by staff; at the same time, however, such areas should not be visible to outpatients or the public.

Providing for the Companion

Patients often bring a friend or relative to their appointment. Companions provide support and distraction. They are someone to talk with; someone whose mere presence is comforting. For patients who may be unable to dress themselves, companions are a great help. When patients are emotionally distraught, companions can act as an intermediary between the patient and staff delivering care. Although most companions sit and wait for the patient in an outer waiting room, companions who accompany patients throughout the diagnostic and treatment experience need to be accommodated:

- Provide at least one dressing room that is large enough to accommodate both the patient and a companion.

- Provide enough chairs in the gowned waiting room for companions.

- In examination and treatment rooms provide comfortable chairs for the companion and the patient, when possible.

- If companions are not allowed to stay in the treatment room, provide a comfortable waiting area for them.

- For those companions remaining in a waiting room, provide access to public telephones, rest rooms, a water fountain, and vending machines.

Conclusion

Whether patients are coming for an annual physical or for radiation therapy, the visit to a diagnostic and treatment area can be a stressful one. However, by designing these areas with patients and visitors in mind, the stress can be reduced. By attending to physical comfort (such as the temperature of an examination room), social contact (like the need to signal for help inside a bathroom), and symbolic meaning (such as the placement of a photomural on the wall of an x-ray room), the health care facility conveys respect and concern for the patient's needs.

Design Review Questions

Special Needs of the Patient

☐ Does the facility anticipate patients' anxieties by providing pretreatment education for new patients undergoing complex or intimidating procedures?

☐ Are destinations located in a sequence that allows patients to move easily from space to space?[1-4]

☐ Are routes and destinations clearly marked?

☐ Are examination and treatment rooms labeled clearly so that patients leaving the area can find their way back?

Undressing and Dressing

☐ Do dressing rooms have lockable doors?[5]

☐ Have devices been installed on the room door to indicate when the dressing room is occupied?[2]

☐ Do curtains or doors on dressing cubicles provide complete visual privacy?

☐ Are nearby bathroom facilities and water fountains available to patients who are gowned?[5,6]

☐ Can a patient travel from the dressing room to the gowned waiting area to the examination or treatment room without going into public circulation space?

☐ Is at least one dressing room or cubicle large enough to accommodate someone in a wheelchair and a companion?[6]

☐ Are dressing areas that are also waiting rooms large enough for patients to wait in comfortably?[7]

☐ Have comfortable chairs been provided?[6,7]

☐ Has a small stool or other piece of furniture been provided to help those who have difficulty bending over to tie their shoes?[6,7]

☐ Is the dressing room kept slightly warmer than the rest of the facility?[6,7]

☐ Has a mirror been installed in the dressing room that can be seen by wheelchair users, short people, and tall people?

☐ Are dressing rooms carpeted?

☐ Are there hooks and shelves in easily reached places for hanging clothes and storing personal items?

Notes

Design that Cares: Planning Health Facilities for Patients and Visitors, by Janet R. Carpman, Myron A. Grant, and Deborah A. Simmons. ©1986 by American Hospital Publishing, Inc.

☐ Are dressing rooms adequately lit?

☐ Are patients provided some mechanism, such as a call button or visual access, to communicate with staff?[6]

☐ If patients cannot securely lock their belongings in the dressing room, has a locker or carry-along bag system been provided?[8,9]

☐ If lockers are provided, are they in an area where visual surveillance can be maintained?[8,9]

☐ If a bag system is instituted, have personnel been trained to help patients keep track of their belongings?[8,9]

☐ If the patient undresses and dresses in the examination room, is there a privacy curtain to screen the view from the door, are hooks and shelves provided in easily reached locations, and is there a mirror that can be used by short and tall people as well as wheelchair users?

Gowned Waiting

☐ If patients are asked to wait in a gowned waiting area, are sex-segregated rooms available or does the facility provide a modest hospital gown or a robe?[8,9]

☐ Are there enough seats for patients and several companions in the gowned waiting area?

Diagnostic and Treatment Rooms

Maintaining Privacy

☐ Are examination or treatment room doors, examination tables, and privacy curtains positioned so that the patient is not exposed to people in the hallway when the doors are opened?[7]

☐ Have privacy curtains been provided in examination and treatment rooms where appropriate, and have staff been encouraged to use them?

☐ Are control monitors kept out of the view of the casual passerby?[2]

☐ Are examination and treatment rooms acoustically private?[2]

☐ Have sound-attenuating materials been used to insulate pipes and duct work in the examination and treatment rooms?[2]

☐ Has a separate, private recovery room been provided for patients needing time to rest after a treatment?[11]

☐ When treatment such as renal dialysis is carried out in an open ward, has a private examination room been provided?[5]

Notes_____

Design that Cares: Planning Health Facilities for Patients and Visitors, by Janet R. Carpman, Myron A. Grant, and Deborah A. Simmons. ©1986 by American Hospital Publishing, Inc.

Patient Comfort
- [ ] When possible, are two comfortable chairs available in each examination or treatment room?
- [ ] Is a night-light provided for patients who are being treated in the dark?[2]
- [ ] Has patient contact with medical equipment been minimized?[15,16]
- [ ] Does the decor of the treatment room reflect a warm, noninstitutional image?[17]
- [ ] Has relaxing artwork been selected?
- [ ] Have patients been psychologically prepared for their treatment?
- [ ] Are examination, treatment, and gowned waiting rooms kept at a warm enough temperature for patients wearing hospital gowns?[5,11]
- [ ] Has the lighting in procedure areas been designed so the patient is not staring into the light?[16]
- [ ] Where examination or treatment procedures are likely to be stressful, has soft, indirect lighting been provided?[16]
- [ ] Is there sufficient space in the treatment room to accommodate both the patient and the various pieces of medical equipment?
- [ ] Are patients protected from contact with cold medical instruments and equipment?

Providing Distraction
- [ ] Where examination or treatment procedures are likely to be lengthy, are companions able to stay with patients?[4]
- [ ] Where examination or treatment procedures are likely to be lengthy, are television, radio, musical tapes, and current magazines available?[5]
- [ ] When privacy is not a problem, are there windows into the hallway or the outdoors?[15,17,20]
- [ ] Does the examination or treatment room have artwork on the walls and/or ceilings?[15,17,20]

Notes _____

Design that Cares: Planning Health Facilities for Patients and Visitors, by Janet R. Carpman, Myron A. Grant, and Deborah A. Simmons. ©1986 by American Hospital Publishing, Inc.

☐ While patients are in an examination or treatment room, is there some way for them to communicate with a staff member?

☐ When monitors are used during the treatment process, are they within view of the patient?[15]

☐ Have other sorts of distraction been considered, such as olfactory records?

Some General Considerations

Satisfying Bodily Functions

☐ Are wheelchair-accessible toilets, drinking fountains, and public telephones available and conveniently placed for patients and their companions?[2,7,11]

☐ Are wheelchair-accessible toilets, drinking fountains, and public telephones located so that gowned patients do not have to go into public areas and companions do not have to go into the treatment area to use them?[2,7,11]

Facilitating Contact between Patient and Staff

☐ Are all waiting areas under constant visual supervision of staff?[1]

☐ Are call buttons visible and reachable in all examination, treatment, patient toilet, and dressing rooms?[16]

Accommodating Both Inpatients and Outpatients

☐ Has the facility made an effort to separate inpatients from outpatients?[1]

☐ Have accommodations been made for those inpatients on stretchers or in wheelchairs who are waiting for treatment?[2]

☐ Have the lights and ceiling of the inpatient waiting room been designed to be nonglaring and visually interesting?

Notes _____

Design that Cares: Planning Health Facilities for Patients and Visitors, by Janet R. Carpman, Myron A. Grant, and Deborah A. Simmons. ©1986 by American Hospital Publishing, Inc.

Providing for the Companion

☐ Has at least one dressing room been made large enough to accommodate both the patient and a companion?

☐ Have enough chairs been provided in gowned waiting areas for companions?

☐ When possible, have comfortable chairs been provided in examination and treatment rooms for both patient and companion?

☐ If companions are not allowed in the treatment room, have comfortable waiting areas been provided for them?

☐ Is there access to public telephones, rest rooms, a drinking fountain, and vending machines for companions remaining in the waiting area?

Notes_____

Design that Cares: Planning Health Facilities for Patients and Visitors, by Janet R. Carpman, Myron A. Grant, and Deborah A. Simmons. ©1986 by American Hospital Publishing, Inc.

References

1. Kebart, R. C. Innovative designs for a diagnostic radiology department. *Radiologic Technology*. 1974 Jan.-Feb. 45(4):260-66.

2. Conway, D. J., Zeisel, J., and others. Radiation therapy centers: social and behavioral issues for design. Unpublished research report, Engineering Design Branch, National Institutes of Health, Bethesda, MD, 1977 July.

3. Green, A. Changes in care call for design flexibility. *Hospitals*. 1976 Feb. 1. 50(3):67-69.

4. Simple, efficient departmental design suits functions, growth of nuclear medicine. *Hospitals*. 1977 May 16. 51(10):30-32.

5. Ringoir, S. Design and function of a hospital artificial kidney centre. *International Journal of Artificial Organs*. 1980 May. 3(3):134-35.

6. Lindheim, R. *Uncoupling the Radiology System*. Chicago: Hospital Research and Educational Trust, 1971.

7. Burgun, J. A. Construction considerations for ambulatory care facilities. *Hospitals*. 1976 Feb. 1. 50(3):79-84.

8. Reizenstein, J. E., and Grant, M. A. Patient activities and schematic design preferences. Unpublished research report #2, Patient and Visitor Participation Project, Office of Hospital Planning, Research and Development, University of Michigan, Ann Arbor, 1981.

9. Reizenstein, J. E., Grant, M. A., and Vaitkus, M. A. Visitor activities and schematic design preferences. Unpublished research report #4, Patient and Visitor Participation Project, Office of Hospital Planning, Research and Development, University of Michigan, Ann Arbor, 1981.

10. Reizenstein, J. E., and Grant, M. A. Patient and visitor issues: currently unmet needs and suggested solutions. Unpublished report #4a, Patient and Visitor Participation Project, Office of Hospital Planning, Research and Development, University of Michigan, Ann Arbor, 1981.

11. Altman, W. CAT scanning and patient inconvenience. *New England Journal of Medicine*. 1977 July 28. 297(4):226-27.

12. Rueter, L. Providing room to care. *Hospitals*. 1974 Feb. 16. 48(4):62-65.

13. Zilm, F., Brimhall, D., and Ryan, D. Ambulatory care survey paves way to the future. *Hospitals*. 1978 June 1. 52(11):79-83.

14. Hayward, D. G., and Gates, L. B. Lighting affects the social character of a space. Working paper, Environmental Institute, University of Massachusetts, Amherst, 1981.

15. Zubatkin, A. Psychological impact of medical equipment on patients. *Journal of Clinical Engineering*. 1980 July-Sept. 5(3):250-55.

16. Langan, J., Wagner, H., and Buchanan, J. Design concepts of a nuclear medicine department. *Journal of Nuclear Medicine*. 1979 Oct. 20(10):1093-94.

17. Radiation unit improves patient access and comfort. *Hospitals.* 1980 Sept. 16. 53(18):57-58.

18. Chaikin, A., Derlega, V., and Miller, S. Effects of room environment on self-disclosure in a counseling analogue. *Journal of Counseling Psychology.* 1976 Sept. 23(5):479-81.

19. Olds, A. Psychological considerations of humanizing the physical environment of pediatric outpatient and hospital settings. In: Gellert, E., editor. *Psychosocial Aspects of Pediatric Care.* New York: Grove and Stratton, 1978.

20. Oberlander, R. Beauty in a hospital aids the cure. *Hospitals.* 1979 Mar. 16. 53(6):74-75.

Chapter 6

Inpatient Rooms and Baths

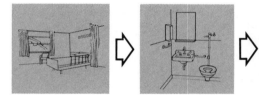

Patient Room   Patient Bathroom   ICU Patient Room

Unlike the variety of settings people enjoy during the course of a day at home, at work, and in the community, hospital patients spend the majority of their time in one room. It becomes their bedroom, living room, dining room, doctor's office, parlor, and sometimes even their bathroom. This chapter discusses how acute care inpatient rooms can be designed to meet the needs of patients and visitors for privacy, physical comfort, and easy communication among themselves and with the health care staff (see also chapter 8).

This chapter also covers the inpatient bathroom, a space that needs to be designed with special care because patients may be weak from recent surgery or medical treatment and would have difficulty using conventional bathroom facilities. Safety features, wheelchair-accessibility, ease of use, and space for nurses to assist are discussed. Finally, the chapter looks at intensive care units and some design features that can make these typically intimidating technological environments a bit more humane, such as providing for some patient privacy, reducing sensory overload and emotional deprivation, attending to patients' desires about lighting and temperature, and providing for family members' needs.

Acute Care Inpatient Rooms

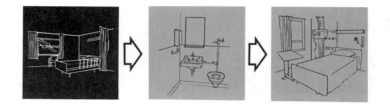

Size

The optimal size of private or semiprivate acute care patient rooms is a topic of great controversy and is frequently debated by medical and nursing staff, by hospital planners, and by designers.[1] In addition, room size is often subject to federal and/or state regulations. Government regulations are usually framed only in minimum square footages and may be based on outdated or misleading information. As a result, many people think these regulations need to be supplemented by performance criteria on the requirements of patients, visitors, and staff and by a systematic process for projecting space needs.[2]

Unfortunately, as with so many hospital design features, there is little systematic evaluation of how rooms of different sizes function in different hospitals. Typically, design decision makers may use the minimum standards or doggedly attempt to create their own optimum room designs without drawing on the experience of other similar facilities. As Research Box #1 shows, the University of Michigan Hospitals looked into the question of room size, using full-size mock-up rooms.

Every facility is likely to have somewhat different requirements for patient room size. A hospital may have been built many years ago and remain constrained by the original construction. Others may be limited by cost or building codes, whereas still others feel the need to provide more than the typical area. In acknowledging this variety of needs and approaches, we offer a few performance criteria for sizing rooms, rather than recommending specific dimensions. Facilities can follow the criteria that best suit their needs and with their designers and medical and nursing staff come up with a workable room size.[2]

To size acute care rooms to satisfy the space-related needs of patients and visitors:

- Provide circulation space, so that medical emergency teams and equipment can easily gain access to the patient.

- Provide space for a wardrobe, bedside stand, overbed table, patient chair, and visitor chair, in addition to the bed.

- Provide space and an unobstructed circulation area to ensure access for wheelchairs, rolling I.V. poles, and walkers.

- Provide space in private rooms to accommodate cots for overnight visitors (see chapter 8).

- Provide circulation area around the beds so that visitors can place their chairs on either side of the patient's bed.

Research Box #1: Using Full Scale Mock-ups as a Design Tool

Designing an optimally sized patient room and bath is critically important for reasons of both health and cost. A patient's life may depend on the ability of staff to perform emergency procedures in these spaces. Furthermore, because these designs may be repeated hundreds of times in a health care facility and because there can be a significant difference between the amount of space *estimated* to accommodate equipment and procedures and the *actual* amount needed, it may be cost-effective to construct full scale mock-ups, run simulation exercises with hospital staff and patients, evaluate the results, and modify the design accordingly. Researchers and designers at the University of Michigan Hospitals did just that.[3]

Full scale mock-ups were built of a private room and bath, a semiprivate room and bath, and an intensive care room. The purpose was to evaluate each room under a variety of common health care delivery situations. Twenty-seven different scenarios (for example, movement of the patient from the bed; using the sink, toilet, and shower; and providing emergency treatment) were simulated. Given the initial design of these spaces, the researchers found that, on the whole, the rooms were too small and that fixed equipment or furniture was inefficiently placed. Evaluations of the scenarios documented a variety of problems, including difficulty encountered when maneuvering a stretcher around a staff sink, insufficient room for staff performing emergency procedures at the head and the foot of the patient bed, and the need to move room furniture, including the other patient's bed, when transferring a patient to and from bed. Problems were also found pertaining to patients' and visitors' needs. Room designs were modified in accordance with these findings.

Number of Occupants

No longer are the multiple-bed, open wards inspired by Florence Nightingale the norm for patients in U.S. hospitals. Patients want more privacy and noise control today. Now many hospitals provide only private rooms, whereas others provide both private and semiprivate rooms in addition to small suites of three or four beds. With the increasing use of private rooms, we might assume that all patients expect or desire the privacy these rooms offer, but this is not always the case. For example, one study found that even if cost were no object, 45 percent would choose a private room, 48 percent would choose a semiprivate room, and 7 percent would prefer a multiple-bed room.[4]

The fact that approximately half the patients in this study said they would choose a semiprivate room, even if cost were no object, may surprise some designers and planners, because privacy seems to be such an unusual and desirable commodity in hospitals. However, it seems many people are willing to trade privacy for company. Many patients enjoy having someone close by—someone to talk with during their hospital stay.

In addition, some patients fear what would happen if they had a medical emergency. They feel more secure knowing there is another human being nearby who could call for help, rather than depending on a call button or the chance a nurse might happen by when needed. It seems advisable, then, to consider providing both private and semiprivate rooms within the hospital. For patients hospitalized for extended periods of time, such as rehabilitation patients, suites of three or four beds may provide much needed social contact.

Accommodating Privacy

The relationship of various elements within the patient room (the bed, views from a window, the doorway, and the bathroom) affects the patient's privacy and comfort. In determining the optimal arrangements of elements, it is important to consider the patient's preferences because they may differ from the preferences of the health care staff.

Visual Privacy

One area of potential conflict between patient and staff is the ease with which the patient can see into and be seen from the hallway. Although patients may like having a view into the hallway, they don't necessarily want people looking in on them.

For patients, a door or interior window (between the room and the hallway) can provide a visual link between their rather confined room and the busy corridor. While looking out, they may feel more a part of the rest of the hospital and enjoy the opportunity to people-watch. For staff, the door and interior window can provide easy visual monitoring of the patient.

Likewise, the location of the bathroom can permit or block the view of the patient's head for anyone passing by. If the bathroom is located on the hallway wall and is in between the patient bed and the hallway, then the patients' head will be blocked from view. In this case, privacy for the patient results in a lack of visual access for the nurse.

One study that showed patients alternative room arrangements found that patients preferred the bathroom on the hallway wall in order to maximize the exterior view. In this study, patients said they would like an interior window only if they could manipulate the shade or curtain covering.[5]

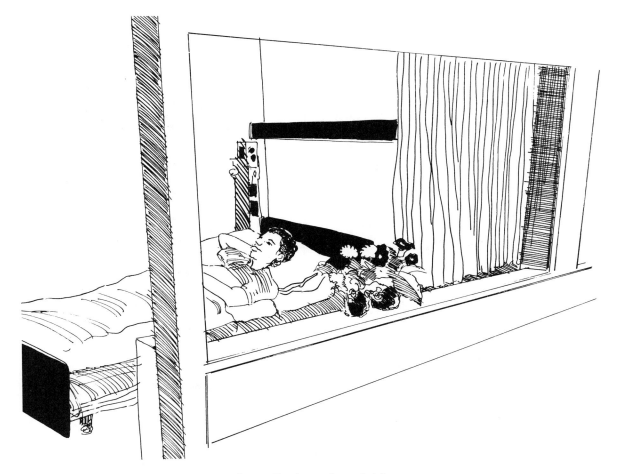

Hallway windows can be pleasant for patients and useful for nurses, provided that patients can manipulate the window covering.

Concern about unwanted exposure also surfaced in a study of patient room layouts. When given a choice, patients preferred to have the foot rather than the head of their bed positioned in line with the doorway. Again, they did not want to be viewed by everyone passing by.[5]

Patients are also concerned about the arrangements of beds within a semiprivate room. Whether beds are placed next to each other (side-by-side) or facing each other (toe-to-toe), issues of choice and territory arise. In one study, patients preferred the side-by-side arrangement because they would not have to look at the other patient.

However, they also recognized a major disadvantage of this arrangement: One patient would tend to claim the window as his or her "territory," and the other patient would tend to claim the door area.[5]

Although the toe-to-toe arrangement provides more equitable territories, some respondents didn't like the idea of patients facing each other. Some patients said that they would not want someone "staring" at them all the time. Others pointed out that one patient's light might shine in the other's eyes.[5]

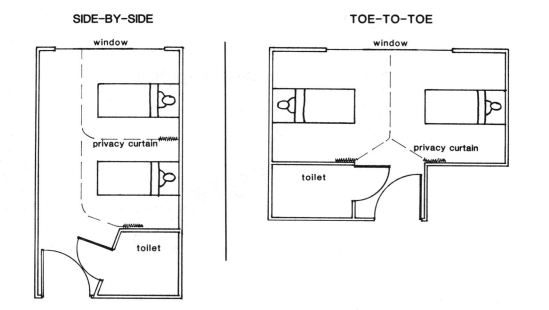

Side-by-side and toe-to-toe arrangements are two possible ways for beds to be placed in a semiprivate room.

Some new approaches to the design of semiprivate patient rooms combine the best features of side-by-side and toe-to-toe arrangements in trapezoid or diamond-shaped rooms, where beds are positioned at 90 degrees to one another. In these designs, both patients have equal access to the door and to the window.[6,7]

Privacy curtains, used by almost all patients during the course of their hospitalization, also reflect concern about unwanted exposure. As one study found, cubicle curtains are pulled for a variety of reasons, including using the bedpan, being examined or treated, dressing or undressing, sleeping, receiving a bed bath, talking with visitors, and blocking out light.[8] Although few patients in this study thought the cubicle curtain provided much privacy, being able to manipulate it was very important to them.

One way of returning some degree of control to hospitalized patients, who otherwise might relinquish much of their usual autonomy, is to let them regulate visual access to and from their bed. A cubicle curtain is one way to provide this control, but many nonambulatory patients (such as rehabilitation patients or orthopedic patients in traction) have to depend on hospital staff to open and close the curtain. A motorized curtain, however, can enable nonambulatory patients to decide when they want visual privacy and to achieve it without leaving the bed. Motorized curtains can be operated by staff, yet they free the staff from having to continually open and close curtains. Although motorized curtains tend to be costly, some require little maintenance.

To sum up, in designing an inpatient room to maximize patient control over privacy, a number of design elements should be considered:[5]

- If there is a window from the patient room to the hallway, give the patient the means to manipulate the covering over this window.

- If a side-by-side semiprivate room scheme is chosen, be attentive to potential difficulties including the view from the window for the bed closer to the hallway and the lack of clear territory for visitors.

- If a toe-to-toe semiprivate room scheme is chosen, enable patients to control their views of each other and make sure that the bed light of one patient does not shine in the eyes of the other.

- To maximize the outside view and to minimize visual intrusion by passersby, locate the bathroom on the hallway wall rather than on the exterior wall.

- Place the doorway in line with the foot of the bed, rather than in line with the head of the bed.

- Consider providing motorized cubicle curtains in areas (not including ICUs) where patients are most likely to be nonambulatory and hospitalized for extended periods of time.

Acoustical Privacy

Another type of privacy that is often at a premium in patient rooms is acoustical privacy—the ability of the patient and family to talk together without being overheard. Acoustical privacy is naturally more difficult to achieve in semiprivate rooms or suites than in private rooms. Although patients and visitors can attempt to keep their voices low or to discuss private matters only when the other patient is out of the room, a lack of acoustical privacy can be stressful. It is often difficult for patients and visitors to choose another setting for private conversation within the health care facility, because lobbies, lounges, waiting areas, and the cafeteria are likely to be crowded.

Sound also travels between the patient's room and such surrounding spaces as other patient rooms, hallways, or waiting areas. Consequently, private information may be inadvertently overheard. Sound-attenuating material between patient rooms (such as wall insulation) and within rooms (such as carpeting and other absorptive surfaces) can help alleviate this problem. If possible, locate patients who are hard of hearing in the patient rooms near noisy areas like nurses' stations. Also, locate other noisy activity areas away from the patient rooms. Ask patients to keep their doors closed when privacy is at issue and ask staff to avoid conversations directly outside patient rooms.

Design guidelines for achieving acoustical privacy within patient rooms include:

- Use sound-attenuating materials in patient room walls.

- Locate only quiet functions near the patient rooms.

- Look into the use of sound-absorbing materials within the patient room.

- Acoustically contain the nurse and physician work areas on the patient floor.

An Outside View

Views to the outdoors are particularly important to patients. Looking out the window gives them something to do, helps orient them to the time of day, season, and weather, and, depending on the nature of the view, provides a source of pleasure.[9-11] Having a pleasant, natural view can also be therapeutic (see chapter 7).[12]

The importance of an outside view was illustrated in a study where patients were given a choice between an interior window (the bath was located on the outside wall of the room) and a large exterior window with an outside view (the bath was located on the hallway side of the room). The latter arrangement was less private for patients using the bathroom, because they might be seen by people in the hallway. It also did not permit a view to hallway activity, yet it was preferred by the vast majority (over 71 percent). The availability of a generous outside view greatly outweighed both the desire to have a view into the hallway and the greater toilet-related privacy offered by the other arrangement.[5]

Consequently, it seems prudent to design patient rooms with a view to the outside. But providing just any window is not sufficient. How the window is designed, the type of view, and whether the window can be covered are also important considerations (see Research Box #2):

- Provide windows as large as possible.

- Position windows so that a bedridden patient can see both the sky and the ground.[13]

- If possible, provide views of activity going on at street level.[13]

- Make sure that visual access to the window is unobstructed by furniture, vents, or oversized sills.[13]

- Provide window coverings that can be easily manipulated by patients and visitors.

- Provide window coverings that enable the room to be completely darkened at night if the patient so desires.

Research Box #2: Providing Windows in the Patient Room

In a study of windows in rehabilitation units, one researcher found a significant relationship between windows and patient well-being.[13] In the first phase of this study patients were asked to rate a number of pictures of the hospital environment showing different types of window openings. They were also asked to complete a number of descriptive sentences relating to their perception of windows in their own hospital unit. The second phase of the study included observation of behavior within the various units as well as interviews with patients who had previously completed the questionnaire.

By analyzing responses to the questionnaire and the interview, the researcher was able to describe the role of windows in patient well-being and then to recommend desirable window designs. Design guidelines regarding the availability of meaningful views from windows, the transmission of daylight, optimal height for the window sill, window orientation, and covering were made. For instance, the researcher recommends that windows overlook street-level activity, that windows and sills be positioned near enough to the floor (no more than 36 inches or 91.4 cm) to allow immobile or wheelchair-bound patients to have a maximum view, and, whenever possible, to have vertical rather than horizontal windows.

The study also revealed the importance of "surrogate" views (wall murals, photographs, pictures) when "ideal" natural views are not available and pointed out that plants in the inpatient room are often used as substitutes if natural views are not available.

Inpatient Room Furnishings

Not only do patients have little variety in the settings they encounter during hospitalization, they also find that within the main setting of their room, there are few alternative places to sit or lie down during the course of a day. The patient's bed and chair are the most frequently used design features. Accordingly, bed and chair design greatly affect patient comfort.

Patient Bed and Chair

Patients who spend long periods of time in bed must conduct a variety of activities without getting up. They must be able to adjust the bed and to move the overbed table in order to eat; to manipulate the bed so that they can comfortably get to sleep; to adjust it so they can read, talk, find a comfortable position for television watching, and reach, dial, and hold the telephone. To facilitate these tasks, the bed's various buttons and switches must be easy to understand and manipulate. Even so, it may be helpful for staff members to point out and demonstrate these devices to new patients.

The following are a set of guidelines for the design and selection of patient bed controls:[14,15]

- Provide controls for the bed, nurse call, light, and television that are easily understood and operable by patients who are lying flat or sitting upright. Controls need to be lighted for nighttime use.

- Provide controls that patients can operate with either hand, because one hand may be injured or immobilized.

- If controls are to be used by patients who have difficulty with hand manipulation, provide pressure-sensitive control buttons.

- Place the telephone so that it can be easily reached and manipulated with either hand.

- Provide controls that are easily operated by patients seated in a chair next to or near the bed.

Patient chairs are often used as an alternative place for reading, eating, and watching television. A visitor may sit in a chair for hours talking or just watching the patient sleep. For all the use patient chairs receive, you might expect them to be designed as carefully as patient beds, with special attention given to extra comfort and physical support. Unfortunately, patient chairs that satisfy all the criteria are extremely rare. In addition to the following criteria for patient and visitors, staff requirements for ease of movement, cleaning, and maintenance need to be considered along with cost and appearance (see also chapter 8):[14,15]

- Select a chair that will be comfortable for long or short periods of time.

- Select patient chairs that provide neck and lumbar support, are easy to get in and out of, have sturdy and comfortable arms, and can be moved easily.

- Select chairs that are wide enough to accommodate heavy patients.

- Select chairs that enable patients to elevate their feet.

- Select chair covering materials that are not only easily cleaned but also comfortable to sit on.

- Since the size, weight, and physical condition of patients vary, consider purchasing a chair that can adjust to satisfy numerous support and configuration demands.

Storage for Belongings

When people stay in a hotel, hospital, or other unfamiliar and relatively impersonal place for a period of time, they often bring along a few personal possessions to make the strange environment more homelike. Despite the fact that almost all the patients' basic needs for food, clothing, communication, and even diversion are provided for in most hospitals, patients tend to bring a number of possessions anyway. In an effort to cheer up the patient, visitors may bring even more things.

Not surprisingly, clothing is the most common type of belonging brought to the hospital.[16] Most patients have shoes, socks, shirts, pants, a bathrobe, slippers, and underwear with them. In areas that have cold winters, they also bring a coat or jacket, boots, gloves, and often a scarf, hat, or sweater. Although clothing storage is more of a problem in winter, adequate storage is needed year round for basic items. There are also personal differences; the hospital must accommodate patients who bring two pairs of underwear and pajamas as well as those who bring ten, or it must limit what can be brought.

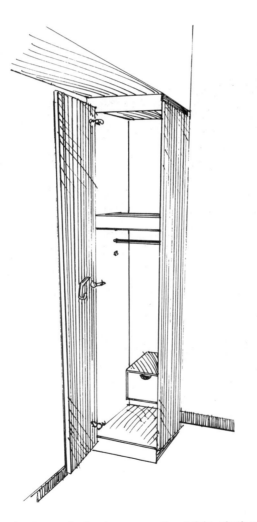

This well-designed patient wardrobe has an adjustable clothes rod, a drawer, clothes hooks, and space for a suitcase, shoes, and boots.

Hospital patients also bring toiletries with them. The variety of toiletries brought and the size of different patients' collections may vary enormously. At the very least, there should be space available for the patient to store a comb, brush, toothbrush, toothpaste, shaving equipment, shampoo, deodorant, cologne or after-shave lotion, and, for women, makeup and lotion.

Space will be needed for reading material, writing supplies, and perhaps a radio. These are the kinds of items that visitors most often bring, along with flowers, greeting cards, knicknacks, and food. It is important that space be available for items brought by visitors who come to the hospital hoping to contribute to the patient's well-being by brightening up the environment.

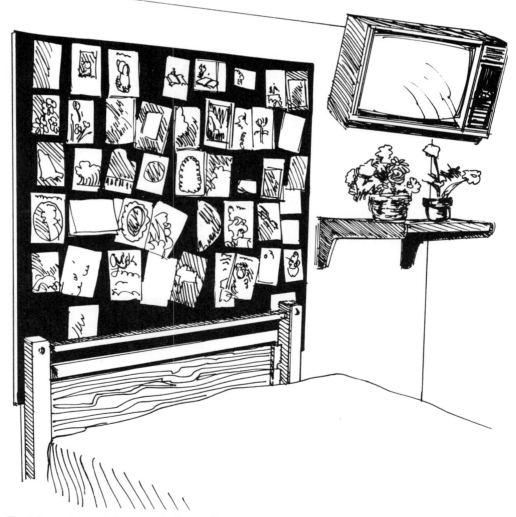

Tackboards and flower shelves allow patients to display cards, gifts, and mementos.

Regardless of who brought the items, if there is not adequate space for storage, they will get in the way of health care staff. Thus adequate and appropriate storage space for all patient belongings is needed for the staff to work efficiently. In addition to the patient wardrobe, the overbed table and bedside stand provide this needed space. Because patients tend to be debilitated in some way and many are elderly with arthritic hands, all storage areas need to be designed for patients' special access needs. Handles on drawers need to be easy to grasp. Drawers and doors should require little effort to push and pull. In designing and selecting storage areas, the following should be considered:[3,14,15]

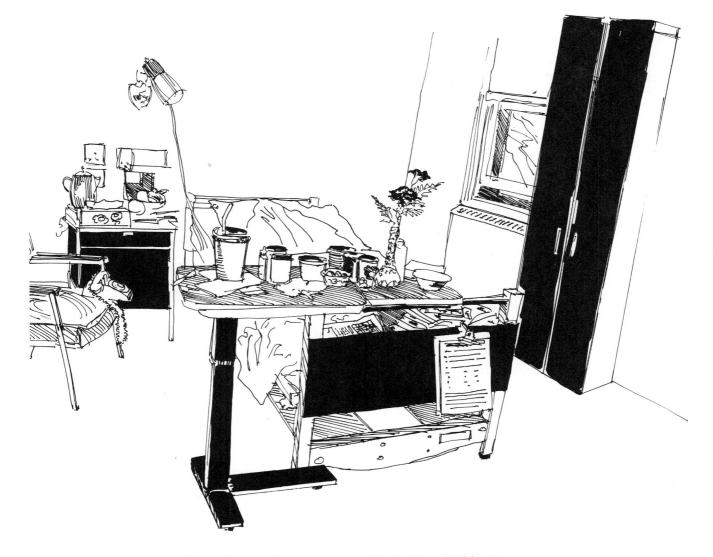

Because things tend to pile up in a patient room, provide shelf and table top surfaces, if possible, in addition to a wardrobe.

Overbed Table

- Provide an overbed table that the patient with arthritis or limited dexterity can easily adjust to various heights.

- Make sure that the overbed table is stable and cannot be tipped over easily.

- Provide storage space inside the overbed table, with easy access from both sides.

- Provide an adjustable mirror in the overbed table that can be easily used from either side.

- Make sure the drawer and mirror are easily manipulated by people with arthritis or limited dexterity.

- Select an overbed table that can be easily used as a writing surface while the patient is seated in a chair.

Bedside Stand

- Select bedside stands that can easily be moved so the bedridden patient can reach the top surface and drawers.

- Select bedside stands with drawers that open easily by patients with arthritic hands or limited dexterity.

Wardrobe[17]

- Design or select wardrobes with sufficient capacity to store winter outerwear, shoes or boots, some clothing, underwear, a suitcase, and other small possessions.

- Provide a small lockable drawer within the wardrobe.

- Select opening and closing hardware that can be used easily by people with arthritic hands or limited dexterity.

- Place the clothes rod at a height that can be reached by wheelchair-bound patients. One alternative is to make the clothes rod adjustable so that it can be used either at wheelchair or standing height.

- Place the wardrobe within the room in a position that does not impede circulation or other room functions.

- Place a few hooks inside the wardrobe for bathrobes and other clothing.

Other Storage[16]

- Provide a tackboard so that patients can display cards and mementos.

- Provide a shelf for displaying flowers and other personal items. Make sure this shelf is sufficiently wide and has enough vertical clearance to accommodate large flower arrangements. It needs to be positioned so that it will not be bumped, and it should have no sharp corners.

- Provide hooks for visitors' coats behind the door or in some other unobtrusive location.

Patient Television

In the hospital, television helps pass the time, provides company for lonely patients, and helps distract patients from their problems. For many patients, it matters less what program is being watched than that television is available to help satisfy these important needs. Television also serves a social function: It provides an activity that patients can enjoy with family and friends.[18]

In most health care facilities, the question of whether or not to provide television in the patient room has given way to the question of what type of television to select. Currently, two types of televisions are often used: large, wall-mounted or ceiling-suspended models and small personal-size models usually suspended on arms. There are advantages and disadvantages associated with both. A study at the University of Michigan compared preferences of patients and nurses for these two types of television.[18]

Although patients were split on their stated preferences (40 percent preferred the wall television, 37 percent preferred the arm television), and a large proportion, 23 percent, couldn't decide which was preferable, nurses strongly preferred the

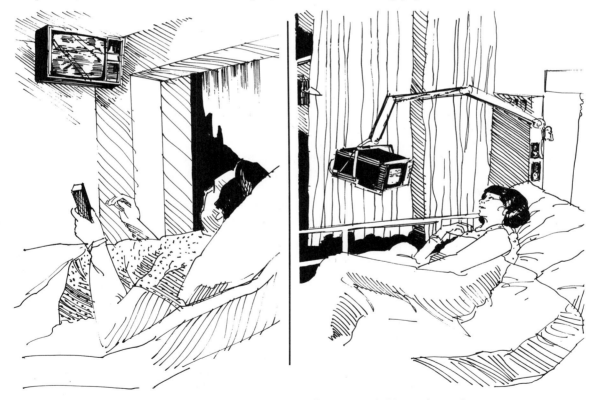

In the past, patient TVs were ceiling-hung or wall-mounted. Now, they often come on a flexible arm. Each type has advantages and disadvantages.

larger wall-mounted television because it did not get in their way as much as the small television did.

Other advantages of the large television were that it accommodated viewing by groups (a patient and several visitors) and was easier to see. However, some patients found the large television less preferable because it was difficult to watch in a comfortable position, especially when their physical condition didn't allow them to be prone. Some patients also reported that the other patient's privacy curtain could be pulled in front of the large television, blocking their view.

Those who preferred the small arm-mounted television liked its closeness to the patient's face, its relative quiet, its ease of adjustment, and the fact that privacy curtains couldn't block it. The small set was more likely to get in the way of staff, however; some patients said its screen was too small to see easily, and others said it sometimes got in their way, too.

Noise from either a small or large television needs to be controlled so that it does not bother other patients. One way of minimizing this problem is to provide personal audio devices such as pillow speakers or earphones.

Another important issue is that of television sharing. Differences in preference for television programs, watching times, and volume preference make many patients unwilling to share a television with another patient. Consequently, to avoid potential problems, it is advisable to provide one television per patient.

Clocks

With the activities and demands of their everyday lives temporarily suspended, time passes slowly for many inpatients. Most patients want to know the time, for keeping track of schedules for medical procedures, medications, visiting hours, television programs, and the like. Because patients are often discouraged from bringing valuable watches or clocks into the hospital with them, clocks need to be provided within the patient room.

- Place a clock in each patient room so that it is visible from the bed, yet not directly in the patient's line of sight.

- If analog rather than digital clocks are used, select clocks with numbers, hour, minute, and second hands readable from the bed.

- Use 12-hour clocks in patient rooms, rather than 24-hour clocks.

- If possible, select clocks that are noninstitutional looking.

Artwork

Patients like to have pleasant and interesting things to look at while bedridden. Most like to look outside, watch television, and enjoy their get well cards. Many patients also like to have some artwork in their room. Although patients have a degree of control over other views (they can close the shades or turn off the television), and have some variety in what they see (views change with the weather and time of day, television channels can be flipped, bulletin board displays can be altered), artwork usually remains static. If they happen to like the piece of art in their room, there may be no complaint. But if they do not, it may add to the stress they are already experiencing.[19]

Because artwork displayed in the patient room has the potential for being a source of pleasure and even for being somewhat therapeutic, it is important to select art that patients like to look at. But can subjective preferences be generalized? Are there certain characteristics of artwork that make it widely appealing to hospitalized patients? The study described in Research Box #3 suggests that patients prefer artwork depicting natural subjects and settings and that representational styles are preferred over abstractions.[20]

Research Box #3: Surveying Inpatient Preferences for Hospital Room Artwork

In order to provide information to be used by people selecting artwork for the new University of Michigan Hospitals, a Patient and Visitor Participation Project study sought to discover patients' relative preferences for different types of artwork.[20] Seventy-one images were used. These represented a wide range of artwork styles that were available for purchase as reproductions and that had been selected as realistic possibilities for the hospital's art collection.

Images selected from manufacturers' catalogs were photographed in color, printed in 3½-inch by 5-inch (8.9 cm by 12.7 cm) format, and mounted individually on white paper in a looseleaf binder. Nearly 300 randomly selected inpatients were interviewed about their preferences for these images. For each image, they were asked if they would definitely, probably, probably not, or definitely not choose to hang it in their own patient room.

Despite the diversity of images (subjects, settings, and styles) and of inpatients (illnesses, lengths of stay, ages, and education), patients' preferences were quite consistent. Images they liked best had natural subjects or settings (animals, water, valleys, mountains, farmland) and were rendered in a representational style. They preferred pictures to posters and liked texturally complex and somewhat organic images. Less favorably rated were pictures of people, urban scenes, still lifes, building interiors, sport scenes, and abstractions. Patients' spontaneous comments reinforced their choices.

The researchers interpreted these findings to mean that hospital inpatients want to look at images far removed from their current situation— images that help them mentally escape to a more natural, peaceful, beautiful setting. Most of the patients in this study shunned abstract art and commented that they did not want to look at a piece of art they could not understand.[21]

Although this study is limited, the findings are strong and held for the most part, regardless of differences in age, sex, or education. Most patients saw artwork as something that could make a positive difference in their hospital stay.

Some hospitals operate their inpatient artwork program on the principle that patients should be able to choose the art they look at. These hospitals have an "art cart" containing a collection of framed art reproductions. Volunteers or staff members periodically take the art cart to patients who make their selections. This way, long-term patients do not have to look at a piece of art they don't care for, and they can enjoy some variety at the same time.

In selecting artwork for inpatient rooms, try to:

- Adopt an "art cart" program so that patients are periodically given choices about the artwork in their room.[20]

- In conjunction with an art cart program, locate the artwork hanging mechanism so the artwork can be seen from the patient's bed.[20]

- Emphasize natural subjects and settings such as water and landscapes.[20]

- Emphasize representational over abstract art.[20,21]

- Emphasize photographs or paintings rather than posters with words.

- Emphasize images that are texturally complex.[20]

- When appropriate, consider mobiles as an artwork alternative for some patient rooms.[20]

- De-emphasize images of urban scenes, portraits, muted or dark colors, and poster art with words.[20]

Color and Lighting

Color and lighting are useful design devices for making inpatient rooms less institutional and more homelike (see also chapter 8). Color has been discussed widely in hospital design literature. Although many authors agree that "hospital white" and "hospital green" should be avoided, arguments have been made for both the use of "cool" colors (green and blue) and "warm" colors (red, pink, coral, and orange) with little apparent agreement or solid research to support either position.[22-25] Consequently, how color is used in the hospital environment and how it affects patients are particularly fruitful areas for further research.

Lighting also contributes to comfort, ambience, and task accomplishment in the patient room. Various activities require specific lighting features. For instance, an examination requires that the patient's body or part of the body be well illuminated by a light source that minimizes shadows and is as close to natural light as possible. (One alternative is to provide a large, diffuse field of light that illuminates the whole bed.) Nursing staff need a general room light so that the patient can be visually monitored from the hall or from just inside the room. Night-lights for nocturnal monitoring are often required by code. Housekeeping staff require lighting that is bright enough to expose hidden areas that need cleaning.

The patients' and visitors' concerns involve ambience and nonmedical functions. They need low lighting for watching television or talking quietly, task lighting over the bed for reading or writing, medium-level lighting for more animated conversation with a number of visitors, and a dim night-light for late visits to the bathroom. Because their lighting needs are varied, it makes sense to design a flexible system that offers several different light sources, each adjustable by multiple switching or a dimmer. This system should include controls at the patient's bedside.

Lighting can make a room look larger or smaller; can emphasize certain features of the room, such as setting off an alcove or highlighting a particular part of the decor; and can make sick patients look more healthy or healthy ones look sick. The following considerations are important when designing a lighting system:

- Provide general room lighting adjustable by multiple switching and/or rheostats. Make sure illumination levels can be adjusted for the time of day, amount of sunshine in the room, the task being attempted, and the patient's vision.[26]

- Place lighting controls within easy reach of both staff and patients.

- Provide a reading light above or close to the patient's bed. Select lighting fixtures that allow the patient to adjust the light upward and downward.[27,28]

- Provide a night-light that illuminates the path between the patient's bed and the bathroom.

- Avoid examination or general room lighting that may cast unflattering shadows or give an unnatural tone to the patient's skin.

- Provide examination and general room lighting that has color characteristics as close as possible to natural daylight.

- Provide some indirect lighting in patient rooms so that patients and visitors are not forced to deal with lights that are too bright.[27,29]

- Consider using a mix of fluorescent and incandescent lighting.[29]

Accommodating Visitors

Now that it is understood that visitors provide valuable emotional and physical support, institutions are involving families in patient care to a greater degree. Visitors may spend hours sitting with the patient, talking, reading, playing games, or just being there to help if needed. They may adjust the patient's pillows, pull the privacy curtain, manipulate the lighting, get fresh water, assist the patient in using the bathroom and occasionally represent the patient in communicating with staff. Design and policies that neglect visitors' needs can only add stress to an already stressful situation. Visitors' requirements include a comfortable chair positioned within easy conversational distance of the bedridden patient, storage space for coats and gifts, provisions for staying overnight if necessary, and space and policies that allow them to share mealtimes with the patient.

Providing for Mealtime

For most people, mealtimes are social times. Many patients find institutional food so disappointing that eating it in bed, alone, can turn what is usually a pleasant situation into a depressing one. To make mealtimes more enjoyable, many patients would like company.[4] In addition to policies that permit them to eat in the patient room, visitors need a comfortable place to sit and a tray or table to eat from.

Providing a Place to Spend the Night

There are many times when a patient might want a family member to stay overnight, such as the fearful night before surgery or nights of pain. This is a particularly desirable option for patients in private rooms who do not want to be alone or who tend not to "bother" staff for what they need.

Having visitors spend the night in the inpatient room on a cot or fold-down couch may not be appropriate for all patients, such as those in a semiprivate room or ward. However, when patients in one University of Michigan study were asked if they would like a family member or friend to be able to spend the night, over 85 percent responded positively.[4] Chapter 9 covers this issue in more detail.

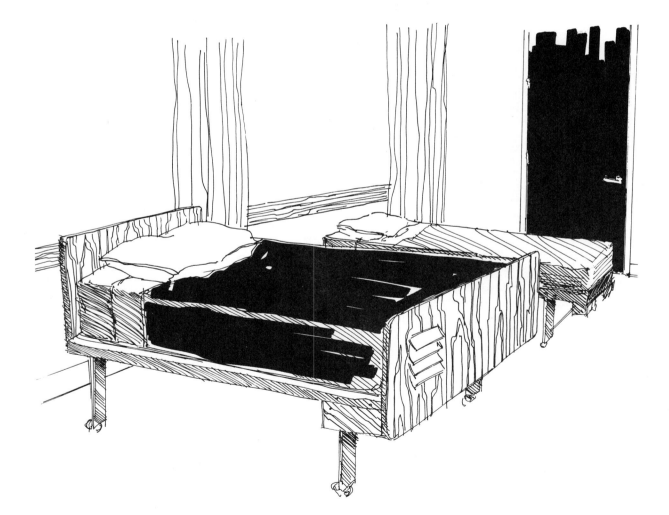

One option for enabling companions to stay overnight with the patient is a rollaway bed or cot in the patient's room.

Inpatient Bathrooms

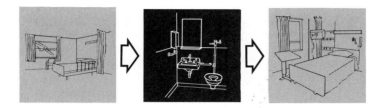

Because of the weakened state of most inpatients, the bathroom for acute care patients requires some special design features (see also chapter 8). Some states require these features by code.

There should be easy wheelchair access from the room threshold to the sink, toilet, and shower. The bathroom door swing should allow adequate clearance, instead of blocking the path to the toilet or sink, as it does in some hospitals.

Because a patient may become ill while inside the bathroom, the door must open outwards in an emergency. Pivot hinges and latch sets that allow doors to be swung either inward or outward are particularly useful.

In addition, there should be space in the bathroom so that staff can assist patients. For nighttime use, a small night-light and illuminated switch may be helpful. The bathroom should be well ventilated and should also be insulated from the surrounding spaces to help ensure acoustical privacy.

Sink Area

The sink area will be used for grooming activities like washing, shaving, combing hair, putting on makeup, and putting in contact lenses. To accommodate these activities patients will need a sink, mirror, storage area, trash receptacle, electrical outlets, and towel racks. The following guidelines apply to the design of this area:

- To accommodate ambulatory as well as wheelchair-bound patients, make sure the sink is at least 34½ inches (87.6 cm) and no more than 36½ inches (92.9 cm) high.[30]

- Select sinks with smooth undersides that are free from obstructions.[30]

- Make sure exposed pipes are insulated to prevent burns and other injuries.[30]

- Select a sink large enough to hold a small basin.

- Select water control levers or knobs that can be reached and operated by patients with little strength or grasping ability.

- Make sure water control levers or knobs are labeled clearly.

- Position the mirror so that it can be seen by tall ambulatory patients as well as by wheelchair-bound, short, or sitting patients.

- Provide electric outlets in close, yet safe, proximity to the sink and mirror, so that hairdryers and shavers can easily be used. Position these in compliance with codes and at a height that can be reached by wheelchair-bound or sitting patients.

- Provide storage shelves that are large enough to hold patients' toiletries and that do not have sharp corners.[16]

- Place shelves within easy reach of someone seated in a wheelchair.[3]

- Install towel racks close to the sink and large enough to hold a washcloth and face towel for each patient.

Shower Area

For many patients, taking a bath or shower can be invigorating, relaxing, or even therapeutic. The shower can be a frightening place, however, for a patient newly ambulatory after a long stay in bed. Thus, safety is a major requirement in shower design. It is important to accommodate those who need staff assistance, as well as those who can shower independently or with a few aids. The following are some suggested considerations:

- Install nonslip flooring.[3,30]

- Provide a portable or foldable seat for those who cannot stand while showering.[3,30]

- Provide a shower seat that is comfortable and nonslippery.

- Allow space in the shower area for two nurses to assist a patient.

- Design the shower area so that a patient can move directly from a wheelchair to the shower seat.

- Select and place grab bars that will support a patient's weight as he or she rises from a shower seat, transfers from a wheelchair, or stands.

- Select shower controls and a shower head operable by patients with little strength or grasping ability.

- Select shower controls that can be easily read and understood by patients standing about three feet away.

- Make sure the shower controls and the nozzle can be reached from both sitting and standing positions.[30]

- Provide a hand-held shower head.[3,30]

- Place the emergency call cord within easy reach of a seated or standing patient, or one who has fallen.

- Place the soap dish and space for shampoo within easy reach of a seated or standing patient.

- Provide hooks for clothing and towels close to the shower but outside the spray area.[3]

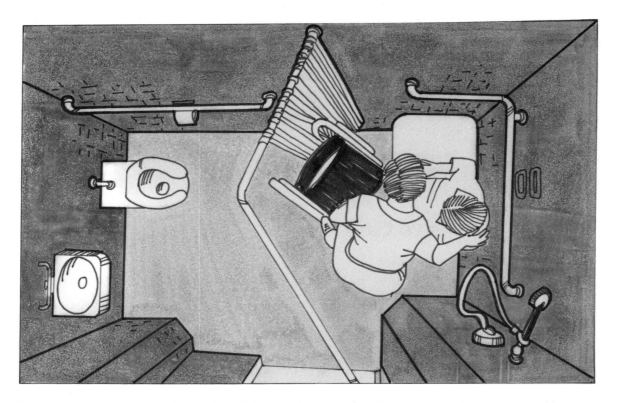

Patient showers need to be designed for safety, wheelchair-access, and nursing assistance. They should contain grab bars, nonslip flooring, and shower controls that are easy to understand and manipulate.

Toilet Area

Key considerations when designing inpatient toilet areas are safety, ease of reaching for and manipulating such items as the toilet paper dispenser or flushing lever, ease of sitting on and rising from the toilet, and the ability of the space to accommodate nurses if they are needed. Specific guidelines include:

- Provide adequate space in front of and directly alongside the toilet for two nurses to assist the patient in transferring from a wheelchair.[30]

- Design the area so that a patient can sit on the toilet and use the sink.

- Provide grab bars as support for sitting and rising.[3]

- Select toilets that are comfortable for elderly patients and high enough (at least 18 inches/45.7 cm) to facilitate easy wheelchair transfer.

- Position the toilet paper dispenser within easy reach of a person seated on the toilet.[3]

- Position the toilet flushing lever within easy reach of a person seated on the toilet.[3,30]

- Select a toilet flushing lever that can be operated by patients with little strength or grasping ability.[3,30]

- Locate an emergency nurse call cord so that it can be easily reached from the toilet.

- Provide a storage area that can be easily reached from the toilet for ointments, suppositories, and other necessary medical items.[30]

Intensive Care Unit

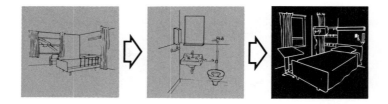

For patients and family members, time spent in an intensive care unit (ICU) is likely to be one of the most physiologically and emotionally stressful periods of their lives. For many, ICUs represent a place where people die. Although this is obviously not always the case, the fears surrounding an ICU are pervasive and real. Design can act together with medical technology, health care staff, and hospital policies to create intensive care units that are humane places for patients and their families.

Patient Needs

Patients admitted to an ICU are experiencing a life-threatening illness that necessitates the use of specialized medical technologies. Even though their physical need for immediate life support may be met by these technologies, studies show that ICU patients need emotional support because they may feel helpless, confused, and afraid. Furthermore, their emotional stress can be magnified by other strains associated with the ICU experience. Perhaps for the first time in their adult lives, all major decisions are being made for them. They lie in what seem like glass-enclosed fishbowls where they are constantly monitored by medical staff and noisy machines that they don't understand.

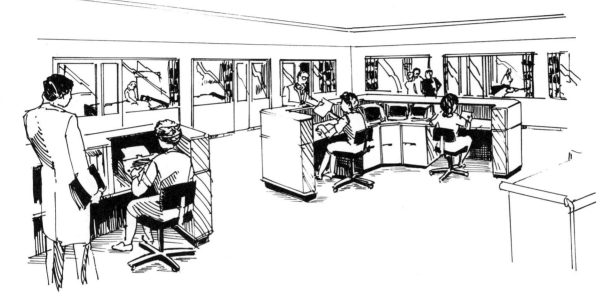

Careful attention is required in ICUs to minimize the harsh effects of the bright, noisy, highly technical environment.

Providing for Privacy

Because ICU patients need constant medical care, these units are often designed for easy visual monitoring and quick access. This makes good medical sense, but if the monitoring is not properly executed, patients may feel exposed and robbed of their privacy. By following a few guidelines, however, increased privacy can be maintained without diminishing good medical care:

- Consider installing solid partitions or walls to separate patients from one another when appropriate.[32]

- Make sure that, upon request, patients can be visually shielded from outside view.[33]

- Provide acoustical privacy for patients so that they can have confidential conversations with medical personnel and with their families.[33]

- To ensure confidentiality and decrease anxiety, provide a space away from, but near, the patient area for doctors to confer. This will decrease the likelihood of others overhearing these conversations.[33]

- Provide auditory, visual, and olfactory privacy for patients using the bedpan or commode, and make sure this equipment is stored out of sight.[33]

Sensory Overload and Emotional Deprivation

The intensive care unit is dominated by medical equipment. An ICU seems to be filled with tubes, wires, I.V.s, bright lights, monitoring equipment, respirators, and other pieces of machinery. It is awash with noise and activity. For patients, all of this activity may create an overwhelming environment in which their senses are seemingly bombarded with noise, light, and, in many cases, pain. Separated from family members and emotionally threatened by the very medical technology that is saving their life, patients may be deprived of much needed human contact and emotional support.

The stresses created by the equipment-related sensory overload and the minimal amount of contact allowed with family have been linked to something called "intensive care unit syndrome." This syndrome is characterized by hallucinations, delusions, psychotic episodes, and sleep disturbances that cannot be traced directly to the illness itself.[34,35] Patients who experience ICU syndrome are far more likely to forget much of their stay in the ICU, misjudge the length of their stay, and be disoriented about the time of day or day of the week than those who do not experience this syndrome. There is some evidence that the incidence of ICU syndrome can be reduced by careful attention to design details (see Research Box #4).[34,35] By providing a less threatening environment (for example, limiting the patient's contact with medical equipment), increasing the patient's contact with others, and providing windows and other orienting devices, the health care facility can limit ICU syndrome. The following design suggestions may help:

- Provide a large clock and calendar in clear view, but not directly in front of, each patient.[36]

- Make sure each patient has a clear and comfortable view of the outside and that this view includes sky and ground.[11,32-34,37]

- Provide ways for patients and nurses to keep each other within view.[33,38]

- Encourage visits by family members by providing comfortable bedside chairs.[33]

- When patients are well enough to receive and make phone calls, provide a phone within easy reach of the bed so that patients can maintain contact with the outside world.[33]

- Use sound-absorbing materials in the ICU patient room and surrounding staff areas to minimize noise.

- Whenever possible, minimize patient contact with medical machinery, store unused equipment out of sight, reduce the cluttered appearance of tubes and wires, and locate monitoring equipment out of the direct line of sight of patients.[33,39]

● Create a less institutional atmosphere by allowing patients to display personal possessions or cards by their bedsides and by providing paintings and other interesting things to look at.[33]

Research Box #4: Providing Windows in the ICU Patient Room

Although it would be difficult in a residential environment to find windowless bedrooms or living rooms, it has been relatively common to find such rooms within health care facilities outside the United States. To examine the effects of windowless ICUs on patients, researchers at Norfolk and Norwich Hospital in England compared patients assigned to windowless and daylit rooms.[34] Patients staying at least 48 hours in the ICU were asked to complete a questionnaire regarding their stay at the hospital. Questionnaire items examined patients' memories of their stay within the ICU, incidences of hallucinations or delusions, problems with sleep, and an estimation of time spent within the ICU.

The results of this questionnaire provide a strong argument for inclusion of windows within the ICU environment. While 91 percent of those patients who stayed in daylit rooms remembered their discharge from the unit, only 73 percent of those in the windowless unit remembered this event. Where 40 percent of those in the daylit rooms believed that they had been oriented as to the time of day, only 9 percent of those assigned to windowless rooms believed that this was true. Those patients in windowless rooms were also much more likely to experience negative psychological episodes than were those in daylit rooms. Those in windowless environments were more likely to experience hallucinations (48 percent compared with 23 percent), visual disturbances (23 percent as opposed to 16 percent), and sleep disturbances (25 percent compared with 16 percent) than were those in daylit rooms.

Although the disturbances examined in this study are commonly experienced by ICU patients, it is clear from these results that the rate of incidence can be considerably lowered if windows are provided in ICU patient rooms.

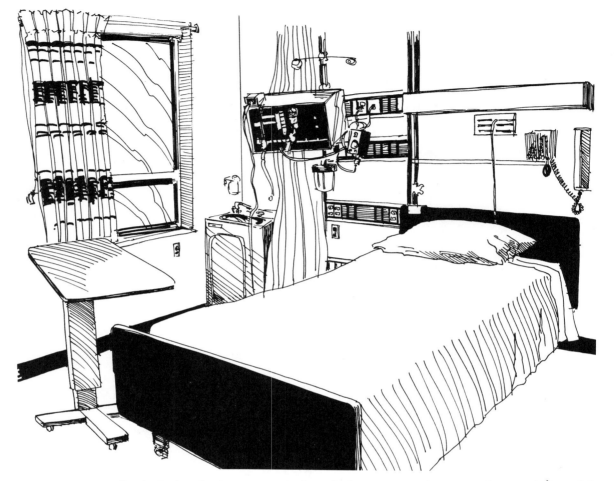

Such design features as exterior windows, acoustic separation, and cheerful colors can be used to soften an otherwise harsh ICU patient room.

Providing a Comfortable Environment

Intensive care patients are often in pain and may find it difficult to position themselves comfortably. They may also have a hard time sleeping. Consequently, attention needs to be paid to lighting levels, lighting quality, temperature, humidity, and the patient's ability to manipulate these systems from the bed. In addition, the design of patient furniture may facilitate both physical and psychological comfort.

- Provide window shades, light dimmers, and double switching on grouped fluorescent fixtures so that patients can adjust lighting to a comfortable level.[33]

- Provide lenses and shades for light fixtures that allow a nonglaring, comfortable quality of light.[33]

- Avoid a situation where lighting from the nurses' station disturbs patients trying to rest.[33]

- Position night-lights so that nursing staff can monitor sleeping patients without disturbing their rest.[33]

- Keep ICU patient rooms at temperatures that reflect the low activity levels of patients.[33]

- Consider maintaining a relative humidity level of 50 percent in patient areas.[32]

- Place a comfortable chair near the patient's bed.[33]

Visitor Needs

Family members of ICU patients suffer great stress. They are worried about the welfare of their loved one and a questionable future. They often feel helpless as they are forced to deal with death or incapacitating illness. They frequently must alter familiar patterns and roles, such as when adult children are faced with making decisions for their parents.

In addition, although visitors want to help and comfort the patient, they are usually allowed only very short visits. Yet they must stay close to the unit in case things take a turn for the worse. Their plight is one of frustration and worry. To make the situation worse, ICU visitors are often forced to wait in hallways or overcrowded and underventilated waiting rooms.

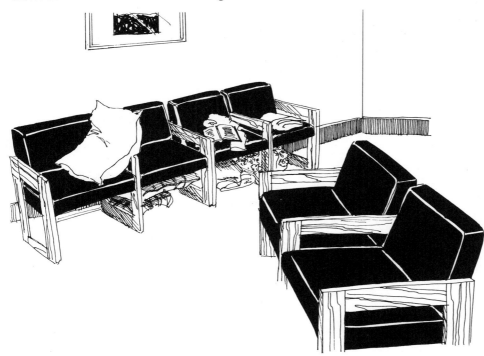

ICU waiting areas should be designed for sleeping, because companions of the ICU patient will often sleep there to be close to the patient at all times. Providing a couch would allow a visitor to rest more comfortably.

When a patient dies, a special consultation or grieving room adjacent to the ICU waiting room should be available, where family members can cope with their loss in private. (Consultation and grieving rooms are discussed in chapter 9.)

Hospitals must not dismiss the emotional needs of family members, who are an important ingredient in the patient's care. The nurturing and support that patients receive from their families are therapeutic and can help them regain health.[40]

Once a hospital recognizes the importance of visitors as an integral part of the total care of the patient, time and resources can be devoted to help care for their emotional and physical needs. For example, at Washoe Medical Center in Reno, Nevada, the concept of "intensive care for relatives" was developed in response to this need.[41] Washoe's trained personnel work directly with family members, helping them understand medical procedures, giving needed emotional support, and, when necessary, helping them begin a healthy grieving process. The program minimizes the potential conflict over policy issues between medical staff and family, allowing everyone to participate in the care of the patient.

Providing emotional support for family members is essential, but they also need a comfortable place to wait, a quiet place to spend the night, a place to be alone, and direct access to information about the patient. (For details on waiting room design, see chapter 4.)

Conclusion

This chapter focused on the inpatient room and bath, the areas most heavily used by patients admitted to a hospital. Again, issues of physical comfort (such as the ability of the bedridden patient to reach and manipulate the nurse call), social contact (such as the ease with which a patient and visitor can hold a private conversation within a shared room), and symbolic meaning (such as the presence and use of privacy curtains) help illustrate how design features can contribute to the patient's well-being and reinforce the caring attitudes shown by staff.

Design Review Questions

Acute Care Inpatient Rooms

Size

☐ Has serious thought been given to making full-scale mock-ups in order to systematically evaluate the designs of acute and intensive care patient rooms?

☐ Has circulation space been provided so that medical emergency teams and equipment can easily reach the patient?

☐ Has space been provided for the bed, a wardrobe, bedside stand, overbed table, patient chair, and visitor chair?

☐ Has space been provided for unobstructed circulation for wheelchairs, rolling I.V. poles, and walkers?

☐ In private rooms, has space been provided to accommodate overnight cots for visitors?

☐ Has sufficient space been provided around the bed so that visitors can place their chairs on either side of the patient's bed?

Number of Occupants

☐ Are both private and semiprivate rooms available?[4]

☐ For those patients who are hospitalized for extended periods of time and who may need social contact, are three-bed and four-bed suites available?[4]

Accommodating Privacy

☐ If there is a window from the patient room to the hallway, has the patient been given the means to manipulate its covering?[5]

☐ If a side-by-side bed scheme is chosen for semiprivate rooms, have potential difficulties been considered, such as the outside view from the bed closest to the hallway and unclear territory for visitors?[5]

☐ If a toe-to-toe double room scheme is chosen, have potential difficulties been considered, such as the patients' views of each other and the bed light of one patient shining in the eyes of the other?[5]

☐ Has the bathroom been located on the hallway wall, rather than on the exterior wall?[5]

Notes

Design that Cares: Planning Health Facilities for Patients and Visitors, by Janet R. Carpman, Myron A. Grant, and Deborah A. Simmons. ©1986 by American Hospital Publishing, Inc.

☐ Has the doorway been placed in line with the foot of the bed, rather than with the head?[5]

☐ Has the facility considered providing motorized cubicle curtains in areas (not including ICUs) where patients are most likely to be nonambulatory and hospitalized for extended periods of time?[5]

☐ Have sound-attenuating materials been used in patient room walls?

☐ Have only quiet functions been located near the patient rooms?

☐ Has the use of sound-absorbing materials within the patient room been investigated?

☐ Have nurse and physician work areas on the patient floor been acoustically contained?

An Outside View

☐ Are the windows as large as possible?

☐ Are the windows positioned so that a bedridden patient can see both the sky and the ground?[13]

☐ If possible, have views been provided of activity going on at street level?[13]

☐ Is visual access to the window unobstructed?[13]

☐ Are the window coverings easily manipulated by patients and visitors?

☐ Do the window coverings allow the room to be completely darkened at night?

Inpatient Room Furnishings

Patient Bed and Chair[14,15]

☐ Are controls for the bed, nurse call, light, and television easily understood and operable by patients who are lying flat or sitting upright?

☐ Are controls lighted for nighttime use?

☐ Can controls be operated with either hand?

☐ Are pressure-sensitive control buttons available for those who have difficulty with hand manipulation?

☐ Can the telephone be easily reached and manipulated with either hand?

☐ Can patients seated in a chair by the bed easily operate the controls?

Notes _____

Design that Cares: Planning Health Facilities for Patients and Visitors, by Janet R. Carpman, Myron A. Grant, and Deborah A. Simmons. ©1986 by American Hospital Publishing, Inc.

☐ Are patient chairs comfortable for both long and short periods of time?

☐ Do patient chairs provide neck and lumbar support?

☐ Are patient chairs easy to get in and out of?

☐ Do patient chairs have sturdy and comfortable arms?

☐ Can patient chairs be moved easily?

☐ Are the chairs wide enough to accommodate heavy patients?

☐ Can patients elevate their feet while sitting in the chair?

☐ Are chair-covering materials easily cleaned and comfortable to sit on?

☐ Can the chair be adjusted to satisfy the requirements of patients who vary in size, weight, and physical condition?

Storage for Belongings

Overbed Table[3,14,15]

☐ Can the overbed table be easily adjusted to various heights by patients with arthritis or limited dexterity?

☐ Is the overbed table stable?

☐ Is there storage space inside the overbed table, with easy access from both sides?

☐ Is there an adjustable mirror in the overbed table that can be used from either side?

☐ Are the drawer and mirror easy to manipulate for people with arthritis or limited dexterity?

☐ Can the overbed table be used as a writing surface when the patient is sitting in a chair?

Bedside Stand[3,14,15]

☐ Can bedside stands be easily moved to maintain the bedridden patient's ease of access to the top surface and drawers?

☐ Are the drawers of the bedside table easy to open for people with arthritis or limited dexterity?

Notes _____

Design that Cares: Planning Health Facilities for Patients and Visitors, by Janet R. Carpman, Myron A. Grant, and Deborah A. Simmons. ©1986 by American Hospital Publishing, Inc.

Wardrobe[17]
- [ ] Do wardrobes have sufficient capacity to store winter outerwear, shoes or boots, some clothing, underwear, a suitcase, and other small possessions?
- [ ] Is there a small lockable drawer within the wardrobe?
- [ ] Can the wardrobe be easily opened and closed by people with arthritis or limited dexterity?
- [ ] Can the clothes rod be adjusted to be accessible by wheelchair-bound patients?
- [ ] Does the placement of the wardrobe not impede circulation or other room functions?
- [ ] Are hooks available inside the wardrobe for bathrobes and other clothing?

Other Storage[16]
- [ ] Has a tackboard been provided so that patients can display cards and mementos?
- [ ] Is there a shelf for displaying flowers and other personal items?
- [ ] Is the flower shelf sufficiently wide and does it have enough vertical clearance to accommodate large flower arrangements?
- [ ] Has the flower shelf been positioned so that it will not be bumped?
- [ ] Does the flower shelf have no sharp corners?
- [ ] Are hooks for visitors' coats behind the door or in some other unobstructive location?

Patient Television
- [ ] Are two televisions provided in semiprivate rooms?
- [ ] Are personal audio devices provided, such as pillow speakers or earphones?

Clocks
- [ ] Has a clock been placed in each patient room? Is it visible from the bed, yet not directly in the patient's line of sight?
- [ ] If analog clocks are used, do they have clear numbers, as well as hour, minute, and second hands that are readable from the bed?
- [ ] Are all patient clocks 12-hour rather than 24-hour clocks?
- [ ] Are the clocks noninstitutional looking?

Notes

Design that Cares: Planning Health Facilities for Patients and Visitors, by Janet R. Carpman, Myron A. Grant, and Deborah A. Simmons. ©1986 by American Hospital Publishing, Inc.

Artwork

☐ Has an "art cart" program been adopted so that patients are periodically given choices about the artwork in their room?[20]

☐ Have locations for hanging artwork been selected so that the artwork can be seen from the patient's bed?[20]

☐ Have natural subjects and settings been emphasized?[20]

☐ Has representational art, rather than abstract art, been emphasized?[20,21]

☐ Have photographs or reproductions of paintings been emphasized?[20]

☐ Have texturally complex images been emphasized?[20]

☐ When appropriate, have mobiles been considered as an artwork alternative for some patient rooms?[20]

☐ Have images of urban scenes been de-emphasized?[20]

☐ Have portraits been de-emphasized?[20]

☐ Have muted or dark colors been de-emphasized?[20]

☐ Has poster art with words been de-emphasized?[20]

Color and Lighting

☐ Can illumination levels be adjusted for the time of day, amount of sunshine in a room, and the task being attempted?[26]

☐ Are lighting controls placed within easy reach of both staff and patients?

☐ Has a reading light been provided above or close to the patient's bed?[27,28]

☐ Do light fixtures allow the patient to adjust the light upward and downward?[27,28]

☐ Is there a night-light that illuminates the path between the patient's bed and the bathroom?

☐ Has lighting that may cast shadows or an unnatural tone to the patient's skin been avoided?

☐ Has examination and general room lighting been provided that has color characteristics as close as possible to natural daylight?

☐ Has indirect lighting been provided in patient rooms so that patients and visitors are not forced to deal with lights that are too bright?[27,29]

☐ Has a mix of fluorescent and incandescent lighting been considered?[29]

Notes _____

Design that Cares: Planning Health Facilities for Patients and Visitors, by Janet R. Carpman, Myron A. Grant, and Deborah A. Simmons. ©1986 by American Hospital Publishing, Inc.

Accommodating Visitors

Providing for Mealtime

☐ Are visitors allowed to eat meals with patients?[4]

☐ Is there a comfortable place to sit, with a tray or table for visitors to eat from?[4]

Providing a Place to Spend the Night
(See chapter 9.)

Inpatient Bathrooms

☐ Does the threshold allow easy wheelchair access?

☐ Can the bathroom door be opened from the outside?

☐ For nighttime use, are a night-light and illuminated switch available?

☐ Is the bathroom well-ventilated and also insulated from surrounding spaces to help ensure acoustical privacy?

Sink Area

☐ Is the sink at least 34½ inches (87.6 cm) and no more than 36½ inches (92.7 cm) high?[30]

☐ Are sink undersides smooth and free from obstructions?[30]

☐ Are exposed pipes insulated to prevent burns and other injuries?[30]

☐ Is the sink large enough to accommodate a small basin?

☐ Can water control levers or knobs be reached and operated by patients with little strength or grasping ability?

☐ Are water control levers or knobs labeled clearly?

☐ Is the mirror positioned so that it can be seen by tall or ambulatory patients as well as wheelchair-bound, short, or sitting patients?

☐ Are electric outlets in close, yet safe, proximity to the sink and mirror, so that hairdryers and shavers can be used easily?

☐ Are electric outlets positioned so they can be reached by wheelchair-bound or seated patients?

☐ Are storage shelves large enough to hold patients' toiletries?[16]

Notes _____

Design that Cares: Planning Health Facilities for Patients and Visitors, by Janet R. Carpman, Myron A. Grant, and Deborah A. Simmons. ©1986 by American Hospital Publishing, Inc.

☐ Are storage shelves free from sharp corners?[16]

☐ Are shelves positioned so that they can be easily reached by someone seated in a wheelchair?[3]

☐ Are towel racks large enough to hold a washcloth and face towel for each patient?

Shower Area

☐ Has nonslip flooring been installed?[3,30]

☐ Is a portable or foldable seat available for those who cannot stand while showering?[3,30]

☐ Is the shower seat comfortable and nonslippery?

☐ Has space been provided in the shower area for two nurses to assist the patient?

☐ Is the shower area designed so that a patient can move directly from a wheelchair to a shower seat?

☐ Will grab bars support a patient's weight, as needed, while the patient is rising from a shower seat, transferring from a wheelchair, and standing?

☐ Are shower controls and the shower head operable by patients with little strength or grasping ability?

☐ Can shower controls be easily read and understood by patients standing about three feet away?

☐ Can shower controls and the nozzle be reached from both sitting and standing positions?[30]

☐ Is a hand-held shower head provided?[3,30]

☐ Is the emergency call cord within easy reach of a seated or standing patient or one who has fallen?

☐ Are a soap dish and a space for shampoo within easy reach of a seated or standing patient?

☐ Have hooks for clothing and towels been provided in close proximity to the shower but outside the spray area?[3]

Notes _____

Design that Cares: Planning Health Facilities for Patients and Visitors, by Janet R. Carpman, Myron A. Grant, and Deborah A. Simmons. ©1986 by American Hospital Publishing, Inc.

Toilet Area

☐ Has adequate space been provided in front of and directly alongside the toilet for two nurses to assist the patient when transferring from a wheelchair?[30]

☐ Is the area designed so that a patient can sit on the toilet and use the sink?

☐ Are grab bars provided as support for sitting and rising?

☐ Are toilets high enough to facilitate easy wheelchair transfer and comfortable use by elderly patients?

☐ Is the toilet paper dispenser within easy reach of a person seated on the toilet?[3]

☐ Is the toilet flushing lever positioned within easy reach of a person seated on the toilet?[3,30]

☐ Can the toilet flushing lever be operated by patients with little strength or grasping ability?[3,30]

☐ Is an emergency nurse call cord easily reached from the toilet?

☐ Has a storage area been provided for ointments, suppositories, and other necessary medical items? Is it easily reached from the toilet?[30]

Intensive Care Unit

Patient Needs

Providing for Privacy

☐ Have solid partitions or walls to separate patients from one another been considered?[32]

☐ Can patients, upon request, be shielded from outside view?[33]

☐ Is acoustical privacy provided for patients so that they can have confidential conversations with medical personnel and with their families?[33]

☐ To ensure confidentiality and decrease anxiety, has space been provided away from, but near, the patient area for doctors to confer?[33]

☐ Is auditory, visual, and olfactory privacy provided for patients using the bedpan or commode? Is this equipment stored out of sight?[33]

Sensory Overload and Emotional Deprivation

☐ Are a large clock and a calendar in clear view but not directly in front of each patient?[36]

☐ Does each patient have a clear and comfortable view to the outside, and does this view include sky and ground?[11,32-34,37]

Notes_____

Design that Cares: Planning Health Facilities for Patients and Visitors, by Janet R. Carpman, Myron A. Grant, and Deborah A. Simmons. ©1986 by American Hospital Publishing, Inc.

☐ Are ways provided for patients and nurses to keep each other within view?[33,38]

☐ Are visits by family members encouraged by providing comfortable bedside chairs?[33]

☐ When a patient is well enough to receive and make phone calls, is a phone within easy reach of the bed?[33]

☐ Have sound absorbing materials been used in the ICU patient room and in surrounding staff areas?

☐ Has patient contact with medical machinery been minimized by storing unused equipment out of sight and by locating monitoring equipment out of the patient's direct line of sight when possible?[33,39]

☐ Are patients able to display personal possessions or cards by their bedside?[33]

☐ Have paintings or other artwork been provided?

Providing a Comfortable Environment
☐ Are window shades, light dimmers, and other controls available so that patients can adjust lighting to a comfortable level?[33]

☐ Are all windows and light fixtures glare-free?[33]

☐ Has a situation been avoided where lighting from the nurses' station disturbs patients trying to rest?[33]

☐ Have night-lights been positioned in ways that enable nursing staff to monitor sleeping patients without disturbing their rest?[33]

☐ Are ICU patient rooms kept at temperatures that reflect the low activity levels of patients?[33]

☐ Is a relative humidity level of 50 percent maintained in patient areas?[32]

☐ Is there a comfortable chair near the patient bed?[33]

Visitor Needs
☐ Does each ICU area have its own visitor waiting room? (For details on the design of high stress waiting areas, see chapter 4.)

☐ Has consideration been given to allowing family members to participate in patient care?

☐ Does each ICU area have its own private consultation or grieving room? (For details on the design of consultation or grieving rooms, see chapter 9.)

Notes _____

Design that Cares: Planning Health Facilities for Patients and Visitors, by Janet R. Carpman, Myron A. Grant, and Deborah A. Simmons. ©1986 by American Hospital Publishing, Inc.

References

1. U.S. Department of Health and Human Services. *Guidelines for Construction and Equipment of Hospital and Medical Facilities.* Washington, DC: U.S. Government Printing Office, 1984.

2. Hayward, C., and members of the AIA Committee on Architecture for Health, Programming Subcommittee. *A Generic Process for Projecting Health Care Space Needs.* Washington, DC: AIA Committee, 1985 Oct.

3. King, J., Marans, R. A., and Solomon, L. A. *Pre-Construction Evaluation: A Report on the Full Scale Mock-Up and Evaluation of Hospital Rooms.* Ann Arbor: Architectural Research Laboratory, University of Michigan, 1982.

4. Reizenstein, J. E., and Grant, M. A. Patient activities and schematic design preferences. Unpublished research report #2, Patient and Visitor Participation Project, Office of Hospital Planning, Research and Development, University of Michigan, Ann Arbor, 1981.

5. Reizenstein, J. E., and Grant, M. A. Schematic design of the inpatient room. Unpublished research report #1, Patient and Visitor Participation Project, Office of Hospital Planning, Research and Development, University of Michigan, Ann Arbor, 1981.

6. Barker, M. People-oriented design. *Hospitals Forum.* 1985 July-Aug. pp. 35-36.

7. Prototype hospital room provides privacy and amenities. *Contract.* 1985 Feb. pp. 92-93.

8. Reizenstein, J. E., and Grant, M. A. Color, cubicle curtains, handrails. Unpublished research report #23, Patient and Visitor Participation Project, Office of Hospital Planning, Research and Development, University of Michigan, Ann Arbor, 1983.

9. Alexander, M. E. No windows. *Lancet.* 1973 Mar. 10. 1(7802):549.

10. Collins, B. L. *Windows and People: A Literature Survey.* Washington, DC: U.S. Government Printing Office, 1975.

11. Keep, P. J. Stimulus deprivation in windowless rooms. *Anesthesia.* 1977 July-Aug. 32(7):598-602.

12. Ulrich, R. S. View through a window may influence recovery from surgery. *Science.* 1984 Apr. 27. 224(4647):420-21.

13. Verderber, S. F. Windowness and human behavior in the hospital rehabilitation environment. Ph.D. dissertation, University of Michigan, Ann Arbor, 1982. Available from UMI, 300 N. Zeeb Road, Ann Arbor, Michigan 48106.

14. Carpman, J. R., and Grant, M. A. Hospital patient room furnishings mock-ups. Unpublished research report #25, Patient and Visitor Participation Project, Office of Hospital Planning, Research and Development, University of Michigan, Ann Arbor, 1984.

15. Solomon, L. A., and Gaudette, R. Adult general hospital bed and furniture evaluation. Unpublished report, Office of Hospital Planning, Research and Development, University of Michigan, Ann Arbor, 1984.

16. Reizenstein, J. E., Vaitkus, M. A., and Grant, M. A. Patient belongings. Unpublished research report #9, Patient and Visitor Participation Project, Office of Hospital Planning, Research and Development, University of Michigan, Ann Arbor, 1982.

17. Reizenstein, J. E., and Grant, M. A. *From Hospital Research to Hospital Design.* Patient and Visitor Participation Project, Office of Hospital Planning, Research and Development, University of Michigan, Ann Arbor, 1982.

18. Carpman, J. R., and Grant, M. A. TVs in hospitals: behavior and preferences. Unpublished research report #11, Patient and Visitor Participation Project; Office of Hospital Planning, Research and Development; University of Michigan, Ann Arbor, 1984.

19. Baron, J. H., and Greene, L. Art in hospitals. *British Medical Journal.* 1984 Dec. 289(22):1731-37.

20. Carpman, J. R., and Grant, M. A. Inpatient preferences for hospital room artwork. Unpublished research report #32, Patient and Visitor Participation Project, Office of the Replacement Hospital Program, University of Michigan, Ann Arbor, 1984.

21. Miller, D. B., and Goldman, L. Selecting paintings for the nursing home. *Nursing Homes.* 1984 Jan.-Feb. pp. 12-16.

22. Birren, F. Human response to color and light. *Hospitals.* 1979 July 16. 53(14):93-96.

23. Edwards, K. The environment inside the hospital. *Practitioner.* 1979 June. 222(1332):746-51.

24. Chaney, P. S. Decor reflects environmental psychology. *Hospitals.* 1973 June 1. 47(11):61-66.

25. Rabin, M. Medical-facility colors reduce patient stress. *Contract.* 1981 Feb. 23(2):78-83.

26. Hayward, D. G. Psychological factors in the use of light and lighting in buildings. In: Lang, J., Burnette, C., and others, editors. *Designing for Human Behavior: Architecture and the Behavioral Sciences.* Stroudsburg, PA: Dowden, Hutchinson and Ross, Inc., 1974.

27. Rosenfeld, N. Indirect lighting improves outlook for everyone. *Modern Hospital.* 1971 Aug. 117(2):78-80.

28. Lam, W. M. C. *Perception and Lighting as Formgivers for Architecture.* New York: McGraw-Hill, Inc., 1977.

29. Boyce, P. R. *Human Factors in Lighting.* New York: Macmillan Publishing Co., 1981.

30. Kira, A. *The Bathroom.* New York: Bantam Books, 1977.

31. A slightly serious look at a serious problem: hospital design and policy versus patient comfort. *Medical Journal of Australia.* 1974 Aug. 2(8):301-2.

32. Hickler, F. D. Symposium on design and function of the operating room suite and special areas. *Journal of Anesthesiology.* 1969 Aug. 31(2):103-6.

33. Clipson, C. W., and Wehrer, J. J. *Planning for Cardiac Care: A Guide to the Planning and Design of Cardiac Care Facilities.* Ann Arbor, MI: Health Administration Press, 1973.

34. Keep, P. J., James, J., and Inman, M. Windows in the intensive therapy unit. *Anesthesia.* 1980 Mar. 35(3):257-62.

35. Gowan, N. J. The perceptual world of the intensive care unit: an overview of some environmental considerations in the helping relationship. *Heart and Lung.* 1979 Mar.-Apr. 8(2):340-44.

36. Kornfeld, D. S. The hospital environment: its impact on the patient. *Advances in Psychosomatic Medicine.* 1972. 8:252-70.

37. Popkin, S. Form must follow function. *Michigan Hospitals.* 1980 Sept. 16(9):9-11.

38. Sturdavant, M. Intensive nursing service in circular and rectangular units compared. *Hospitals.* 1960 July 16. 34(14):46-48, 71-78.

39. Zubatkin, A. D. Psychological impact of medical equipment on patients. *Journal of Clinical Engineering.* 1980 July-Sept. 5(3):250-55.

40. Molter, N. C. Needs of relatives of critically ill patients: a descriptive study. *Heart and Lung.* 1979 Mar.-Apr. 8(2):332-39.

41. Hoover, M. J. Intensive care for relatives. *Hospitals.* 1979 July 16. 53(14):219-22.

Chapter 7

Gaining Access to Nature

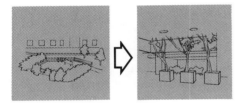

Outdoor Spaces   **Nature Indoors**

For most of us, nature holds deep meaning: it is a place of refuge, peace and tranquility, and a symbol of life and growth.[1,2] It is not surprising, then, that people gain a great deal of pleasure from contact with nature. We surround ourselves with plants, we hang photographs and paintings of natural scenes, we go to mountains and seashores as a way of "getting away from it all." Research findings support this sense of the importance of nature. Evidence of the pleasure associated with nature emerges from a number of empirical studies examining preferences, in which participants consistently preferred photographs of natural views dominated by vegetation or water over unblighted urban scenes.[3-5]

However, the benefits reaped from natural scenes go beyond simple pleasure. Laboratory studies involving both stressed and nonstressed people have shown that simply viewing photographs of nature reduced anxiety and increased levels of relaxation.[6,7] These studies suggest that the availability of nature, in the form of views from windows as well as accessible outdoor spaces, can be restorative. According to one researcher, if an individual is stressed, viewing an attractive natural scene will be soothing because it can "elicit feelings of pleasantness, hold interest, and block or reduce stressful thoughts."[3]

Health Care Facility Outdoor Spaces

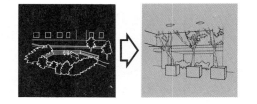

Outdoor spaces—especially courtyards, rooftop gardens, or "vest pocket" parks—provide needed relief and respite. Natural settings provide soothing and inviting opportunities to "get away," at least pyschologically, from the pressures inside the health care facility. In addition, an attractive outdoor space has important symbolic value, giving the health care facility a positive image and showing both users and the community that the facility is sensitive to the needs of its users, and understands that comfort and beauty, as well as technical competence, are part of the healing process (see Research Box #1).

There are numerous outdoor functions a health care facility can accommodate if appropriate space and conditions are available. If one large, optimally located space is not available, it may be advantageous to provide several smaller spaces that relate well to the building areas they are near. For instance, exterior space near the cafeteria could accommodate staff and visitors having lunch outside during warm weather. An outdoor area near a major public space like the main lobby would be appropriate for a children's play area and for a walking and sitting park for visitors. Quiet, protected, easily accessible areas near inpatient units would provide opportunities for bedridden and ambulatory patients to get outside.

The patients, visitors, and staff who are likely to use an outdoor courtyard or park at a health care facility are diverse in age and physical ability. Although it might seem surprising, even inpatients are likely to be frequent users of an outdoor space. In one study, 91 percent of the inpatients sampled at a tertiary care hospital said that they would like to use an outdoor space planned for walking or sitting.[5] Because more than two-thirds of these patients reported walking to at least one place—from 25 feet (7.5 meters) to well over 1,000 feet (300 meters) from their rooms—their use of an outdoor space seems likely. The fact that many patients are eager for a change of scene makes it all the more probable that they will go outdoors, given good weather and an outdoor space that can accommodate their special needs.

Research Box #1:
Evaluating a Hospital Park

Recognizing that staff, patients, and visitors need a quiet place to escape from hospital stress, Bellevue Hospital in New York City built a park.[8] The park, cut off from the noise of the city by an earth berm, was designed to provide year-round use. With benches, walkways, a fountain, and an amphitheater, the park was designed to facilitate both solitude and social activities.

To evaluate the park design, environmental design researchers interviewed patients, staff, and visitors using the park one month after its opening and again approximately one year later. To supplement the interview data, "head counts" of the number of people using the park were also made.

Those interviewed overwhelmingly endorsed the park. When given a choice between the park and other amenities, 98 percent reported that they would not like anything else in its place. Participants in the study reported using the park repeatedly; they found that the park "re-energized" them and that it was a relaxing and comfortable place to spend time. The establishment of the park was also seen as evidence that the hospital cared for staff, patients, and visitors.

Finally, the evaluation documented that active use of the park wasn't necessary for people to benefit from its existence. Just walking by the park was found to be relaxing. For these "visual" users, the park served as a focal point, a pleasant place for one's mind to wander. From these interviews, it was concluded that the park benefited a much larger group than just those who entered it.

The desire to use a courtyard is not limited to ambulatory patients. At one hospital, for example, patients on gurneys and in wheelchairs have such a strong desire to be outside that they are frequently seen on the front entrance sidewalk during warm months, quite close to passing traffic. However, an outdoor space that serves a wide range of inpatients, outpatients, and visitors has design requirements not necessarily met by a typical urban courtyard. In addition, outdoor areas that will be used as play spaces for children—both sick and well—have particular design requirements.[9-13] This broad spectrum of would-be users, therefore, requires an unusual set of design guidelines to be considered in designing an outdoor space.

Designing Outdoor Spaces for Health Care Facilities

Even though people enjoy contact with nature and enjoy an outdoor space associated with a health care facility, not all outdoor spaces are equal; it is not enough merely to plant a few trees and set down a bench or two. Just as most people hold strong preferences for natural settings over urban scenes, some natural areas are preferred over others. After reviewing the results of a number of studies in environmental perception, researchers have described characteristics of places that are highly preferred—places that provide a degree of complexity and a sense of enclosure, yet are also understandable and harmoniously composed.[14,15]

When people look at a scene, they seek a sense of involvement and a richness that gives them reason to continue viewing.[14,15] For instance, a densely planted area provides greater visual interest than a sparsely planted one. It provides more to view and a greater variety of textures. Similarly, an area of lawn with people sitting or walking is more interesting to look at than an area planted with ground cover that prevents people from using it.[16]

People also have strong preferences about what they like to look at.[4] For instance, in one study, scenes with a greater number of trees were consistently rated higher than those with fewer trees. The ratings increased in a linear fashion as the number of trees increased. Trees were seen as a source of visual interest as well as a source of beauty, shade, and color. Absence of planting was characterized as "bare" and "boring" by some respondents.[17]

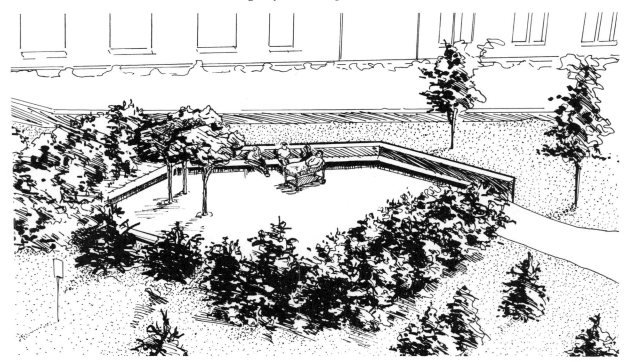

Accessible outdoor space is highly valued by patients, visitors, and staff.

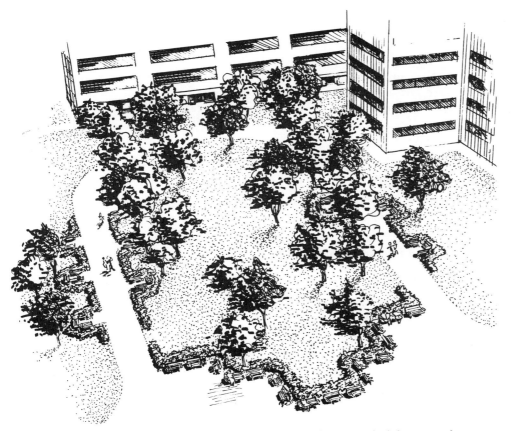

One study showed that when given a choice, patients and visitors prefer densely planted outdoor spaces. They also like to have many possible places to sit and the option to sit and talk privately or to sit out in the open and people-watch.

It has been theorized that people enjoy a sense of enclosure when they are outdoors.[14,15] A seating area surrounded by trees, adjacent to an open circulation or activity area, provides a sense of enclosure. It allows users to look through the perimeter trees to a highly visible open space; it allows them to be one of the observers rather than the observed. Although the mere presence of vegetation is appreciated, the fact that trees and other planting materials are arranged in a way that gives a sense of enclosure is also very important.

In one study, where patients and visitors were asked to choose among private seating areas surrounded by shrubs, trees, or both shrubs and trees, they preferred the greatest vegetation possible.[17] The option showing "shrubs and trees" was most preferred, "trees only" was a close second choice, and "shrubs only" was the third choice. This preference for enclosure was also affirmed in a study of seating behavior in hospital courtyards, where one of the most popular areas to sit—particularly with couples looking for privacy—was screened by a planter.[16]

People like spaces that are understandable, where there is no question how one element relates to another. People tend not to enjoy things that "float" or seem disconnected and alone, like single trees in planters.[18]

When designing an outdoor space for a health care facility:

- Provide as many trees as possible.

- Provide a hierarchy of seating arrangements and locations, ranging from public to private.

- Plant trees and shrubs adjacent to seating to give people a sense of enclosure and privacy.

- Choose trees and shrubs that will provide outdoor spaces with different colors and fragrances throughout the year.

- Design comfortable seating areas as settings for conversation and people-watching.

- Where appropriate, provide some open lawn for active use.[16]

- Keep in mind that some patients and people in nearby buildings will only experience the outdoor space as it is seen from the inside.

- Avoid paving materials, such as brick, that will give wheelchair users a bumpy or uneven ride.

Although these principles will prove valuable in developing a design, each site has its own particular attributes and limitations that must be taken into consideration. The design of a park that works well in one area may be inappropriate for a different site. The needs and preferences of a particular group of users also may differ significantly from one area to another. Consequently, we suggest that a participatory approach to outdoor space design be considered (see Research Box #2). Paying heed to the preferences of future users allows design decision makers to develop a plan that will balance human preferences with site demands and other constraints (see chapter 10).

Research Box #2: Enabling Users to Participate in the Design of an Outdoor Courtyard

In designing outdoor spaces, each site comes with a slightly different set of parameters. Each site has built-in limitations and features that will make it a unique place to be; each site requires an individual design approach. But along with site-specific parameters such as size, climate, and adjacent spaces, the design needs to consider the particular characteristics and preferences of its eventual users.

As part of an ongoing research effort at the University of Michigan Hospitals, a study was conducted about design elements of an outdoor courtyard.[12] Two hundred randomly sampled patients and visitors were interviewed concerning their preferences for different planting densities, seating arrangements, and other issues. As part of the interview process, patients and visitors examined a series of black and white photographs showing various outdoor spaces and indicated their preferences.

These photographs were taken of a specially constructed architectural model and showed different design alternatives for the proposed courtyard. Participants rated 27 photos on a 1-to-5 scale indicating how much they thought they would like to go to the place shown in the photo.

The responses showed that patients and visitors preferred:

Dense rather than sparse tree plantings

Having an opportunity to choose from among several different seating options

Being able to sit directly or diagonally across from the person they were talking with, rather than on benches arranged in a straight line

Private seating areas surrounded by both shrubs and trees, rather than by little or no vegetation

Benches with both armrests and backs

The findings of the study allowed researchers to make a number of design recommendations based directly on the eventual users' preferences.

Location and Access

People can use an outdoor space only if they know it exists and can travel to it easily. One study comparing the uses of different hospital courtyards found that the most frequently used courtyard was visible from a main circulation area.[16] Courtyards that could be seen and entered only from a particular medical unit were not as widely used. Thus, the location of the outdoor space and its adjacency to other spaces or buildings will affect how readily patients and visitors use it:[16]

- Provide visual access to the outdoor space from the main public spaces and circulation areas.

- Whenever possible, provide direct access to the outdoor space from public areas.

- Consider promoting outdoor spaces by placing them prominently on maps and including them on tours of the facility.

Many users of a health care facility's outdoor space will be physically impaired. They may have difficulty walking or have limited upper body strength. They may be in a wheelchair or on crutches. They may feel unsure about their ability to travel far on their own and need a degree of security before they will venture outside. To provide access to the outdoor space a number of design features should be considered:[16]

- Avoid using heavy doors that may be difficult to open or that have a raised threshold which may be difficult to negotiate in a wheelchair.

- At outdoor space entrances, consider using automatic doors to ensure easy access by those who are mobility-impaired.

- Avoid using self-locking doors.

- Provide visual access to the outdoor space, so patients can see what the space looks like and decide whether they feel up to making the journey.

Walkways

Walkways should be constructed to encourage visits to the facility's outdoor spaces by a variety of users. It is easy to imagine an outdoor space in which narrow, bricked pathways wind around, climbing over small hills and descending into sunken areas. However, these design elements would subject a recent surgical or orthopedic patient to unnecessary discomfort. Long distances, steep grades, or uneven surfaces may even tax the physical abilities of many ambulatory patients. In order to accommodate all users, circulation surfaces should allow wheeled equipment to proceed easily. There should also be some physical support like a handrail in order to make it easier for frail patients to get some outdoor exercise. In addition, there should be places where nonambulatory patients can situate themselves close to friends seated on benches, without feeling conspicuous.

To facilitate use of outdoor walkways, a number of design features should be considered:

- Provide walkway surfaces that can be easily and smoothly negotiated by stretchers, gurneys, wheelchairs, strollers, and other wheeled equipment. Avoid brick and other uneven surfaces.[16]

- Provide surface grading that is as level as possible, so manual wheelchair users can wheel themselves around and frail patients can walk easily.

- Avoid ramps at doorways that inhibit movement of a patient in a wheelchair or on a gurney.[16]

- Provide a continuous handrail along walkways on sloped and flat grades.

- If metal handrails are used, coat them with plastic or vinyl so that they are not slippery when wet.[19]

- Make walkways wide enough for two gurneys to pass each other and for three or four people to walk side by side.

- In those regions where winter weather is a problem, consider various means for ice and snow removal on walkways, including melting devices below the surface.

Seating

Patients, visitors, and staff will use an outdoor area for a variety of reasons. Some need solitude. Some need a place to hold a private conversation. Others need a comfortable place to have lunch with companions. Given the wide variety of potential activities, users of outdoor space will appreciate having an opportunity to choose among several seating options. The kind of seating options available will determine how much perceived privacy is present or how easily a conversation can be held. For example, to converse comfortably, people prefer to sit directly or diagonally across from the person they are talking to. With a single straight bench, people are forced to turn their bodies or heads awkwardly in order to talk. Conversations are made much easier when two or three benches face one another, at a comfortable distance.

Seating orientation may affect comfort as well. Seats should be oriented to allow users to take advantage of or to shield themselves from the sun at different times of the day. Some patients may be particularly bothered by wind and cooler temperatures. Seating for them should be sheltered from the wind and placed in maximum sunlight.[16]

The following are guidelines for the design of outdoor seating arrangements (see also chapter 8):

- Provide a variety of seat types ranging from chairs to benches.

- Provide some seating that will usually be in sun and some that will usually be in shade. In addition, provide some seating that will be sheltered from wind.[16]

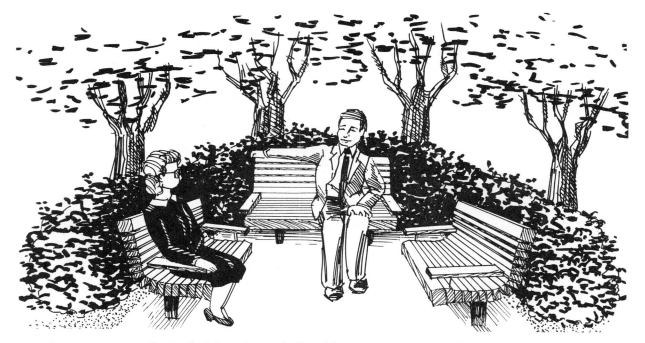

Seats that face inward, like this, create a cozy setting for conversation.

● Provide some seating along major circulation paths, so sitters can people-watch.

● Provide some seating that gives users a feeling of enclosure and separation from the mainstream.

● Provide some seating that allows for groups of five or six and some seating for one or two.

● If possible, provide some seating around tables.[16]

● Provide places for patients on stretchers or in wheelchairs to situate themselves among seating for ambulatory people. Make these areas accessible from a major walkway.

● If possible, provide seating that users can arrange in groups or move to a more comfortable location.

● Provide seating that enables people to easily see and talk with each other.

Bench size and design are also important considerations. How seating is designed (for example, how high it is, and whether it has armrests or a back) will affect how comfortable and useful it is. Some ambulatory patients, especially older ones, have trouble getting up from low seating. Benches with backs give needed support, and armrests will help these users lower themselves comfortably and rise easily and safely.

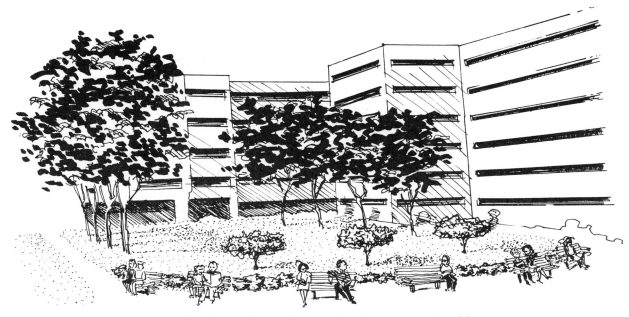

Benches arranged along major circulation paths provide good opportunities for people-watching.

The scale or size of outdoor furniture should be comfortable. For instance, when shown pictures of small, medium, and large benches, respondents in one study rejected the small bench (holding one to three people) as "too small."[17] Some respondents felt that this bench might force them to sit uncomfortably close to someone else. The large benches (holding six or seven) were rejected as "too large." Respondents felt comfortable only with the medium-size bench (holding three to five people). It should be noted, however, that preferences for sitting in individual chairs were not examined.

The bench material also makes a difference. A bench that looks comfortable is more likely to be used than one that looks hard, hot in the summer, or cold in the winter. In one study, when patients and visitors were shown drawings of six bench designs of various materials (wood, concrete, and wire mesh), with various types of back support and the presence or absence of armrests, their perceptions of comfort became clear.[17] The two most-preferred styles were made of wood and had backrests, whereas the concrete bench without arms or backrest was one of the least preferred designs.

The following are suggestions to consider when selecting seating for outdoor areas:

- Provide seating with backs and armrests.
- Provide seating that allows an elderly person or someone with little flexibility and strength to sit and rise easily.
- Provide seating that is comfortable for an hour or more at a time.
- Consider seating materials other than concrete.
- Provide seating that is considered attractive by patients and visitors.

Research Box #3: Evaluating Various Outdoor Seating Options

Several seating types were considered for the central courtyard being designed for the new University of Michigan Replacement Hospital Program. In order to make an informed decision, planners needed information about user perceptions of comfort and aesthetics.[20] This information would be combined with facts about maintenance, cost, and other factors in contributing to the final decision about selection of outdoor seating.

Four seats were considered: two wire mesh outdoor chairs and two wooden outdoor chairs. Seat A was portable white metal mesh, seat B was curved wood with metal arms, seat C was heavy, dark green wire mesh, and seat D was curved wood with wooden arms.

The four seats were placed in the cafeteria of the existing hospital. Patients, visitors, and staff were all asked to sit in the four chairs and fill out a short questionnaire. The questionnaire asked the 320 participants to indicate their preferences for the various seats, on the basis of comfort and aesthetics. They were also asked a number of background questions. Seat D (curved wood with wooden arms) was the overwhelming favorite. It ranked consistently high on the various comfort and aesthetic criteria as well as on an overall evaluation question. The researchers recommended that only this seat be selected for the central courtyard.

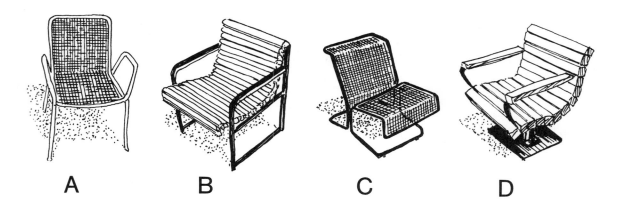

A **B** **C** **D**

See Research Box #3: These four chairs were evaluated for comfort and aesthetics before outdoor furniture was chosen for a central courtyard.

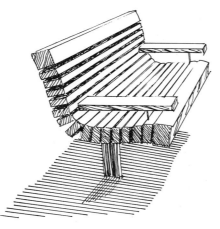

A well-designed bench for use in outdoor spaces of a health care facility should look inviting, feel comfortable, provide good back support, and have arms to assist people in sitting down and in rising.

Amenities

Outdoor spaces of health care facilities provide places to sit, relax, talk with friends, and perhaps eat lunch. They are places of great activity as well as settings for solitude. In designing outdoor spaces to meet these diverse uses, design decision makers should also consider the need to support a number of everyday activities, such as getting a drink of water and properly disposing of trash. Some suggestions for accommodating these mundane, yet important, functions include:

- Provide drinking fountains that can be used by children and persons in wheelchairs, as well as by ambulatory adults.

- Provide trash receptacles that are attractive yet obvious about their function.

- Consider providing kiosks or other devices for information sharing.

Special Considerations

In addition to the needs already described, issues relating to safety and long-term use of the space need to be considered, including medical emergencies, security, maintenance, conflicting uses, and weather conditions.

A facility that encourages patients and visitors to use outdoor space must take precautions for medical emergencies occurring outdoors. An emergency phone system should be available for people outdoors to call for help. The facility may also consider providing some form of supervision for patients, because many patients who would benefit from visiting an outdoor area may not be able to leave the unit without a nurse in attendance.[16]

Although the outdoor space of a health care facility is likely to be more heavily used during the day, the area may also be used at night. Unfortunately, at night, mugging and rape become potential problems in some areas. By following some simple principles, however, planners can design outdoor spaces to discourage crime.[21] Lighting should be carefully considered so that there are no unlit potential hiding places. The location and shape of plantings are critical for the same reason.

In order to encourage use and keep a positive image, maintenance needs to be as simple and inexpensive as possible. The selection of plant materials, the design of landscape architectural details, and the provision of a watering system require careful consideration to facilitate ease and completeness of maintenance.

Outdoor spaces make particularly good places for large gatherings. If a stage or other open area has been included in the design, the outdoor area can more easily function as a meeting place for special health care facility occasions as well as for community events. Remember to place electrical outlets near special staging areas.

Conflicting user needs are a potential problem in any space. One area of potential conflict is between those who want to be social and those who want to be quiet. Fountains are one type of design feature that may help ensure acoustical privacy in the midst of a public setting.

Facilities located in snowy climates will find that winter weather may discourage active use of the outdoor space. However, there will always be people who use it in all weather, if only in transit. Icy patches can be treacherous for the physically able as well as for disabled people and should be prevented by regular snow removal or the installation of melting devices.

Bringing the Outdoors In

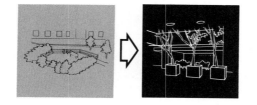

Nature is not limited to the outdoors. Atriums, greenhouses, planters, and window boxes all allow constant greening of the indoor environment. In shopping malls, hotels, and hospitals, nature has become an integral part of interior design, ranging from a few potted plants to trees and hanging vines. Providing a "green" interior has even become the trademark and a key element of the marketing strategy of a major hotel chain. Its advertisements beckon the traveler to enjoy the beach and golf course during the day and the lush green of the hotel atrium at night.

Bringing nature indoors holds similar psychological benefits to gaining access to nature outdoors. Plants are soothing and restful. Plants, especially flowering ones, represent life, growth, and hope. They can provide interest and diversion.[22-24] The number of people who bring plants or flowers to sick friends or relatives as gifts is an indication of the powerful symbolic value of plants.[25]

Plants have been used as a therapeutic tool for a wide variety of patients, including psychiatric, pediatric, geriatric, and rehabilitation patients. Horticultural therapy gives patients a link with life and a sense of being needed. It also provides the opportunity for physical activity and social interaction. For those with visual impairments, especially the elderly, it provides an absorbing activity that does not strain their eyes.[26-29]

Plants do have their limitations. They are not appropriate in every space, and they present maintenance problems. Because they catch dust and provide a moist growing environment within their soil, plants should not be placed in sterile environments such as surgical suites and recovery rooms.[30] Also, it is possible that funds allocated for the maintenance of indoor plantings may be cut suddenly if the administration is not firmly committed to a landscaped interior.

Views from Windows

Views of attractive outdoor spaces are important, especially if the viewer is unable to go outside. If there is at least visual access to an outdoor space, a greater number of users will benefit from it.[16] Attractive views provide relief and pleasure. And, there is evidence that pleasant views can increase the patient's sense of well-being and decrease recovery time and the need for pain-relief medication (see Research Box #4). Outdoor views remind the viewer of the season, time of day, and weather. These are important "reality cues" for long-term, critically ill inpatients.

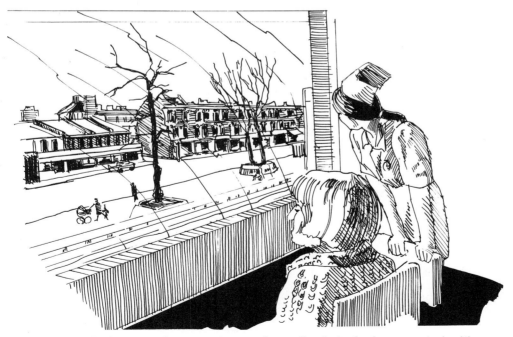

Views from windows are important ways for patients to feel connected with the rest of the world.

Research Box #4: Studying Impacts of Outside Views on Recovery

For many patients and visitors, access to a courtyard or park-like space may be quite limited. This does not mean, however, that nature loses its importance or that its therapeutic benefits should be ignored. Unfortunately, few studies have explored the importance to hospital patients of the view from their windows.

However, one study of surgery patients examined the restorative value of the view from a window.[31] Specifically, records were compared of postoperative gallbladder surgery patients. One group stayed in rooms with a view of a small stand of trees while the other group had a view of a brick wall. To make sure that differences could be attributed to the window view, patients were matched in terms of age, sex, floor level, and other variables. In all, 23 pairs of patients were included in the study.

Patient records were examined to ascertain the number of minor complications, dose and number of pain relief medications taken, dose and number of tranquilizers taken, length of hospitalization, and the nurses' general comments. Differences between the tree-view and wall-view groups were found in four out of the five measures. Patients in wall-view rooms stayed in the hospital longer, were given more moderate and strong pain relief medication, suffered a greater number of minor complications, and received a greater number of negative comments from the nursing staff.

Although this study compared reactions to two dramatically different views, it shows that something as simple as the view from a window can affect patient well-being.

Conclusion

Whether indoors or out, nature has therapeutic value. It provides a comfortable and restful retreat, which is especially important in the stress-filled health care environment. Providing access to nature is not only beneficial, it is necessary. It is not a luxury or an optional "add-on" feature. It is an integral part of a humane and caring environment.

Design Review Questions

Health Care Facility Outdoor Spaces

☐ Has the entire site surrounding the health care facility been evaluated for its potential use as accessible outdoor space?

☐ Have the needs for both active and passive types of outdoor space been considered?

☐ Have the outdoor space needs of all users been considered, including ambulatory and nonambulatory patients, visitors, staff, children, and elderly people?

Designing Outdoor Spaces for Health Care Facilities

☐ Has the outdoor space been designed to have as many trees and shrubs as possible?

☐ Has a hierarchy of seating arrangements and locations been provided, ranging from public to private?

☐ Have trees and shrubs been arranged to give people a sense of enclosure and privacy?

☐ Have trees, shrubs, and flowers been chosen that will provide outdoor spaces with different colors and fragrances throughout the year?

☐ Have plantings and bench arrangements been designed to provide comfortable settings for conversation and people-watching?

☐ Where appropriate, has some open lawn been provided for active use?[16]

☐ Has the outdoor space been designed to appeal to patients and others who can only see it from the inside?

☐ Have paving materials such as brick been avoided so as not to give wheelchair users a bumpy ride?

Location and Access[16]

☐ Has visual access to the outdoor space been provided from the main public and circulation spaces?

☐ When possible, has direct access been provided to the outdoor space from a major public area?

☐ Are outdoor spaces included in facility tours?

☐ Do outdoor spaces appear prominently on maps?

Notes

Design that Cares: Planning Health Facilities for Patients and Visitors, by Janet R. Carpman, Myron A. Grant, and Deborah A. Simmons. ©1986 by American Hospital Publishing, Inc.

☐ Have heavy or self-locking doors been avoided?

☐ Have automatic doors been considered for outdoor space entrances to ensure easy access by the mobility-impaired?

☐ Is visual access provided to the outdoor space so patients can see what the space looks like and decide whether they feel up to making the journey?

Walkways

☐ Can sidewalk surfaces be easily and smoothly negotiated by stretchers, gurneys, wheelchairs, strollers, and other wheeled equipment?[16]

☐ Are sidewalks graded with minimal slopes so that users of manual wheelchairs can wheel themselves around the area?

☐ Have ramps been avoided at doorways, because these would inhibit the movement of a patient in a wheelchair or on a gurney?[16]

☐ Has a continuous handrail been provided along walkways on both sloped and flat grades?

☐ If metal handrails are used, have they been coated with plastic or vinyl so that they are not slippery when wet?[19]

☐ Are walkways wide enough for two gurneys to pass each other or for three or four people to walk side by side?

☐ In those regions where winter weather is a problem, have various means been considered for ice and snow removal on walkways?

Seating

☐ Has a variety of seat types been provided, ranging from chairs to benches?

☐ Have seats been oriented in various directions to allow users to take advantage of or to shield themselves from the sun at different times of the day?[16]

☐ Do people have a choice of sitting in the sun or in the shade?[16]

☐ Have some seats been placed along major circulation paths, so that sitters can people-watch?

☐ Have some seats been placed so that users are given a feeling of enclosure and separation from the mainstream?

☐ Are seating arrangements provided that accommodate groups of different sizes?

☐ If possible, has some seating been provided around tables?[16]

Notes

☐ Are places available in seating areas for patients on gurneys, stretchers, or in wheelchairs?

☐ Has some seating been provided that can be rearranged into suitable groups?

☐ Do some seating arrangements make it easy for people to talk in small groups?

☐ Does the seating have backs and armrests?

☐ Does the seating allow an elderly person or someone with little flexibility and strength to sit and rise easily?

☐ Is the seating comfortable to sit on for an hour or more at a time?

☐ Has concrete seating material been avoided?

☐ Is the seating attractive to patients and visitors?

Amenities

☐ Can drinking fountains be used by children and people in wheelchairs as well as by ambulatory adults?

☐ Are attractive trash receptacles available?

☐ Have kiosks or other devices for information-sharing been provided?

Special Considerations

☐ Has an emergency communication system been provided in outdoor spaces used by patients?

☐ Has adequate lighting been provided to discourage crime?

☐ Have trees and shrubs been selected and arranged so that they do not provide muggers with places to hide?[21]

☐ Has the need for a large public gathering and presentation area been considered?

☐ Have outdoor electrical outlets been provided at stage or presentation areas?

Bringing the Outdoors In

☐ As appropriate, have plants been used as a therapeutic tool for patients?[26-29]

Views from Windows

☐ Have the windows in patient rooms, lounges, waiting areas, lobbies, food services areas, and corridors been designed to maximize exterior views?

Notes _____

Design that Cares: Planning Health Facilities for Patients and Visitors, by Janet R. Carpman, Myron A. Grant, and Deborah A. Simmons. ©1986 by American Hospital Publishing, Inc.

References

1. Alexander, C., Ishikawa, S., and Silverstein, M. *A Pattern Language.* New York: Oxford University Press, 1977.

2. Wohlwill, J. F. The concept of nature: a psychologist's view. In: Altman, I., and Wohlwill, J. F., editors. *Human Behavior and Environment: Advances in Theory and Research,* Vol. 6. New York: Plenum Press, 1983.

3. Ulrich, R. S. Aesthetic and affective response to natural environment. In: Altman, I., and Wohlwill, J. F., editors. *Human Behavior and Environment: Advances in Theory and Research,* Vol. 6. New York: Plenum Press, 1983.

4. Kaplan, R. The role of nature in the urban context. In: Altman, I., and Wohlwill, J. F., editors. *Human Behavior and Environment: Advances in Theory and Research,* Vol. 6. New York: Plenum Press, 1983.

5. Reizenstein, J. E., and Grant, M. A. Patient activities and schematic design preferences. Unpublished research report #2, Patient and Visitor Participation Project, Office of Hospital Planning, Research and Development, University of Michigan, Ann Arbor, 1981.

6. Ulrich, R. S. Visual landscapes and psychological well-being. *Landscape Research.* 1979 Spring. 4(1):17-23.

7. Ulrich, R.S. Natural versus urban scenes: some psychological effects. *Environment and Behavior.* 1981 Sept. 13(5):523-56.

8. Olsen, R. V. A user evaluation of a hospital park. Unpublished report, Environmental Design Program, Bellevue Hospital Center, New York, no date.

9. Henneberry, J., and Robertson, P. Free in the sun: an outdoor program in a health care setting. *Children's Health Care.* 1983 Summer. 12(1):37-40.

10. Alcock, D. Developing an outdoor playground. *Dimensions in Health Service.* 1978. 55:32-37.

11. Moore, G., Cohen, U., and McGinty, T. *Planning and Design Guidelines: Child Care Centers and Outdoor Play Environments.* (7 vols.) Milwaukee: University of Wisconsin, Milwaukee, Center for Architecture and Urban Planning Research, 1979.

12. Moore, G., Cohen, U., and others. *Designing Environments for Handicapped Children.* New York: Educational Facilities Laboratory, 1979.

13. Olds, A., and Daniels, P. *Child Health Care Facilities: Design Guidelines and Literature Review.* Washington, DC: Association for the Care of Children's Health, forthcoming.

14. Kaplan, S., and Kaplan, R., editors. *Humanscape: Environments for People.* Belmont, CA: Duxbury Press, 1978.

15. Kaplan, S., and Kaplan, R. *Cognition and Environment: Functioning in an Uncertain World.* New York: Praeger, 1983.

16. Paine, R. Design guidelines for hospital open space: case studies of three hospitals. Master's thesis, University of California, Berkeley, 1984.

17. Reizenstein, J. E., and Grant, M. A. Patient and visitor preferences for outdoor courtyard design. Unpublished research report #10, Patient and Visitor Participation Project, Office of Hospital Planning, Research and Development, University of Michigan, Ann Arbor, 1981.

18. Grant, M. A. Structured participatory input. Master's thesis, University of Michigan, Ann Arbor, 1979.

19. Koncelik, J. A. *Designing the Open Nursing Home.* Stroudsburg, PA: Dowden, Hutchinson and Ross, 1976.

20. Reizenstein, J. E., and Grant, M. A. Outdoor seating evaluation. Unpublished research report #22, Patient and Visitor Participation Project, Office of Hospital Planning, Research and Development, University of Michigan, Ann Arbor, 1983.

21. Newman, O. *Design Guidelines for Creating Defensible Space.* Washington, DC: U.S. Government Printing Office, 1975.

22. McDuffie, R. F. The greening of interiors. *Interior Landscape Industry.* 1984 June. 1(6):29-31.

23. Hughes, E. F., and Bryden, M. C. The development of an occupational therapy program in a solarium area. *Canadian Journal of Occupational Therapy.* 1983 Feb. 50(1):15-19.

24. Wasserman, B. Greening the corner where you are. *Dental Management.* 1974 Dec. 14(12):65-71.

25. Reizenstein, J. E., Vaitkus, M. A., and Grant, M. A. Patient belongings. Unpublished research report #9, Patient and Visitor Participation Project, Office of Hospital Planning, Research and Development, University of Michigan, Ann Arbor, 1982.

26. Relf, P. D. Horticulture as a recreational activity. *Journal—American Health Care Association.* 1978 Sept. 4(5):68-71.

27. Flourney, R. L. Gardening as therapy: treatment activities for psychiatric patients. *Hospital and Community Psychiatry.* 1975 Feb. 26(2):75-76.

28. Sullivan, M. E. Horticultural therapy: the role gardening plays in healing. *Journal—American Health Care Association.* 1979 May 5(3):3-8.

29. Spelfogel, B., and Modrzakowski, M. Curative factors in horticultural therapy in a hospital setting. *Hospital and Community Psychiatry.* 1980 Aug. 31(8):572-73.

30. Schultz, J. K. Plants in OR harbor potential contaminants. *Association of Operating Room Nurses Journal.* 1979 Apr. 29(5):898-99.

31. Ulrich, R. S. View through a window may influence recovery from surgery. *Science.* 1984 Apr. 27. 224(4647):420-21.

Chapter 8

Special Users

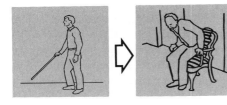

Impaired Users   Elderly Users

Thus far in the book, we have pointed out some special needs of disabled and elderly users of health care facilities. Although this information appears throughout the text, we feel that it is important to summarize the needs of some specific groups—mobility-impaired, hearing-impaired, and vision-impaired users—and to expand upon the needs of elderly patients and visitors.

Users with Impairments

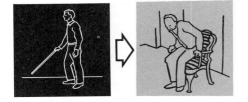

Statistics identify more than 13 million people in the United States with hearing impairments, more than 11 million with vision impairments, more than 30 million with mobility problems, and more than 27 million who are over 65.[1-3] Add to these the countless numbers of people who are temporarily handicapped at any given time, whether due to injury, pregnancy, illness, or postoperative recovery and the like, and you have a tremendous demand for supportive design.

Indeed, design that is enabling for handicapped persons usually helps, and rarely inconveniences, able-bodied persons too. As one architectural journal put it, automatic doors relieve everyone of manual effort, grab bars in showers protect everyone from falls, telephone volume controls help everyone hear better in a noisy environment, "talking" exit signs aid everyone's evacuation of a building.[1]

Mobility-Impaired Users

In addition to showing humanitarian concern, health care facilities need to accommodate their mobility-impaired users because of two major trends. First, as we described in chapter 1, the population is living longer, and as a result, hospitalized patients may be older and frailer than in the past. A concurrent trend resulting from the use of diagnosis-related groups (DRGs) as a basis for third-party payment is that hospital lengths of stay are becoming shorter and many patients who once would be hospitalized are now being treated as outpatients. As a result, users of outpatient facilities may also be sicker and weaker than before and more likely to be mobility-impaired. In addition, persons with sprained ankles or with bad backs and those on walkers or in leg casts are *temporarily* mobility-impaired.

To meet the needs of these users, health care facilities should provide handrails along circulation routes, provide resting areas with seats along long corridors, and provide more wheelchair-accessible toilet facilities than currently required by code.

Unfortunately, planning health facilities that meet the needs of patients and visitors with particular impairments is not a simple matter of following relevant building codes. The American National Standards Institute developed the first handicapped accessibility standard (known as ANSI A117.1) in 1961, renewed it in 1971, expanded it in 1980, and renewed it again in 1986. Many, but not all, states have adopted the ANSI standard for their codes. In addition to state codes, there are two federal codes: the Minimum Guidelines of the Architectural and Transportation Barriers Compliance Board (1982) and the Uniform Federal Accessibility Standard (1984). Each of these codes differs in some respects. Although the intent—to provide environmental access to disabled as well as able-bodied persons—tends to be widely agreed upon, details of the codes themselves and the ways they can be applied are subject to much debate.[1,4] For those interested in more detailed information on design for accessibility, many useful reference books are available.[5,6]

Hearing-Impaired Users

There are an estimated 13.4 million Americans suffering from hearing impairments.[3] For hearing-impaired persons, the critical factor is not the measurable amount of hearing loss, but rather the limitations on verbal communication skills that result.[7] For the hearing-impaired person, the communication that is so important to human interaction is often severely limited, and the hearing population is generally uneducated about how to communicate with the hearing-impaired population.[8]

Hearing-impaired patients must be able to communicate with health care staff. Through both policy and design, the health care facility needs to provide the support that will make this communication possible. Health care staff need to be educated about the special communication problems of the hearing-impaired. Interpreters should be available within the facility or on call. Various methods of communication may be used, including sign language, TDD (telecommunications device for the deaf), lipreading, handwritten notes, supplemental hearing devices, or any combination of these. One solution for large organizations is to establish a central office that supervises services for hearing-impaired patients. In these ways, most hearing-impaired individuals will be able to communicate with the health care staff. In addition,

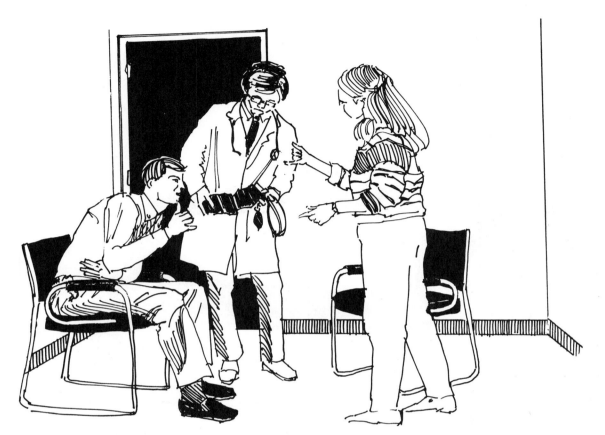

Communication is essential in times of crisis. In the emergency room, a qualified interpreter can relay critical information between the medical staff and a deaf patient who "signs."

the design of the facility—its lighting, sound attenuation, and availability of visual cues—is an important factor in providing access to communication.

Because hearing-impaired persons rely heavily upon their sense of sight, it is crucial to develop environments that enhance visual cues. This includes providing as much natural light as possible, avoiding backlighting or illuminating from behind, and locating light sources to avoid throwing shadows on speakers or interpreters. Signage that is easily understood and readily available, as well as other written or graphic information, is essential. And because many of these users may not be able to hear a fire alarm or other warning signal, such alternatives as flashing lights, vibrators, and variable-intensity fans should be considered.[3]

Not all hearing-impaired users are totally deaf; many depend upon hearing aids for communication. Consequently, it is important that background noise levels and vibrations be reduced to a minimum and that certain frequencies of sound be controlled.[3]

A number of communication devices are available and should be considered. They include telecommunications devices that transmit typed conversations via phone lines (TDDs), closed-circuit television systems for communicating messages, vibrating pagers, and telephone amplifiers compatible with hearing aids.

Telecommunications Devices for the Deaf (TDDs) allow "conversations" over telephone lines. Some TDDs are equipped with a scroll printout, as well as a light-emitting diode (LED). TDDs are appropriate for use in admitting areas, emergency rooms, and numerous other health care facility spaces.

Assigning deaf patients to rooms near the activity hub of an inpatient unit is another way the health care facility can meet these users' needs for information. Rooms near the nursing station tend to be noisy places for hearing patients, but they may provide deaf patients with an opportunity to interact with staff members—something essential for providing them with information and social contact they would otherwise miss.

Vision-Impaired Users

Finding one's way and negotiating obstacles are two major difficulties blind or partially sighted users have in health care facilities. With limited sight or no sight at all, the vision-impaired user is unable to use signs and other wayfinding aids. However, through the use of raised letters, engraved signs, braille, sharply contrasting colors, audible signals, and tactile guides such as textured strips, the ease of wayfinding can be increased.[9,10] This range of cues is important to provide, because only around 20 to 25 percent of the blind population in the United States is able to use braille information.[11,12]

In addition, the mobility of vision-impaired users is limited and put in potential danger by obstacles. Pathways obstructed by furniture, equipment, posts, or protrusions from the wall (such as water fountains) are safety hazards. Stairways, roadways, and other structures that may be hazardous to the visually impaired should be marked by tactile warning signals, such as grooves or strips.[9,10,13]

For blind patients and visitors, thoughtfully designed circulation areas can be especially helpful. Hard surfaces on floors, ceilings, and walls of hallways should be avoided, because these surfaces reflect and redirect sounds that are particularly important spatial location cues for blind people. Such hard surfaces can cause a sound, such as conversation, to appear to be on one side of the corridor when it is really on the other, resulting in problems for the blind user. Also, corridors that intersect at right angles are the easiest for blind users to negotiate. Oblique or acute angles are much more difficult to perceive and remember.

Stairs can be treacherous places for blind users. Stair width and tread height need to be consistent; railings should begin at the first step and run continuously, flatten out along landings, and rise or fall again with the next flight. Elevators with speech synthesizers are helpful for blind users, although quite costly. Knowing if the car is going up or down, which button has been pushed, and what floor has been reached helps the blind person avoid confusion, false starts, asking for help, and having to backtrack.

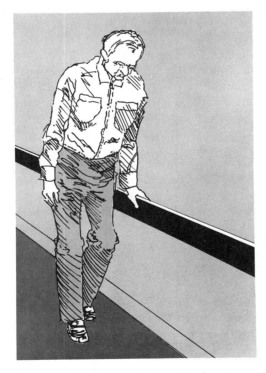

Contrasting color values can help visually-impaired persons distinguish among walls, floors, and handrails.

People who have impaired vision often cannot distinguish subtle variations in color. In order to minimize potential difficulties and dangers, items they come into contact with need to be designed of highly contrasting colors. For instance, clinic registration counters should contrast with the paper forms used, toilet seats should contrast with toilet bowls, and showers or tubs should contrast with the floors and walls around them.

Elderly Users

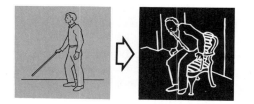

Designing health care facilities that meet the needs of older patients and visitors is an important challenge. Older consumers have particular requirements as a result of the physiological, social, and psychological changes associated with aging. Although a great deal of research has investigated the environmental requirements of aging, most of this has focused on housing or long-term care facilities (especially nursing homes) rather than on health care facilities. Part of the challenge to design decision makers is to extrapolate from this related research to the needs of elderly patients and visitors in both inpatient and outpatient health care settings—something we have done in the design guidelines presented below. Nevertheless, the design-related needs of older patients and visitors clearly deserve special research attention in the future.

Again, one of the significant benefits accruing from considering the design needs of a special segment of the population like the elderly is that in many cases the resulting design becomes even more functional for other users, too. For instance, if corridors are free from windows located at either end, not only will older users not be disturbed by sudden glare but younger users will also be able to see more easily.

Demographics

There were 27.4 million persons in the United States 65 or older in 1983, constituting 11 percent of the U.S. population, with a ratio of 149 women for every 100 men. Despite the increasing longevity of the population, elderly people are still more prone to chronic conditions and are more frequently hospitalized than are younger persons. In 1981, for example, the most frequently occurring chronic conditions among the noninstitutionalized elderly population were arthritis (46 percent), hypertension (38 percent), hearing impairments (28 percent), heart conditions (28 percent), sinusitis (18 percent), visual impairments (14 percent), orthopedic impairments (14 percent), arteriosclerosis (10 percent), and diabetes (8 percent).[2]

About 18 percent of older persons were hospitalized during 1981, compared to about 9 percent of persons under 65. The elderly were more likely than younger persons to have more than one hospital stay per year and to stay in the hospital longer (ten days versus seven days). They also averaged more visits to doctors than did younger persons (six visits versus four).[2]

Physiological and Psychosocial Changes

Physiological changes—usually losses—are characteristic of the normal aging process. Changes in the various systems of the body usually result in reductions in mobility, strength, stamina, visual acuity, hearing, tactile sensitivity, and thermal sensitivity.[14,15] The norm is for the aging person to experience losses in all of these areas rather than having one single disability. It is the combination of physiological changes that often leads to a general sense of vulnerability.[14] More specifically, physiological changes may include the following:

Vision. The lens of the eye thickens, resulting in loss of acuity, narrowing of the visual field, slowed accommodation to temporal or spatial changes in illumination, sensitivity to glare, and some loss of color differentiation.[16] Three times as much task lighting may be necessary for an older person to perceive and discriminate small detail than would be required for a younger person.[17] In addition, the upward gaze may be limited, resulting in difficulties for the older person in reading signs. Use of bifocal or trifocal lenses can lead to visual blurring or double images and can have serious safety implications for stair use.[18]

Hearing. Hearing becomes less acute, especially in the higher frequency range on which speech and other signals (such as bells and fire and smoke sirens) depend for their clarity. This is known as *presbycusis.* Auditory distortion may result, and there may be less ability to filter out extraneous sounds, as in discerning one voice from a background of competing sounds or voices.[14-16,18,19]

Tactile and Thermal Sensitivity. There are declines in sensitivity to pain and temperature. Elderly people are less aware of dangerous changes in temperature and, at the same time, less able to tolerate such changes. There is increased susceptibility to hypothermia, the lowering of body temperature to potentially fatal levels. If older people are aware of temperature changes, as most are, they are likely to prefer more warmth in winter, to be less able to endure heat in summer, and to be particularly uncomfortable in drafts. Older people may also experience a sensation of insufficient air in buildings with sealed windows.[14]

Mobility. Older persons may have slower movement, reduced strength and stamina, stooped posture, difficulty walking and turning, and stiff joints. Loss of balance and dizzy spells may result as side effects from certain medications.[14,18]

Memory and Learning. Aging does not impair intelligence per se, but the speed with which information is processed, stored, summoned, and expressed may decline.[14] Short-term memory deficits, longer times required to learn new information, requirements for more repetitions, and longer times required to process sensory information may be characteristics associated with aging.[18] In addition, older people may have increasing difficulty creating new mental images of unfamiliar settings, leading to wayfinding problems.[14]

The aging person experiences a number of psychological and social changes as well as physiological ones, and environmental design needs to be supportive of these, too. Older patients and visitors may be suffering from bereavement, social isolation, feelings of uselessness, or an inability to cope with rapidly changing environmental circumstances, such as a move from their home of many years. Social and psychological needs include choice about when to be private and when to be social, access to information, a sense of control, identity, and independence, and assurance of personal safety and security.[20]

Design Principles

To lessen the difficulties that the older patient or visitor experiences, the designed environment can provide some appropriate forms of physical assistance, psychological support, and behavior cues.[14] The key is to understand the needs of this special user group and to respond appropriately through design and related policies.

It is likely that more elderly patients will be at least temporary wheelchair users than younger patients and that when hospitalized, older patients will have longer lengths of stay. This, in addition to their vulnerability, makes the functional nature of the design of the facility and of all the objects within it even more important than usual. However, the physical environment needs to achieve a delicate balance between being supportive of physiological and psychosocial needs and maintaining a healthy degree of challenge.[15]

The following principles, adapted for health facilities used by the public, have been suggested as a guide for providing appropriate environments for aged users.[15]

Safety. Safety features should not only guard against the possibility of accidental injury but also afford patients and visitors a sense of confidence that they can negotiate the space themselves.[20] Slipping and falling, blacking out in unobserved areas, bumping into furnishings with sharp edges, tripping over unseen low obstructions, and other dangers are real hazards faced by elderly users. Rounded corners and edges on all furnishings, carefully designed (even recessed) bed rails, and walls with sufficient surface texture to help prevent hands from slipping are important to consider in health care environments designed especially for the elderly.[15]

Independence. In the face of increasing physical difficulties after many years spent as competent adults, most elderly people highly value their independence and appreciate design features and policies that support their competence.

Access. Whether or not patients or visitors are wheelchair bound or ambulatory, it is essential that features of the environment enable them to have independent access. Sidewalks should be smooth in texture, free of steep slopes, and wide enough to allow two wheelchair users to pass comfortably. Outdoor seating areas should be designed to be wheelchair accessible, so that users can sit with others or transfer comfortably to a bench. Transitions between exterior and interior spaces should be free of steps and steep ramps. In addition to having wheelchair-accessible circulation on the inside, elderly users should also be able to reach and manipulate switches, call buttons, the telephone, and the like.[15,16]

Management of Sound and Light. It is not enough to provide sufficient quantities of sound and light, because the deterioration of hearing and vision of most elderly people requires some special adjustment of these environmental features. Sound and light must be carefully designed and managed in order to support older patients and visitors in their everyday needs to hear and see.[15]

Control over Social Contact. Whenever possible, elderly patients and visitors should have control over the types of social situations they participate in. They should be able to choose when to have contact with others and when to be alone.

Implications for Design

A large number of design guidelines that have appeared in the literature on aging and environments can be appropriately adapted to health care settings. Most of these guidelines pertain to environmental features that appear throughout a health care facility, rather than being unique to a specific area. Accordingly, in this chapter features such as lighting, color, and seating will be discussed separately, with only the inpatient room and bath described as unique spaces. The guidelines also distinguish between environmental areas or features that are designed to be used exclusively by older patients, such as a geriatric hospital unit, and those features that will be used by patients and visitors of all ages.

Safety Systems
Safety systems refer to such emergency warning devices as fire alarms, as well as to ways of reducing potential dangers within everyday situations:

- Determine a minimum radius for the edges of all hard surfaces and protrusions that might cause injuries in any spaces targeted for elderly patients and visitors. (The more a corner or edge is rounded, the broader the impact area and the more dispersed the force of the blow.)[17]

- Make sure that visual warning devices such as exit signs are backed up with a middle-frequency auditory signal to enhance the ability of an older person to locate the exit. In the event of a fire, the vision problems that older people experience may be increased because many signs are placed high up and may be obscured by smoke.[14,15]

Sound

Changes in the hearing of older persons make it much more difficult for them to distinguish among several simultaneous sounds. The environment needs to be designed so that certain sounds—especially conversation—can be heard clearly.

- When possible, reduce ambient background sounds in open public spaces by using baffling materials such as wall hangings, screens, banners, or acoustical panels, as well as by using sound-attenuating materials for walls, floors, and ceilings.[15]

- Avoid "canned" background music, which can make the whole environment seem more uniform and can increase the difficulty of distinguishing one place from another.[15]

Lighting

Two major considerations should influence lighting decisions in health facilities that will be used by elderly patients and visitors: sensitivity to glare and increased adaptation time to move between darkness and light. Glare caused by unshielded artificial lighting and by direct sunlight can be a major problem because it can be visually overwhelming and can temporarily distract older persons, affecting the awareness of their immediate physical environment, as well as their attention span and short-term memory.[14] Entering a bright room from a low-lit corridor can be considered dangerous for older patients because it will take some time for them to adapt to the brightness. Even for a period of time after adaptation, there is likely to be insufficient discrimination of fine details or objects, resulting in the potential for injury (see also chapters 3 and 6).[17]

- Avoid having windows, mirrors, and other bright or reflective surfaces placed at the end of corridors.[14]

- Avoid abrupt changes in illumination levels. For instance, use low-level night lighting in patient rooms and reduce the level of nighttime corridor lighting.[14,18]

- Use indirect lighting whenever possible.[14]

- Consider using carpeting in corridors to reduce both glare and noise.[17]

- Consider lighting the first few stairs in a series, because this is where many falls occur.[20]

- Select warm-toned lighting if possible. Cool fluorescents not only are unflattering but also emphasize the blue-green tones most difficult for elderly persons to perceive.[17]

- Shield all light sources so that bare bulbs are not visible.[17,20]

- Attempt to reduce disturbing glare by fitting all windows with some means of light reduction, such as reflective glass, shades, blinds, or drapes.[17,20]

Color

In addition to thickening, the lens of the aging eye gradually changes color. Instead of being clear, it becomes yellowish-brown, slightly altering the older person's perception of certain colors. Colors of similar intensity or brightness are more difficult to differentiate, especially when viewed under constant lighting conditions or against similarly textured or reflective surfaces. Different pastels, very dark colors, and combinations of blues and greens can be especially difficult to distinguish within their color group.[14] Pure tones or primary colors are likely to be easiest for elderly users to recognize and name, whereas off-whites and pale grays may appear drab.[21]

In environments for elderly users, color can be used to organize a series of rooms so that they appear to be grouped in some way; it can signify change, suggest outlines or emphasize contours, signal an alert, or work as a background surface on which a focal object can be easily distinguished. It can also camouflage certain spaces or areas.[21]

Although color is often thought of as a useful nonverbal cue for finding one's way through an environment, color coding is not likely to be effective in environments used by elderly persons. As one gerontologist has noted, color coding is a relatively abstract idea, and with memory impairments, elderly people may not be able to rely on those portions of memory that support abstract reasoning. Because recognition memory is often intact, orientation may be better served by objects, signs, and action (see also chapter 3).[21]

Some suggested guidelines pertaining to the use of color in health facilities used by elderly patients include the following:

- Consider color in conjunction with lighting. (Dim lighting may wash out some colors, whereas direct or bright lighting may intensify others.)[21]

- Consider color in conjunction with texture. (Very smooth textures can make colors appear lighter, and uneven surfaces make most colors appear darker.)[21]

- Emphasize changes in planes—such as the intersections of walls and floors or the treads and risers of stairs—with highly contrasting colors.[14,16]

- Be extremely careful with the use of patterns. These can be confusing to elderly users. (Broad stripes on a floor can appear to be steps, stripes on a wall can appear to be bars, and wavy patterns can appear to be in motion, causing unsteadiness.) If patterns are to be used at all, it may be more effective to use them along one wall only, like a mural, rather than using them repetitively.[21]

- Use contrasting colors on design components in order to make them stand out for the elderly patient or visitor. Such components might include bathroom fixtures, grab bars, doors, door frames, latches, knobs, and switches.[18]

Texture

Because so many elderly users experience losses of both vision and hearing, texture used in design can be quite effective. In addition to braille, other textural markers such as shape coding of handrails (notches or grooves cut into the handrail to identify location) or changes in the textural surfaces of walls can be used. Textures need to be sufficiently different so that users do not become confused by them.[15]

- Consider the use of texture to identify different locations within the health care facility.[15]

- Avoid surfaces that are so reflective that they cause glare.[17]

- Provide wall surfaces with enough texture to enable elderly persons to use them to steady themselves.[15,17]

- Avoid wall surfaces that are so abrasive that they will injure those who rub up against them.[17]

Hardware

Gerontologists explain that architectural hardware plays two important roles in facility design. It can actually facilitate or impede use by persons with handicaps, and it can convey a symbolic message (usually false) of personal incompetence to users "long before their infirmities reach a point where they *do* inhibit environmental use."[15] Once again, supportive design features such as hardware can help facilitate use and feelings of competence on the part of *all* users, handicapped or not.

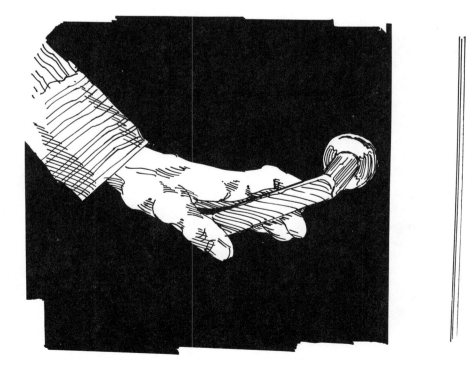

Lever handles are easier for arthritic hands to manipulate than are doorknobs.

- Provide hardware—such as lever and push-type handles—that can be operated with one hand and that does not require twisting, turning, or excessive strength.[14]

- Provide door hinges or opening devices and door closers that require no more than 3 to 5 foot-pounds of pressure to open.[14]

- Provide door closers with a "check-action delay" of 4 to 6 seconds before closing.[14]

Flooring

When knowledgeably selected, flooring materials can prevent the elderly patient or visitor from having to cope with glare or potentially dangerous situations (see also chapter 3):

- Provide carpeting rather than hard flooring whenever possible, because of carpeting's significant glare reduction and safety advantages.[17]

- Where carpeting is not considered appropriate, such as the inpatient room, provide flooring that is resilient, nonglare, and nonslip, even when wet.[15,17]

Seating

Choosing seating for use by older persons in health care facilities is especially important because of the particular needs of these users. They often sit for extended periods of time, have weaker blood circulation, and have more difficulty sitting down on and getting up from chairs. Important considerations are the ease of sitting down on the chair, comfort and support while sitting, and the ease of rising (see also chapters 4, 6, and 7).[14]

Older persons need to be able to center themselves in front of the chair, move their heels underneath it, and sit—rather than fall—down. Chair arms aid this process greatly. A clear space under the front of the chair provides an area for placing the heels. When the front of the chair arms is in the same vertical plane as the front edge of the seat, the strength required to sit down is reduced. Seat height should be just below knee height, and the seat angle should be no more than 4 degrees. A chair seat should never be so high that it lifts the person's feet off the floor, as this can cause damaging interruption of blood flow to the lower legs and feet. Of course, people come in different sizes, so it is difficult to specify an ideal seat height. However, the height that seems to work well for most people is 17 inches (43 cm).[14,15]

Seats that are too hard can cause skin ulcers. One way to test a seat's firmness is to press your fist into the center of the seat, gradually increasing the pressure, until your full weight is on your fist. If your fist is stopped by a board or spring, then the seat is probably too hard to accommodate an older person for an extended period of time.[14]

Skin ulcers can also be caused by moisture against the skin. Even where incontinence is not a problem, it is wise to avoid nonabsorbent upholstery like vinyl, because it prevents the escape of moisture. Some gerontologists recommend that regardless of the potential for incontinence, nonabsorbent upholstery should not be used.[17]

Rising is made easier by the same design features that facilitate sitting down. A chair's arms can help older persons pull themselves to the front of the seat. Then, they can place their heels under their center of gravity and can push up and out if the front of the chair's arms is in the same vertical plane as the front of the seat.[14]

Chair selection guidelines for older patients and visitors include the following:

- Provide a clear space under the front of the chair, so that the user's heels can be placed underneath.[14]

- Select chairs in which the front edge of the chair arms is in the same vertical plane, or extends slightly beyond, the front edge of the seat.[14,15]

- Make sure the seat angle is no more than 4 degrees.[14]

- Avoid seats that are so firm that they will cause skin ulcers.[14]

- Avoid nonabsorbent upholstery whenever possible.[14,17]

- Because the elderly population is somewhat shorter than average, select seating with a height from the floor to the seat's front edge of no more than 17 inches (43 cm).[14,15]

- If tables are used with chairs in places used exclusively by the elderly, select tables that are 31 inches (79 cm) high or that adjust to different heights.[15]

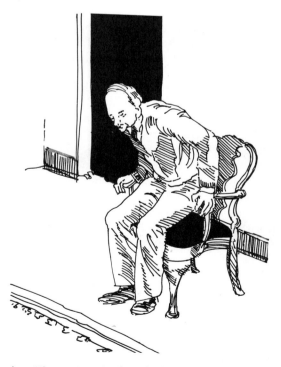

Sitting down and getting up out of a chair can be a difficult task for some elderly patients and visitors. Chairs designed with sturdy armrests and open space under the front edge of the seat can make this task easier.

Heating, Ventilating, and Air Conditioning (HVAC)

The following guidelines suggest ways in which the thermal environment needs to be regulated in order to accommodate the changes in thermal sensitivity likely to be experienced by older patients and visitors:[14]

- Select heating systems capable of maintaining a temperature of 75°F.

- Select cooling systems capable of maintaining a temperature of 78°F.

- Select air-handling systems designed to avoid creating drafty areas.

- Select mechanical ventilation systems that provide approximately 10 air changes per hour.

Wayfinding

Although elderly persons may have a good understanding of familiar complex environments, they are likely to have difficulty creating new mental images. Finding their way through an unfamiliar complex environment may be even more stressful.[14] Architectural and interior designs that emphasize unique, recognizable, and memorable features and areas will help older (and younger) users who may become confused trying to differentiate among many seemingly repetitive elements (see also chapter 3).[15]

To create a system that enables elderly patients and visitors to find their way through the health care facility more easily, consider the following:

- Create memorable "landmarks" throughout the facility, using color, artwork, unique architectural features, plants, and other design elements.[15]

- Provide high contrast between the message and background used on signs. In areas that will be used predominantly by elderly patients and visitors, the use of white symbols on a dark background is recommended.[15]

- Avoid potential sources of glare, such as windows and artificial lighting, in sign design and placement. For example, directories should not have reflective covers.[14,15]

- Pay special attention to type size on signs and notices that will be read by older patients and visitors. Type on signs should be a minimum of 1⁹/₁₆ inches (40 mm) high. Notices to elderly patients and visitors should be printed in large type.[17,18]

- In places used predominantly by older patients and visitors, consider repeating directional signs more frequently than usual.[18]

Circulation

Circulation areas can pose certain difficulties to older users, such as long distances to walk, obstructions within corridors, or level changes that are difficult to see. Design that attends to these users' special needs can result in a safer and more pleasant health care experience (see also chapter 3):

- Minimize the distances to frequently used destinations.[18]

- Provide small rest areas along corridors used heavily by older patients and visitors.[18]

- Provide sufficient storage areas so that carts and other large pieces of medical equipment do not need to be stored in hallways and do not act as obstructions to older users.[18]

- Avoid protrusions from walls that older patients or visitors might bump into.[18]

- Design entrance and exit areas to allow for older users' slower adaptation rates to dark and light.[18]

- Mark glass walls and doors in order to make their presence obvious to older users.[18]

- Consider using contrasting colors to accentuate entrances, exits, merging of corridors, steps, approaches to elevators, ramps, and other changes in level or flooring surfaces.[18]

- Consider using sound signals to indicate when it is safe to enter or exit an elevator. Middle-frequency tones could serve as an additional cue, along with visual signals that indicate arrival. Such sound signals can be especially useful for elderly and visually impaired users.[15]

- Consider a double handrail and kick plate combination in hallways to provide support for older ambulatory users and wheelchair users and also to prevent scuffing. Mount one handrail at 32 inches (81 cm) and the other at approximately 26 inches (66 cm).[17]

Inpatient Room

When elderly persons are hospitalized, the patient room becomes their home for a time. Because these patients are often more vulnerable than others, a supportive environment is especially important (see also chapter 6).

Beds

- Select beds that can be lowered to a normal bed height of 20 inches (51 cm) from the floor to the top of the bedding. This allows for independent dressing, getting in and out of bed, comfortable conversation with a seated visitor, and wheelchair transfer.[15]

- In order to avoid injuries stemming from patients falling and striking the bedrails, rails should be completely retractable.[15]

- Select beds with rounded corners and edges in order to prevent injuries.[17]

Furnishings

- Select furnishings that can help steady an ambulatory patient who needs some physical support.[15,17]

- Avoid tables or bedside stands with white or shiny top surfaces that might lead to excessive reflection or glare. It is likely that glassware, papers, and other items would not be seen on a pure white surface, especially when there is glare.[17]

Telephones

- For older patients, consider selecting inpatient room telephones with illuminated dials or with letters and numerals that greatly contrast with the background. On push-button telephones, buttons should be larger than the standard size, if possible.[17]

- Consider providing telephone speaker devices that assist hearing-aid users and that eliminate interference from ambient noise.[18]

Display

- Make provisions for some display of personal items, such as family photographs, in the older patient's room.[17]

- Allow space to display signs, calendars, and other devices that can help the patient understand the time, place, and activity.[17]

Inpatient Bathroom

As one gerontologist has noted, "As people age, the bathroom becomes a place of danger."[15] Loss of strength and mobility, perceptual difficulties, changes in the performance of tasks, and the privacy implied in bathroom use—all lead to dangers for the older patient. For instance, exposed hot water pipes can cause serious leg burns for wheelchair users, patients can slip and fall when entering or leaving the tub or shower, and toilet grab rails that are incorrectly placed are of little help to a patient in getting on or off the toilet.[15] Design features can help make the inpatient bathroom a safer place (see also chapter 6):

Toilets

- Provide fixture-mounted grab bars or arms, resembling the arms of a chair, on both sides of toilets used by persons needing assistance to lower and raise themselves. (Wall-mounted grab bars are often placed too far away to be useful.)[14,17]

Sinks

- Make sure the waste pipes and hot water feed pipes are inaccessible and wrapped in order to prevent leg burns.[15]

- To make it easy for wheelchair-bound elderly patients to use the sink, consider various alternatives for mounting faucets and water controls, in addition to the traditional back mounting. For instance, side-mounted models are available.[17]

- Clearly mark water controls to indicate hot and cold.[17]

- Select oversized, textured control knobs to enable the older patient to identify and grasp them easily.[17]

Other

- Over bathroom mirrors, use light bulbs that simulate natural light.[14]

- Design towel racks to be extremely strong, so that they can support a patient's weight if necessary.

Conclusion

This chapter has reviewed and expanded on some of the design-related needs of special patients and visitors within a health care facility: mobility-impaired, hearing-impaired, vision-impaired, and elderly users. Attention to the design or selection of a wide variety of design features—from large scale to small scale—can help these users to negotiate the facility safely and independently and as a result to retain a sense of competence. With a focus on wayfinding (such as selecting highly contrasting colors for floors and walls so vision-impaired users can tell where one ends and the other begins), physical comfort (such as selecting chairs with padded, sturdy armrests for elderly users), social contact (such as providing access to TDDs for deaf patients), and symbolic meaning (such as door levers that can be operated by all users), the message that the organization cares about their needs is not likely to be lost on these groups.

Design Review Questions

Users with Impairments

Mobility-Impaired Users

☐ Have handrails been provided along patient and public circulation routes?

☐ Do rest areas with seats occur regularly along long corridors?

☐ Are more wheelchair-accessible toilets provided than are required by code?

Hearing-Impaired Users[3,8]

☐ Has the health care facility provided a variety of communication methods and devices for hearing-impaired users, such as telecommunication devices for the deaf (TDDs)?

☐ In large organizations, is there a staff member responsible for supervising services for hearing-impaired patients?

☐ Are interpreters available, within the facility or on call, to consult with the patients and help them communicate with staff?

☐ Are handwritten messages, drawings, TDDs, and interpreters readily available to assist staff in communicating with hearing-impaired patients in admitting and emergency departments?

☐ Are alternative alarms such as flashing lights, vibrators, and variable-intensity fans available?

☐ Is the facility designed to minimize noise?

☐ Is there a policy to locate deaf inpatients close to the nurses' stations?

Vision-Impaired Users[9,10,13]

☐ Does the wayfinding system include raised letters, braille, audible signals, tactile guides, and highly contrasting colors on floors and walls, treads and risers?

☐ Are pathways free from obstructions, such as furniture and equipment, and protrusions from the wall, such as water fountains?

☐ Have hazards been marked by a tactile warning signal?

☐ Have hard surfaces on floors, walls, and ceilings of hallways been avoided, if possibile?

☐ Do corridors intersect at right angles?

☐ Within a given flight of stairs, is stair width consistent?

Notes

Design that Cares: Planning Health Facilities for Patients and Visitors, by Janet R. Carpman, Myron A. Grant, and Deborah A. Simmons. ©1986 by American Hospital Publishing, Inc.

☐ Within a given flight of stairs, is stair tread height consistent?

☐ Do stair railings begin at the first step, run continuously, flatten out along landings, and rise or fall again with the next flight?

☐ If the budget permits, have speech synthesizers been considered for elevators in multistorey facilities?

☐ Are contrasting colors used to make environmental features easy for vision-impaired people to notice and manipulate?

Elderly Users

Implications for Design

Safety Systems

☐ In spaces targeted for elderly patients and visitors, is there a minimum radius for the corners and edges of all hard surfaces and projections—especially furnishings—in order to help reduce injuries?[17]

☐ Are visual warning devices backed up with middle-frequency auditory signals?[14,15]

Sound[15]

☐ When possible, have ambient background sounds in open public spaces been reduced using sound-attenuating and baffling materials?

☐ Has "canned" background music been avoided, especially in high-use areas?

Lighting

☐ Has the placement of windows, mirrors, and other bright or reflective surfaces been avoided at the end of corridors?[14]

☐ Have abrupt changes in illumination levels been avoided?[14,18]

☐ Has indirect lighting been used whenever possible?[14]

☐ Has the use of carpeting been considered in corridors, to reduce glare and noise?[17]

☐ Has accentuating lighting around the first few stairs in a series been considered, in order to avoid injuries?[20]

☐ When possible, has warm rather than cool-toned lighting been selected?[17]

Notes _____

Design that Cares: Planning Health Facilities for Patients and Visitors, by Janet R. Carpman, Myron A. Grant, and Deborah A. Simmons. ©1986 by American Hospital Publishing, Inc.

☐ Have all light sources been shielded so that bare bulbs are not visible?[17,20]

☐ Has glare reduction been attempted by fitting all windows with some means of light reduction, such as blinds, shades, or reflective glass?[17,20]

Color

☐ Has color been planned in conjunction with lighting?[21]

☐ Has color been planned in conjunction with texture?[21]

☐ Have changes in planes been emphasized with highly contrasting colors?[14,16]

☐ Have patterns been used with caution?[21]

☐ Have contrasting colors been used on design components in order to make them stand out?[18,21]

Texture

☐ Has texture been considered as a means to help identify different locations within the health care facility?[15]

☐ Have reflective and shiny surfaces been avoided, especially on floors and on bathroom fixtures?[17]

☐ Do wall surfaces provide enough texture to enable elderly persons to use them to steady themselves?[15,17]

☐ Have wall surfaces been avoided if they are so abrasive they will cause injury?[17]

Hardware[14]

☐ Can hardware be operated with one hand and without requiring twisting, turning, or excessive strength?

☐ Do door hinges or opening devices and door closers require no more than 3 to 5 foot-pounds of pressure to operate?

☐ Do door closers have a "check-action delay" of 4 to 6 seconds before closing?

Flooring

☐ Whenever possible, has carpeting been provided because of its significant glare reduction, acoustic, and safety advantages?[17]

☐ Where carpeting is not considered appropriate, has flooring been used that is resilient, nonglare, and nonslip, even when wet?[15,17]

Notes_____

Design that Cares: Planning Health Facilities for Patients and Visitors, by Janet R. Carpman, Myron A. Grant, and Deborah A. Simmons. ©1986 by American Hospital Publishing, Inc.

Seating

☐ Have chairs been selected that have a clear space under the front, so that the user's heels can be placed underneath?[14]

☐ Have chairs been selected that have arms that align with the front edge of the chair or extend slightly beyond it?[14,15]

☐ Have chairs been selected with a seat angle no more than 4 degrees?[14]

☐ Have chairs been selected that have comfortably soft, rather than overly firm seats?[14]

☐ Has nonabsorbent upholstery been avoided whenever possible?[14,17]

☐ Is the front edge of the chair at most 17 inches (43 cm) from the floor?[14,15]

☐ In places used exclusively by the elderly, have tables been selected that are 31 inches (79 cm) high or that adjust to different heights?[15]

Heating, Ventilating, and Air Conditioning[14]

☐ Are heating systems capable of maintaining a temperature of 75°F?

☐ Are cooling systems capable of maintaining a temperature of 78°F?

☐ Have air-handling systems been designed to avoid creating drafty areas?

☐ Do mechanical ventilation systems provide approximately 10 air changes per hour?

Wayfinding

☐ Have memorable "landmarks" been created throughout the facility, using color, artwork, unique architectural features, plants, and other design elements?[15]

☐ On signs, is there high contrast between the message and the background?[15]

☐ For signs in areas that will be used predominantly by elderly patients and visitors, have white symbols on a dark background been used?[15]

☐ Has sign design and placement been planned to avoid reflection and glare from lights and windows?[14,15]

☐ Is type at least 1⁹/₁₆ inches (40 mm) high on signs directed to older patients and visitors?[17,18]

☐ Have notices directed to elderly patients and visitors been printed in large type?[17,18]

Notes

Design that Cares: Planning Health Facilities for Patients and Visitors, by Janet R. Carpman, Myron A. Grant, and Deborah A. Simmons. ©1986 by American Hospital Publishing, Inc.

☐ Has consideration been given to repeating directional signs more frequently than usual in places used predominantly by older patients and visitors?

Circulation

☐ Have distances to frequently used destinations been minimized?[18]

☐ Have small rest areas been provided along corridors used heavily by older patients and visitors?[18]

☐ Are circulation areas free of potential obstructions, such as carts and large pieces of medical equipment?[18]

☐ Have protrusions from walls been avoided?[18]

☐ Have entrance and exit areas been designed to allow for older users' slower adaptation rates to dark and light?[18]

☐ Have glass walls and doors been marked to make their presence obvious to older users?[18]

☐ Have contrasting colors been considered to accentuate entrances, exits, merging of corridors, steps, approaches to elevators, ramps, and other changes in level or flooring surface?[18]

☐ Has the use of sound signals been considered to indicate when it is safe to enter or exit an elevator?[15]

☐ Has a double handrail and kick plate combination been considered to provide support for older ambulatory users and wheelchair users and also to prevent scuffing? If so, is one handrail mounted at 32 inches (81 cm) and the other at approximately 26 inches (66 cm)?[17]

Inpatient Room

Beds

☐ Have beds been selected that can be lowered to a normal bed height of 20 inches (51 cm) from the floor to the top of the bedding?[15]

☐ Are bedrails completely retractable, in order to avoid injuries resulting from patients falling against them?[15]

☐ When possible, have beds been selected that have rounded corners and edges on their hard surfaces?[17]

Furnishings

☐ Have furnishings been selected that can help steady an ambulatory patient who needs some physical support?[15,17]

☐ Have tables or bedside stands with white or shiny top surfaces been avoided?[17]

Notes

Design that Cares: Planning Health Facilities for Patients and Visitors, by Janet R. Carpman, Myron A. Grant, and Deborah A. Simmons. ©1986 by American Hospital Publishing, Inc.

Telephones

☐ Do telephones have illuminated dials or letters and numerals that greatly contrast with the background?[17]

☐ On push-button telephones, are buttons larger than standard size?[17]

☐ Has consideration been given to providing telephone speaker devices that assist hearing-aid users and that eliminate interference from ambient noise?[18]

Display[17]

☐ Has provision been made for some display of personal items, such as family photographs?

☐ Is there space for displaying signs, calendars, and other devices to help the patient understand the time, place, and activity?

Inpatient Bathroom

Toilets

☐ Have fixture-mounted grab bars or arms been placed on both sides of toilets used by people needing assistance to lower and raise themselves?[14,17]

Sinks

☐ Are waste pipes and hot water feed pipes inaccessible and wrapped in order to prevent leg burns?[15]

☐ Have various alternatives been considered for mounting faucets and water controls, in order to make it easy for wheelchair-bound elderly patients to use the sink?[17]

☐ Are water controls clearly marked to indicate hot and cold?[17]

☐ Have oversized, textured control knobs been selected, in order to enable the older patient to identify and grasp them easily?[17]

Other

☐ Have light bulbs that simulate natural light been used over bathroom mirrors?[14]

☐ Have towel racks been designed to be strong enough to support a patient's weight if necessary?

Notes

Design that Cares: Planning Health Facilities for Patients and Visitors, by Janet R. Carpman, Myron A. Grant, and Deborah A. Simmons. ©1986 by American Hospital Publishing, Inc.

References

1. Fisher, T. Enabling the disabled. *Progressive Architecture.* 1985 July. pp 13-18.

2. Fowles, D. G. *A Profile of Older Americans, 1984.* Washington, DC: American Association of Retired Persons, U.S. Department of Health and Human Services, Administration on Aging, 1984.

3. Milner, M. Breaking through the deafness barrier: environmental accommodations for hearing impaired people. Unpublished report, Division of Public Services and Design and Construction Department, Washington, DC: Gallaudet College, 1981.

4. Hopf, P., and Raeber, J. *Access for the Handicapped: The Barrier-Free Regulations for Design and Construction in All 50 States.* New York: Van Nostrand Reinhold, 1984.

5. Goldsmith, S. *Designing for the Disabled.* London: RIBA Publications, Ltd., 1977.

6. Robinette, G. *Barrier-Free Exterior Design.* New York: Van Nostrand Reinhold, 1985.

7. Wyatt, H. J. You and your deaf patients. Seminar materials, National Academy of Gallaudet College, Washington, DC, 1983.

8. Carpman, J. R., Grant, M. A., and Norton, C. Needs of the hearing impaired in a hospital setting. Unpublished research report #30, Patient and Visitor Participation Project, Office of Hospital Planning, Research and Development, University of Michigan, Ann Arbor, 1984.

9. Harkness, S. P., and Groom, J. N. *Building Without Barriers for the Disabled.* New York: Watson Guptill, 1976.

10. Zimring, C. M., and Templer, J. Wayfinding and orientation by the visually impaired. *Journal of Environmental Systems.* 1983-1984. 13(4):333-52.

11. Goldish, L. *Braille in the United States: Its Production, Distribution, and Use.* New York: American Foundation for the Blind, 1967.

12. Berkowitz, M., and others. *Reading with Print Limitations: Executive Summary.* Prepared for the National Library Service for the Blind and Physically Handicapped. New York: American Foundation for the Blind, 1979.

13. Genensky, S. M. Design sensitivity: the partially sighted. *Building Operating Management.* 1981 June. 28(6):50-54.

14. American Institute of Architects Foundation. *Design for Aging: An Architect's Guide.* Washington, DC: AIA Press, 1986.

15. Koncelik, J. A. *Aging and the Product Environment.* Stroudsburg, PA: Hutchinson and Ross, 1982.

16. Lawton, M. P. Therapeutic environments for the aged. In: Canter, D., and Canter, S., editors. *Designing for Therapeutic Environments.* New York: John Wiley and Sons, 1979.

17. Koncelik, J. A. *Designing the Open Nursing Home.* Stroudsburg, PA: Dowden, Hutchinson and Ross, 1976.

18. Drader, D. The design of geriatric assessment units: psychosocial considerations. Consulting report, Department of National Health and Welfare, Ottawa, Canada, 1982.

19. Abend, A., and Chen, A. Developing residential design statements for the hearing-impaired elderly. *Environment and Behavior.* 1985 July. 17(4): 475-500.

20. *Facilities for the Elderly in Canada: Design and Environmental Considerations.* Vol. 1, *Geriatric Units in Hospitals.* Ottawa, Canada: Department of National Health and Welfare, 1984.

21. Hiatt, L. G. The color and use of color in environments for older people. *Nursing Homes.* 1981 May-June. 30(3):18-22.

Chapter 9

Special Places and Special Services _____

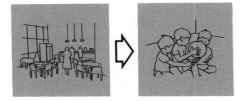

Special Places   Special Services

Throughout this book, we have discussed a number of typical destinations and activities of patients and visitors. For the most part, these have been places and activities that might be found in most health care facilities. This chapter deviates from this path to cover a number of special areas. Some of these are found in all facilities; others exist only in large or specialized care organizations. This chapter examines some policy and design issues that relate to special places and some special services that a facility might consider offering.

Special Places _____

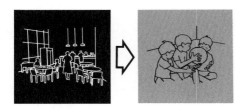

There can be hundreds of spaces within a large health care facility—patient rooms, waiting areas, examination rooms, and others. We have tried to concentrate on those spaces that are most commonly frequented by patients and visitors. However, there are additional spaces that affect how users experience the facility. This section examines the design criteria for consultation and grieving rooms, the emergency department, patient lounges, a patient and visitor library, a chapel, and eating areas.

Consultation and Grieving Rooms

It is important to dedicate space for consultation and grieving in most health care facilities. A family faced with death must have a place to cope in private; a woman who has been raped needs to talk with a social worker alone; and patients faced with a difficult decision about their treatment need a quiet place to discuss their case with a doctor. Consultation and grieving need to be accommodated in nearly all patient care spaces, such as the emergency department, inpatient floors, diagnostic and treatment areas, the surgery area, the labor and delivery area, and intensive care units. If a specific room is not dedicated for this purpose, these activities will continue to occur, but they will occur in public—in the hallway, in the waiting room, or in the semi-private inpatient room—and will invade the privacy of those discussing their problems and those inadvertently overhearing the discussion.

Once the commitment has been made to dedicate space for consultation and grieving, a number of design elements should be considered:[1]

- Provide both visual and acoustical privacy.

- Provide a phone so that the patient or family members can communicate in private.

- Avoid an institutional ambience by selecting subdued colors, carpeting, and table lamps or other types of indirect or incandescent lighting.

- Provide comfortable seating, both chairs and couches.

- Provide adequate ventilation to accommodate both smokers and nonsmokers.

- Provide coat racks or hooks for personal belongings.

- To avoid unnecessary disturbances, place a permanent, movable sign on the door that indicates whether the room is being used.

- Locate grieving and consultation rooms so that people do not have to walk a long way before they can deal with their crisis in private.

- Provide separate grieving and consultation rooms in emergency departments, because there will be high demand for both functions.

Emergency Department

In many ways, the issues involved in the design of an emergency department are similar to those of an outpatient diagnostic and treatment area (see chapter 5). The important difference, however, is the nature of the situation. Most people come to emergency departments with an acute illness or injury. They are under an unusual amount of stress. They may be traveling to the emergency department for the first time, or visiting it in the middle of the night.

Wayfinding

During an emergency, being able to find one's destination is particularly critical. Under stress, neither patients nor their companions have the extra mental energy necessary to deal with confusing traffic patterns during arrival or confusing pedestrian routes once inside the facility. In designing the entrance, therefore, the following factors should be considered (see also chapter 3):[2]

- Provide separate ambulance and ambulatory entrances so that walking patients and visitors do not have to cope with seeing ambulance patients being attended to.

- If there are separate entrances for ambulances and walk-in patients, provide a clear route for cars. Although this can be the same as that for the ambulance during the approach, the two routes should separate before the ambulance drop-off area.

- At or near the entrance area, provide seating for those waiting to be picked up, phones, change machines, and newspaper racks.

Triage, Registration, and Checkout

Triage and registration areas represent the first opportunity for the walk-in patient to be assessed and to receive help. Because confidential information will be discussed here, the environment should provide acoustical privacy. Although attention will be focused on the patient, companions often play an important role, providing information, consent for treatment, and comfort.[3] Provisions should be made for the companion to accompany the patient. The following are some design issues to consider:[2]

- Clearly define the intended order of the reception, registration, and triage process by use of logical physical layout and signage.

- Arrange the triage area or registration desk to ensure that staff have visual access to the entrance.

- Install registration or checkout stations that provide acoustical privacy and visual separation for patients.

- Make sure that at least some portion of the registration or checkout desk is wheelchair-accessible so that those too weak to stand may sit down.

- Provide ample space for triage so that it does not have to take place in the hallway.

- Consider making the triage area large enough for a stretcher.

- If there is more than one triage interview station, provide acoustic separation between them.

- In the triage interview station, provide comfortable chairs for both the patient and a companion.
- Locate a public rest room nearby.

Visitor Waiting Areas

Family and friends who accompany patients to an emergency department may have to wait for hours as tests and examinations are completed. Comfort, privacy, and access to amenities are important considerations in these waiting areas (see also chapter 4):[1,2,4,5]

- Consider providing both smoking and nonsmoking areas.
- Provide an outside view, if possible, but avoid a view of arriving ambulances.
- Locate visitor waiting areas with good visual access to a staff member, so that companions do not feel forgotten.
- Provide rest rooms, telephones, vending machines, and a water fountain near visitor waiting areas.
- Provide a television area and an area away from the television.
- Provide a children's area that is separated from, but visually connected to, the main waiting area (see also chapter 4).
- Provide some seating arranged in small conversational groups.
- Consider providing table lamps for reading.
- Develop a comforting ambience by selecting attractive, comfortable, movable furniture, as well as carpeting, warm colors, plants, and artwork.
- Provide a place to store coats and other personal belongings.
- Consider using an aquarium as a focal point.

Patient Waiting Area

After triage and registration, many emergency departments escort patients into a separate patient waiting area. It should be comfortable and designed to accommodate patients in wheelchairs or on stretchers. Because patients may feel vulnerable and may need emergency assistance, this waiting area should be designed to reassure them that help is available. In designing a patient waiting area, consider the following:[2]

- Locate the patient waiting area with good visual access to a staff area.
- Install an easily identified nurse-call mechanism.
- Locate the patient waiting area near a bathroom.
- If possible, provide an outside view, artwork, plants, and other focal points.

- Consider using cove or incandescent lighting rather than overhead fluorescents.

- Provide reclining seats or some other way for patients to lie down if they need to.

- Select comfortable seats with good upper and lower back support. Seats should be easy to sit on or rise from and should have padded armrests.

Inpatient Lounge

Many inpatients are encouraged to get up from their beds as part of the recovery process. They are more likely to become ambulatory if they have attractive places to go. A patient lounge can serve this purpose. Unfortunately, a patient lounge at the far end of the hall or one shared with another unit may never be discovered or may seem too far away to a patient just beginning to walk again. The location of the lounge is critical. If it is centrally located, close enough to most patients' rooms, they will feel that it is within a comfortable walking distance and will be more likely to make it a destination. The lounge's size is another important issue. Although guidelines on recommended size range from 10 net square feet (.9 square meters) to 50 net square feet (4.5 square meters) per bed on a unit, size should be determined by the activities that will take place within the lounge. If parties and dining are to be encouraged, the room will need more space than one that is designed for merely sitting and reading only (see Research Box #1).[6-8]

Furnishings and entertainment options available within the patient lounge may also affect its use by patients. A lounge that is likely to attract patients will be furnished with comfortable, movable, and durable seating; will contain plants and appealing artwork; will provide a view of the outside; and will offer a variety of entertainment options, such as a television, stereo, pool table, table tennis, or movie screen (see Research Box #2).[7,9-14]

Because the patient lounge will be used by a number of people at a time, subareas within the room should be easily formed using furnishings or dividers.[7,15] In this way, small groups or individuals can comfortably participate in an activity without bothering others. There should also be some way to keep noise inside the lounge so that it will not disturb other patients or staff.

If the health care facility allows smoking, there should be smoking and non-smoking areas within the lounge. The facility also may consider allowing patients to eat their meals in the patient lounge; this will afford them companionship and an additional opportunity to get out of their rooms. If eating in the lounge is desired, tables of appropriate size should be available. (The tables should be stored out of the way when not in use.) Finally, because this is a patient-oriented space, staff will need to be discouraged from using it themselves.

People often want to inspect a social area before they enter it, to see what is going on and who is there. A glass panel in the lounge's door or wall would let patients preview lounge activity, so they can decide whether or not to participate.[16]

Research Box #1:
Evaluating Inpatient Lounges

The patient lounge is a common feature of almost every inpatient floor. It provides an alternative to the patient room, a destination for patients just getting up and around, and a place to socialize. In a study of patient lounges in three different hospitals, researchers at the University of Saskatchewan documented lounge use and other design-related issues.[7] Through interviews with patients, visitors, and various staff (including head nurses and planning personnel), and by compiling a physical features checklist, the researchers found that the patient lounges studied had common problems.

For the most part, patient lounges were found to be:

Too small, given the demand

Too noisy, with noise spilling over into other patient areas

Arranged poorly, with activities such as watching television conflicting with visiting or game playing

Remotely located

Other problems included unattended children, uncomfortable furniture, furniture that could not be easily rearranged, and conflicts between smokers and nonsmokers.

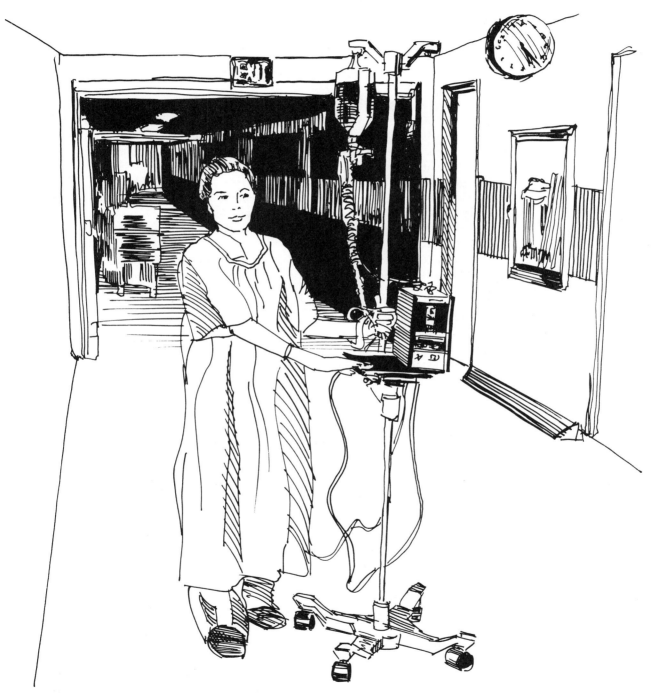

Getting up and moving after surgery is often considered good therapy for the patient. Patients are more likely to walk if there are attractive and interesting places to go.

Research Box #2: Creating Unusual Inpatient Lounges

Researchers at Bellevue Hospital in New York City joined forces with the 3M Company and Berkey K & L Custom Photographic Services to create and evaluate some unique inpatient lounges.[10] They believed that the lounge's design could play a role in enhancing patient morale. They hypothesized that well-designed lounges could lure patients out of their rooms, decreasing passivity and feelings of confinement. Lounges might also decrease boredom and provide an arena for social contact among patients.

The four identically sized lounges they were using measured 441 square feet (39.7 square meters). Each room had two exterior walls with views to Manhattan or the East River. A 10-foot (3-meter) partition wall located in the center of each room subdivided them into two distinct areas. Despite comfortable seating and commanding views, patients did not make much use of the lounges; they found them unattractive and unstimulating.

Two of the four lounges, located at opposite corners of a square floor for surgical patients, were selected for redesign using Scanmurals. Scanmurals are made by a computer-graphics process that enlarges color photographs to full color, floor-to-ceiling images. Accompanying the murals were two audio systems containing two-minute tapes of sounds appropriate to the images.

One lounge became the "Harbor" lounge with murals created from aerial photographs of New York Har-

bor, the East River, the Statue of Liberty, and the lower Manhattan skyline. Patients could push a button to hear sounds of sea gulls, lapping water, tugboats, and foghorns. The other lounge became the "Central Park" lounge, with photographs of the park's lake, a backdrop of the Manhattan skyline, a waterfall, a cluster of trees, and one of the park's ornamental bridges. This tape contained sounds of oars dipping into the lake, horses' hooves on the cobblestones, vendors selling their wares, and a merry-go-round. Both lounges also had park benches and large plants.

Observations of the use of all four lounges were made in the corridors and in the lounges both before and after the Scanmurals were installed. Patients were also interviewed to learn what they thought of the lounges and how often they used them.

The evaluation showed that the Scanmural lounges were very successful for the patients who visited the rooms. Almost all patients reported liking the photomurals and sound systems, and most saw a positive relationship between the lounges and their own morale. The data indicated that the Scanmural lounges were perceived more positively than were the lounges without murals. However, observation data indicated that the effects of the Scanmural lounges on overall patient mobility was no greater than that of installing televisions in each lounge. One reason for this was that most patients who did not use the Scanmural lounges simply did not know about them.

When asked about ways to make the Scanmural lounges more appealing to patients, both patients and staff suggested adding television, providing more comfortable seating, supplying games and magazines, and improving housekeeping. Staff suggested making music available, in the same way airplanes do.

This study makes two important points. First, attractive and interesting patient lounges will be enjoyed by patients, but only if they know the lounges are there. Innovative design must be accompanied by publicity directed to its potential users. Second, lounges designed for a single purpose—in this case, experiencing special sights and sounds—may be less widely appealing than lounges designed to accommodate a number of different activities.

Patient and Visitor Library

Time spent recuperating in a health care facility can be boring. The sense of wasting time or spending time unproductively may aggravate already high levels of stress. Many patients would like to have something to read or an opportunity to learn more about their illness. In one study, nearly 60 percent of the visitors surveyed said they would like to use a reading room within the hospital, and over 80 percent said they would like to learn more about a particular illness.[17] A patient and visitor library can satisfy these desires.

To encourage use, the library should have a quiet and warm ambience, with comfortable, well-lighted places to sit and read. If smoking is allowed, a ventilation system capable of handling cigarette smoke should be installed, and separate smoking and nonsmoking areas should be delineated.

The library should be designed to accommodate wheelchairs, walkers, and rolling I.V. poles. Consequently, sufficient circulation space should be provided between bookshelves, as well as within the reading area. Books should be displayed so that their titles are easily readable and reachable by those with limited mobility. Signs used within the library identifying checkout procedures and book areas should be designed to be legible to people with vision impairments.[18] Many users with vision impairments may need books with large type or other reading aids (see also chapter 8).

To promote patient education, a separate area with cubicles and audiovisual equipment could be made available. Through pamphlets and slide-tape or videotape programs, patients and their companions can learn more about an illness and its reatment. Because a family or a group of patients may wish to view a presentation at the same time, the patient education portion of the library may need a conference room capable of accommodating small groups.

Library and patient education areas can be used only if patients and visitors are aware of their existence. In a study at the University of Michigan Hospitals, for example, nearly a third of the patients interviewed did not know that a patient library was available.[15] An effective system should be developed for conveying information about the library and its services to patients and visitors. In addition, patients' and visitors' knowledge of the library would likely be increased if the library was located along a major circulation route.

Roving library carts, stocked with a variety of titles and taken to patients' bedsides by volunteers, serve two functions. They provide access to library materials for bedridden patients and also provide publicity about the library itself.

Food Service Areas

Patients often evaluate a health care facility, especially a hospital, by the quality of its food.[19] With people becoming more concerned about nutrition, the importance placed on a hospital's food service is bound to increase. From a marketing standpoint, good food service makes good business sense. And it shows the health care facility's sensitivity to the needs of patients and visitors who are away from home and under great stress. Visitors attending sick patients around the clock need nutritious food to sustain them during the ordeal. Ambulatory patients may find drinking coffee with visitors in a cafeteria a pleasant alternative to spending all day in their room.

Often, visitors want to take their meals near patients and resist going elsewhere to eat. In some cases, family members will maintain a vigil by eating in shifts. Given these circumstances, the food service in a large health care facility may be expected to provide meals for a large number of visitors. In one study, 36 percent of the inpatient visitors interviewed reported eating breakfast, 68 percent lunch, and 58 percent dinner in the hospital cafeteria. In addition, 80 percent reported eating snacks in the hospital. The need for some food service is obvious, but there is also a desire for alternatives; of these visitors, 99 percent said that they would use a cafeteria if one were available, 84 percent would use a coffee shop, and 76 percent would use vending machines.[17,20]

The design of a cafeteria or coffee shop will play an important role in whether it is considered a comfortable and pleasant place. Comfortable, movable seats, tables large enough to accommodate cafeteria trays, tables of various sizes to suit groups of different sizes, and subdued lighting all may help to create an inviting atmosphere. A view outside, and perhaps an outdoor courtyard, may also provide a calming focus. As in all public spaces, provision should be made for separate smoking and non-smoking sections.

Food service areas within health care facilities should be designed for mobility-impaired users. Tables should accommodate someone in a wheelchair or with a rolling I.V. pole. The cafeteria line should permit these users to manuever in the line and to see the food selections. Because many using the food service have difficulty with muscle control and spill food easily, dishes should have higher rims than usual. The facility might also consider avoiding flimsy throwaway dishes and trays in favor of more stable dishware and trays.[21] Finally, cafeterias are notoriously noisy places. Every effort should be made to subdue noise by using carpeting and sound-absorbing wall materials and by keeping background noise to a minimum, especially during busy times.[21]

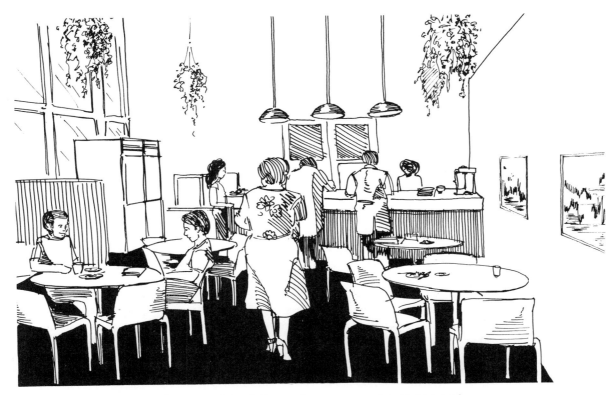

Food service areas are important to visitors who may need a change of scene or a bite to eat.

Chapel

A chapel located within a health care facility serves a special need for some patients and visitors. It will be used individually by those who need time and space alone, as well as for organized services. Given its special function, a chapel should be a comfortable, quiet place with adjustable lighting. Its design and ambience should facilitate quiet thought. As with other public areas, it should be accessible to all patients and visitors, including those in wheelchairs, those with walkers, and those with I.V.s. If the chapel is next to a waiting area, an auditorium, or other similar space, a common flexible wall could allow the chapel's area to expand as needed during scheduled services.

Special Services

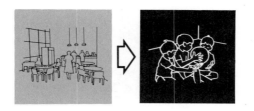

Hospitals and other large health care facilities often become small cities complete with 24-hours-a-day, 7-days-a-week activity. Visitors eat and sleep in the hospital for days or even weeks. During the long hours of waiting, they need emotional and physical support, as well as activities that help take their minds off their worries. Visitors in one study were asked about activities they would participate in if they were at the hospital but unable to be with the patient for a couple of hours. Sixty percent or more said they would enjoy sitting in an outdoor courtyard, walking around the hospital grounds, going to a small mall within the hospital, attending a movie, or using a reading room in the hospital. The most popular activities seem to involve the least amount of effort on the visitor's part. Visitors want a place nearby to sit, chat, walk, or look around.[17]

Given the time many visitors must spend waiting and the number of hours that are spent away from the patient, it is not surprising that visitors want recreational and diversionary activities. Such activities perform many therapeutic functions for the visitor, including relaxation, refreshment, tension release, education, and satisfaction of practical needs.

Overnight Accommodations

Some hospital visitors and outpatients need overnight accommodations. The family members or friends they have come to visit may be very sick and require a long hospital stay, leading the visitors to want to remain close to the hospital over a period of days, weeks, or months (see Research Box #3).

Many visitors are family groups that come from great distances and simply cannot afford to pay hotel or motel fees for any length of time. Some outpatients who come for daily treatment over a one- or two-week period and do not have to be admitted may also need a nearby, inexpensive place to stay.

In its humane concern for patients and visitors, health care facilities with out-of-town outpatients and visitors should provide inexpensive overnight accommodations close to the facility. This temporary housing can become part of the marketing strategy.

Research Box #3: Assessing Visitor Preferences for Overnight Accommodations

To learn what arrangements for overnight accommodations were most desirable, a study was conducted of 102 randomly sampled inpatient visitors at the University of Michigan Hospitals.[22]

The study found that more than 60 percent would be likely to use inexpensive accommodations close to the hospital if these were available. What is considered inexpensive, however, may not overlap with what is available. Visitors' ability to pay for hotel or motel double rooms was limited, as was their desired rate for single rooms. For nearly 60 percent of the visitors interviewed, $15 per night was the maximum they would be willing or able to spend for a single room; 40 percent could afford to pay a maximum of $25 per night for a double. An additional option was a "host home" program, in which people in the surrounding community offer rooms to inpatient visitors at a nominal fee or without charge. Only 40 percent of the visitors surveyed thought that this would be a viable option for them.

This study found that two accommodation options that would be the least expensive for hospitals to provide—hotel or motel discounts and a "host home" program—were likely to provide a partial solution to the accommodations problem. However, any single approach would not satisfy the wide variety of needs and preferences regarding the desired cost and quality of accommodations. Consequently, it was recommended that both of these options be pursued as partial solutions. It was also considered desirable to provide visitors with a variety of options for overnight accommodations, including building or renovating a nearby facility to be owned and operated by the hospital.

There are a number of options being used by facilities around the nation to achieve this objective (see Research Box #4). They include:

1. Allowing visitors to sleep in patient rooms, in most cases on cots or folding beds.
2. Accommodating visitors elsewhere in the complex. Visitors and outpatients can be allowed to sleep in unused rooms, such as those for medical students, residents, nurses, family consultations, or inpatients.
3. Offering a "host home" program in which visitors and outpatients can be given a place to shower and get a good night's sleep in the home of someone in the community, either with or without charge.
4. Building, renovating, leasing, or otherwise providing some type of facility (apartments, motel, room and bath) under the hospital's management.
5. Arranging for a discount program with nearby hotels and motels, with transportation provided by shuttle bus.
6. Encouraging either a for-profit or not-for-profit group to build and operate a hotel facility.

Research Box #4: Studying Overnight Accommodations Provided Nationally

In a study of overnight accommodations for visitors and outpatients, researchers at the University of Michigan Hospitals conducted a telephone survey of teaching and nonteaching hospitals around the country.[23] Eighty hospitals were contacted and surveyed concerning their arrangements, restrictions on use, occupancy rates, services and amenities provided, and cost.

The study indicated that hospitals have only limited involvement in arranging overnight accommodations. A majority (61.3 percent) of the hospitals sampled allowed a visitor to sleep in the patient's room. The next most common type of overnight arrangement (43.8 percent) was the provision of a list of hotels and motels in the area. Discounts to visitors and patients at nearby hotels or motels had been arranged by 13.7 percent of the hospitals, and 17.5 percent of the hospitals had made arrangements with a hotel or apartment complex owned and run by another organization. One-fourth of the sample provided no arrangements for overnight accommodations.

Although the question of how to provide inexpensive accommodations for visitors and outpatients has been before health care facilities for years, it has not been directly addressed by many. Some, however, have made great strides in providing for the needs of these vulnerable groups. A combination of the existing strategies can satisfy a range of circumstances, making the health care experience less stressful for all concerned.

Child Care

Whether or not special facilities are provided, many parents will bring their children to a health care facility. These children, often bored or tired, may annoy other visitors in waiting areas, play in hallways where they get in the way of staff, or make noise that disturbs patients. Parents are often forced to take turns watching the children and being with the patient, a situation that only increases stress.[17]

When asked if child care should be offered in a health care facility, more than 80 percent of the visitors interviewed in one study said yes, and most would be willing to pay for it.[17] Because bringing children to a health care facility is often stressful, it would be helpful to have children happily occupied and supervised for a few hours. Providing child care would not only offer a valued service to visitors but might also provide an incentive for recruiting and retaining nurses and other staff members.

Hair Care

How people feel about their appearance influences their general state of mind, as well as their health. Being a patient does not mean a person ceases to care about personal grooming; in fact, some pampering may go a long way towards increasing a sense of well-being. Thus, the availability of a barber shop or beauty salon may be important, especially for long-term patients. When asked about the desirability of providing hair care services in one large hospital, more than 85 percent of patients and nurses responded positively.[24]

Such hair care service need not be elaborate. For the most part, patients and nurses agreed that hair washing and cutting were the most important services to offer, followed by setting, drying, and shaving. Many patients who need hair care services are not able to travel to a barber shop or beauty salon within the hospital. Hair care services need to be brought to the bedsides of these patients.

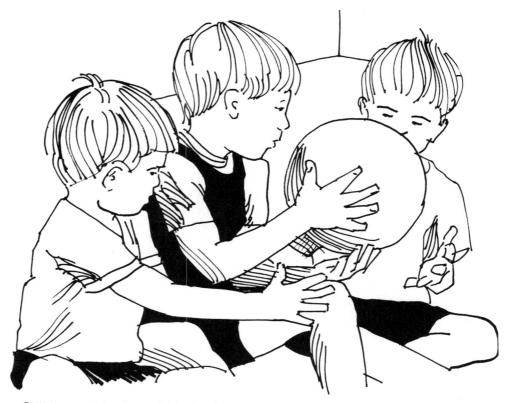

Children will be brought to health care facilities whether or not the facility has planned for their needs. Special children's waiting areas and child care services deserve consideration.

Conclusion

This chapter has described design criteria for some special places that may be present in health care facilities: consultation and grieving rooms, the emergency department, patient lounges, a patient and visitor library, a chapel, and eating areas. It also discusses special services a health care facility might offer, including overnight accommodations, child care, and hair care. Once again, issues related to wayfinding (such as delineating a clear route for automobiles approaching an emergency department), physical comfort (such as providing reclining seats in a patients' emergency department waiting area), social contact (such as designing a patient lounge to accommodate a holiday party), and symbolic meaning (such as showing concern for visitors by providing nearby, inexpensive overnight accommodations) are the key to establishing good relationships between the health care facility and its consumers.

Design Review Questions

Special Places

Consultation and Grieving Rooms[1]

☐ Are consultation and grieving rooms available for patients and their families in all patient care areas?

☐ Are both visual and acoustical privacy provided?

☐ Is a private phone available?

☐ Has a noninstitutional ambience been created?

☐ Have comfortable individual seating and couches been provided?

☐ Has adequate smoke ventilation been provided?

☐ Have coat racks or hooks been provided?

☐ Is there a way of indicating on the door whether or not the room is occupied?

☐ Are grieving and consultation rooms located so that people don't need to walk far to get to them?

☐ Does the emergency department provide both a grieving room and a consultation room?

Emergency Department

Wayfinding[2]

☐ Has the ambulance entrance been visually and acoustically separated from other patient and visitor areas?

☐ Has a clear automobile route to the emergency entrance been provided, with its drop-off area separate from the ambulance drop-off?

☐ Has seating for those waiting to be picked up been provided at or near the entrance?

☐ Are phones, change machines, and newspaper racks available at the entrance?

Triage, Registration, and Checkout[2]

☐ Is the intended order of the registration and triage process clearly reflected in design?

☐ Is there visual access from the front desk to the entrance?

Notes

Design that Cares: Planning Health Facilities for Patients and Visitors, by Janet R. Carpman, Myron A. Grant, and Deborah A. Simmons. ©1986 by American Hospital Publishing, Inc.

- ☐ Is there acoustical privacy during a triage interview?
- ☐ Is there acoustical privacy during registration and checkout?
- ☐ Is some portion of the registration and checkout desk wheelchair-accessible?
- ☐ Has ample space been provided for triage so that it does not have to take place in the hallway?
- ☐ Is the triage area large enough to accommodate a stretcher?
- ☐ If there is more than one triage interview station, has acoustic separation been provided between them?
- ☐ Within the triage interview station, have comfortable chairs been provided for the patient and a companion?
- ☐ Are patient and public bathrooms located nearby?

Visitor Waiting Areas[1-5]
- ☐ Are both smoking and nonsmoking areas provided?
- ☐ Is there an outside view?
- ☐ Is there good visual access between the waiting area and the clerk?
- ☐ Are visitor waiting areas near rest rooms, phones, vending machines, and a water fountain?
- ☐ Has a television been provided?
- ☐ Is there an area away from the distraction of the television?
- ☐ Has a children's area been provided that is separated from but visually connected to the main waiting area?
- ☐ Has some seating been arranged in small conversational groups?
- ☐ Have some table lamps been provided for reading?
- ☐ Has a comforting ambience been developed?
- ☐ Is there a place to store coats and other personal belongings?
- ☐ Has an aquarium or other interesting focal point been considered?

Notes _____

Design that Cares: Planning Health Facilities for Patients and Visitors, by Janet R. Carpman, Myron A. Grant, and Deborah A. Simmons. ©1986 by American Hospital Publishing, Inc.

Patient Waiting Area[2]

☐ Has space been provided for patients in wheelchairs or on gurneys?

☐ Is the patient waiting area visually connected to a staff area?

☐ Has a nurse-call system been provided?

☐ Is the patient waiting area near a bathroom?

☐ If possible, have an outside view, artwork, plants, and other focal points been provided?

☐ Has indirect or incandescent lighting been considered?

☐ Is there a recliner chair or some other way for patients to lie down if they need to?

☐ Is seating easy to sit on and rise from, with good back support and padded armrests?

Inpatient Lounge

☐ Is the inpatient lounge centrally located?[6-8]

☐ Does the size of the lounge accurately reflect the types of activities that will take place in it?[7,8]

☐ Can subspaces within the room be easily formed using furnishings or dividers?[7,15]

☐ Is the lounge designed to accommodate a variety of activities?

☐ If smoking is allowed, have the needs of nonsmokers been addressed?

☐ Is a glass panel provided in the door or wall to allow patients to see in before entering?[16]

☐ Has providing a unique activity or focal point in the lounge been considered?

Patient and Visitor Library

☐ Is the library inviting, with comfortable, well-lighted places to sit and read, reflecting a quiet and warm ambience?

☐ Is the library designed to accommodate people in wheelchairs, those using walkers, and those with rolling I.V. poles?

☐ Is sufficient circulation space provided between bookshelves?

☐ Are books within easy reach of those with limited mobility?

☐ Are books with large type available for those with vision impairments?[18]

Notes _____

Design that Cares: Planning Health Facilities for Patients and Visitors, by Janet R. Carpman, Myron A. Grant, and Deborah A. Simmons. ©1986 by American Hospital Publishing, Inc.

☐ Is a separate area with cubicles and audiovisual equipment available for patient education?

☐ If smoking will occur in the library, is there a nonsmoking area and extra exhaust ventilation?

☐ Is the library located along a major patient circulation route?

☐ Is there a library cart regularly serving patient room areas?

Food Service Areas

☐ Are a cafeteria, a coffee shop, and vending areas available to patients and visitors?

☐ Do food service areas have outside views?

☐ Do tables within food service areas accommodate people in wheelchairs and those with rolling I.V. poles?

☐ Does the cafeteria food line accommodate people in wheelchairs and those with rolling I.V. poles?

☐ Can tables be arranged to accommodate groups of different sizes?

☐ Have efforts been made to subdue noise?[21]

☐ Have stable dishware and trays been provided?[21]

☐ Does the dishware have higher rims than usual?[21]

☐ Has smoking been prohibited, or have separate smoking and nonsmoking areas been provided?

Chapel

☐ Is the chapel a comfortable, quiet space with adjustable light levels?

☐ Is the chapel accessible to persons using wheelchairs, crutches, and I.V. poles?

☐ Has the chapel been located next to a waiting area, auditorium, or similar space and do the two areas share a common flexible wall that can be opened for services?

Notes

Design that Cares: Planning Health Facilities for Patients and Visitors, by Janet R. Carpman, Myron A. Grant, and Deborah A. Simmons. ©1986 by American Hospital Publishing, Inc.

Special Services

Overnight Accommodations

☐ Has the health care facility provided a variety of overnight accommodation alternatives for outpatients and visitors?[22,23]

Child Care

☐ Has a child care service been provided for patients and visitors with children?

Hair Care

☐ Are hair care services available for ambulatory patients and for those who cannot leave their beds?

Notes_____

Design that Cares: Planning Health Facilities for Patients and Visitors, by Janet R. Carpman, Myron A. Grant, and Deborah A. Simmons. ©1986 by American Hospital Publishing, Inc.

References

1. Petersen, R. W. Behavioral criteria: patient and companion needs for reception and waiting areas. Unpublished report, R. W. Petersen and Associates, McMinnville, OR, 1981 July 31.

2. Carpman Associates. St. Joseph Mercy Hospital emergency department behavioral design program. Unpublished report, Carpman Associates, Ann Arbor, MI, 1984.

3. Nicklin, W. M. The role of the family in the emergency department. *Canadian Nurse.* 1979 Apr. 75(4):40-43.

4. Welch, P. Hospital emergency facilities: translating behavioral issues into design. Report, Department of Architecture, Harvard University, Cambridge, 1977.

5. Drury, L. R., and Rosen, P. Multiple use, flexibility key to emergency department planning. *Hospitals.* 1977 July 16. 51(14):201-11.

6. Kenny, C., and Canter, D. Findings from the development of USEP. Report, Department of Psychology, University of Surrey, Guildford, Surrey, 1978 Sept.

7. Hamilton, D. N. Patient lounge study. Unpublished research report #1, Saskatoon Hospital Evaluation Project, University of Saskatchewan, Canada, 1983.

8. Murtha, D. M. Environmental requirements for a community room on a patient care unit: recommendations. Unpublished report, Nurse Utilization Project, St. Mary's Hospital, Milwaukee, WI, 1970.

9. Edwards, K. The environment inside the hospital. *Practitioner.* 1979 June. 222(1332):746-51.

10. Olsen, R. V., Pershing, A., and Winkel, G. A patient and staff evaluation of the Scanmural lounges. Unpublished research report, Environmental Design Program, Bellevue Hospital Center and Environmental Psychology Program, City University of New York, New York, 1984.

11. Bobrow, M. L., and Thomas, J. Achieving quality in hospital design. *Hospital Forum.* 1976 Sept. 19(4):4-6.

12. Noble, A., and Dixon, R. Ward evaluation: St. Thomas Hospital. Unpublished report, Medical Architecture Research Unit, Polytechnic of North London, London, 1977 Dec.

13. Beckman, R. Getting up and getting out: progressive patient care. *Progressive Architecture.* 1974 Nov. 55(11):64-68.

14. Reizenstein, J. E., and Grant, M. A. Spontaneous design suggestions by patients and visitors. Unpublished research report #6, Patient and Visitor Participation Project, Office of Hospital Planning, Research and Development, University of Michigan, Ann Arbor, 1981.

15. Reizenstein, J. E., and Grant, M. A. Patient activities and schematic design preferences. Unpublished research report #2, Patient and Visitor Participation Project, Office of Hospital Planning, Research and Development, University of Michigan, Ann Arbor, 1981.

16. Howell, S., Epp, G., Reizenstein, J., and Albright, C. *Shared Spaces in Housing for the Elderly*. Cambridge, MA: Massachusetts Institute of Technology, Department of Architecture, 1976.

17. Reizenstein, J. E., Grant, M. A., and Vaitkus, M. A. Visitor activities and schematic design preferences. Unpublished research report #4, Patient and Visitor Participation Project, Office of Hospital Planning, Research and Development, University of Michigan, Ann Arbor, 1981.

18. Kamisar, H. Signs for the handicapped patron. In: Pollet, D., and Haskel, P., editors. *Sign Systems for Libraries*. New York: R. R. Bowker Co., 1979.

19. Rose, J. C. Marketing new food services. *Hospitals*. 1983 Aug. 1. 57(15):64-66.

20. Reizenstein, J. E., and Grant, M. A. Hospital patient and visitor issues: currently unmet needs and suggested solutions. Unpublished research report #4a, Patient and Visitor Participation Project, Office of Hospital Planning, Research and Development, University of Michigan, Ann Arbor, 1981.

21. Hiatt, L. G. Architecture for the aged: design for living. *Inland Architect*. 1978 Nov.-Dec. 23:6-17.

22. Reizenstein, J. E., and Grant, M. A. Visitor preferences for overnight accommodations. Unpublished research report #13, Patient and Visitor Participation Project, Office of Hospital Planning, Research and Development, University of Michigan, Ann Arbor, 1982.

23. Carpman, J. R., Grant, M. A., and Simmons, D. A. Overnight accommodations for visitors and outpatients: a nationwide study. *Health Care Strategic Management*. 1984 June. 2(6):9-14.

24. Reizenstein, J. E., and Grant, M. A. Executive summary: patient hair care and storage. Unpublished research report #9, Patient and Visitor Participation Project, Office of Hospital Planning, Research and Development, University of Michigan, Ann Arbor, 1981.

Part 3

Incorporating User Needs and Preferences

Chapter 10

User Participation in Health Care Facility Design_____

Going beyond Guidelines_____

Commissioning a design and construction project is a little bit like buying an expensive new suit. With a building, you may know the approximate number of square feet desired, the functions that must be accommodated, the image to be conveyed, the time frame, and the budget. With a suit, you may know the color, the style, the amount you want to spend, and the size you wear. But chances are you would not walk out of the store until the suit has been altered to fit your exact proportions—the waist may need to be nipped in, the hips let out a bit, the sleeves lengthened. The same is true for the design of a building. A general set of design parameters, even informed guidelines like those presented in this book, must be tailored to the specific needs at hand.

Design guidelines supply information of a general nature, for example, how to arrange cubicles in an admitting area, how to position a window in relation to a patient's bed, and how to locate privacy curtains in an examination room. However, in order to ensure that these guidelines are relevant to a specific problem—such as an admitting area extremely short on space, an older hospital that can't afford to change its windows, or a medical staff that would prefer not to use examination room privacy curtains—it is necessary to supplement general design guidelines with specific design-related information gathered from the people—both staff and patients—who will use the facility. Those who administer and maintain the facility are also likely to want some say in its design.[1]

Users of a health care facility can participate successfully in the design process. Through description and example, this chapter discusses some important contributions users can make, and some practical ways in which this participation can occur.

What Is User Participation in Design?

User participation deals with systematically gathering information about design-related needs and preferences of the facility's eventual users and incorporating this information into the design decision-making process. User participation is desirable for any health care facility design project, small scale or large scale, including interior design, landscape architecture, and architectural design.[2]

Participation in design can encompass a number of quite different activities, from relatively little or no direct user involvement to a great deal of direct involvement. If for some reason direct user participation is not feasible, experienced behavioral consultants might be asked to act as user advocates in the design process. Users themselves can participate by conveying information to designers or researchers about their design-related needs and preferences. Users might be slightly more involved by selecting one of several complete designs. They might participate even more actively by reviewing and commenting on schemes presented by designers (design review). Users might participate in design most fully by taking a stab at offering some design ideas themselves. This participation might occur as a natural outgrowth of design review, if the user feels the proposed design does not work well and suggests an alternative. It could also happen during a full-scale simulation in which users literally manipulate environmental features to best suit their needs.[3,4]

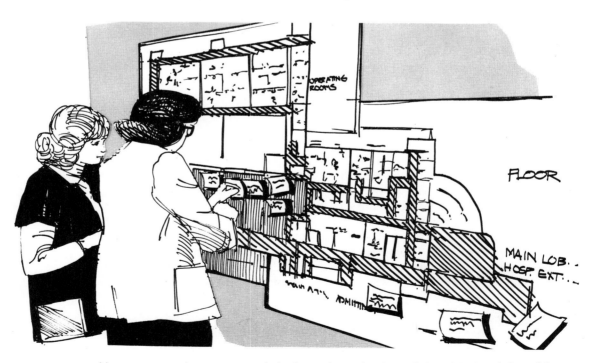

Users can review proposed designs, in order to point out potential problem areas.

Some real-life examples may help clarify what we mean. The examples show that participation can occur throughout the design process and can be achieved using a variety of techniques. All of the following occurred as part of the design process for the University of Michigan Replacement Hospital Program.

1. As part of predesign programming, the staff members in each clinical, hospital, and administrative department were interviewed about their requirements for space, equipment, lighting, finishes, and furnishings. This information was recorded and used to guide design.

2. Before decisions were made about the layout of the acute care inpatient room, including the location of the bathroom and the relationship of beds in a semiprivate room, randomly sampled patients were interviewed using small, three-dimensional models to show the arrangements they preferred. Their preferences, in addition to staff's preferences and other considerations, played an important role in decisions about the eventual layout.

3. When detailed decisions needed to be made about the design of the inpatient bathroom, both staff and recently discharged patients took part in evaluating several full-scale mock-ups. They acted out scenarios (such as a nurse helping a patient into the shower), assessed the degree to which the design of the mock-up worked well, and made suggestions for design changes. The findings from the mock-up studies had a direct impact on the eventual bathroom design.

4. Before interior design decisions were due, working groups composed of key staff members from each department pored over proposed furniture layouts. They tried to envision how each layout would function, debated alternative approaches, and suggested changes. When these suggestions were compatible with other performance criteria, the interior designers modified the designs to incorporate the users' suggestions.

Benefits of Participation

Although it is more complex to orchestrate a participatory design process than it is to have just one or two decision makers, some significant benefits can result.

Participation can help clarify design objectives. With clear objectives stated and relevant constraints in mind, designers are then free to do what they do best; meet these challenges with creative design approaches.[5] Participation can also help relieve users' anxieties about the otherwise unknown changes ahead.[3]

Participation can lead to better design decisions. Without user participation, design decision makers need to rely on their own experience and intuition and on the small body of available written information on health facility design and behavior, much of which is based on opinion rather than on objective data.[6] Without intimate familiarity with what goes on within a given space, design decision makers are far less likely to accommodate the users' needs optimally.[1,3] Participation can bridge the gap between generally relevant approaches and specifically appropriate alternatives. For example, staff participation in the design of a registration and triage area in a community hospital's emergency department led to a different and more workable layout than the one originally proposed.[7]

Participation can lower construction costs. Errors can be avoided, reducing the need for expensive renovation later. The study of parking structure entrances described in chapter 2 illustrates this point. Visitors participated in this study and described their likely behavior in two different design scenarios, showing that one design approach was likely to cause a major traffic congestion problem. Although this design approach was under serious consideration at the time, as a result of the study it was not selected as the design solution. The need for redesign and renovation later was eliminated, as were potential legal and operational costs of injuries due to unsafe conditions.[8]

Participation can stimulate positive behavior and attitudes. When people have been involved in a participatory process, they take better care of the resulting design.[5] They also feel a vested interest in the project, leading perhaps to less staff absenteeism, turnover, theft, or vandalism.[1,3,9] For example, one study of hospital social workers who had participated in a departmental renovation showed that some social workers who had experienced a decrease in office space thought they had received increased space. This was explained as a positive side effect of participation.[10]

Participation can help create a sense of community. A participatory design process often brings people together to talk about common concerns—something rare in segmented or large organizations. This opportunity for persons at different levels, in different roles, or in different departments to work together on an important and challenging task can create at least a temporary sense of teamwork that might otherwise be missing.[1]

Participation provides an opportunity to assess design-related organizational policies. When participants review proposed designs, questions often arise about related policies. For example, the degree to which a clinic's waiting area is overcrowded may be a function of scheduling practices, as well as design. Design and policy need to work in concert to achieve organizational objectives.

Participation can be used as a marketing strategy. Knowing what design features and amenities are important to patients and visitors can help the health care facility attract patients and visitors as consumers. As health care organizations become more aggressive about competing to attract patients, references to such design features as parking, comfort, and attractiveness are likely to appear with greater frequency in marketing materials.[11] Furthermore, the fact that consumers participated in the design process is a marketable feature in itself.[12]

Necessary Conditions

Achieving a fully successful participatory process cannot be guaranteed. A number of conditions are needed in order to achieve maximum benefits from participation.[1]

1. A client who seeks to promote the well-being and morale of its users and who understands the potential benefits of a participatory design process.

2. Designers who place a high value on satisfaction of user needs and who are also knowledgeable about and receptive to user participation.

3. Users who are willing to contribute time, effort, and enthusiasm to the participatory process.

4. A skilled, experienced participation leader who can guide the process.

5. Information aids and tools that are flexible and manipulable to increase the realism of the project and to move it quickly and easily from the verbal to the visual realm.

Selecting Users to Participate

Users are all the people who come into contact with the physical environment. In health care facilities, users include patients, visitors, staff, and administrators, as well as others who use the buildings, such as salespeople and delivery workers. When selecting users to participate in a design process, consider the type and extent of knowledge they bring, their motivation to participate, and how well they may represent the views of others.[3]

Users can be classified into groups according to their role in the facility, such as physicians, patients, or technicians. Relevant user groups may differ with various construction projects. For example, the renovation of a department chairperson's office may only require the participation of that physician and an administrator, whereas the renovation of an obstetrics and gynecology clinic may call for involvement of patients, companions, nurses, clerical staff, physicians, technicians, maintenance staff, housekeeping staff, and administrators.

Both the size of the user group and the frequency of facility use should be considered in selecting participants. To continue the example of the obstetrics and gynecology clinic, in planning user participation in the design of the clinic's renovation, the 12 nurses on duty every day should each have an opportunity to contribute ideas and to review the design's progress, because they will use the renovated clinic so frequently. On the other hand, although more than 25,000 patients visit the clinic each year, a manageable sample of participants could be systematically drawn from this group.

A sample of patients is the preferable approach for two reasons. First, even though a large number of patients use the facility each year, any one individual is likely to use the clinic infrequently. It is not time-effective or cost-effective to involve every patient in the design process, and the potential information that could be gathered is not likely to differ widely within the group. Second, involving only one or two patients would not result in an accurate enough representation of group opinion.

Political power is another consideration when selecting participants. A rule of thumb is that the more powerful the individuals, the more likely it is they will participate in the design process anyway. Even so, it is important that these persons be sought out because they can contribute useful information based on experience, and their approval of the design is often necessary.

At the same time, it is important to seek out the participation and expertise of less powerful user groups. They, too, will have important views of how the facility should be designed. Because they are often the people who are most directly involved in the day-to-day operations, their contributions are critical.

When planning new or renovated facilities, it is not always possible to involve the actual individuals who will be future users. One reason is that there are often so many present and future users that it is not feasible to involve them all. In addition, individuals who occupy specific roles may change between the time a project is planned and the time it is occupied, and they will continue to change throughout occupancy. There is no foolproof solution to this common problem, but it pays to be aware of it before the process begins. One approach is to involve current users who have characteristics similar to those of future users. Another option is to refer to research on users in a similar type of facility.

How Can Participation Occur?

As we described earlier, user participation can occur in a variety of ways. Here we discuss the most common mechanisms for design participation: working groups, systematic research, and consultation by outside experts.

Users' working groups may meet only a few times to resolve specific problems, or they may meet many times over a period of months to contribute ideas and monitor the design's progress. Such groups might represent a particular occupational group, they might represent users from one department, or they might be composed of users from several different departments.

On a small design project, like the renovation of the obstetrics and gynecology clinic described earlier, one or two working groups may suffice. On a large-scale project, like the design of a teaching hospital, there may be a need for many departmental working groups, with some additional groups organized by design issues, such as signs and graphics.

These working groups may visit other related facilities, review the details of proposed design schemes, select from several completed design schemes, or even "try out" a proposed design through simulation. Regardless of the specific way each group functions, it has been found that users can respond to different design alternatives and predict what will work for them.[5]

The working-group format requires that users and design decision makers learn to negotiate with each other as they work toward a final design. It is important that all working-group members have an opportunity to contribute and that the process not be dominated by one or two particularly powerful individuals. Otherwise, the

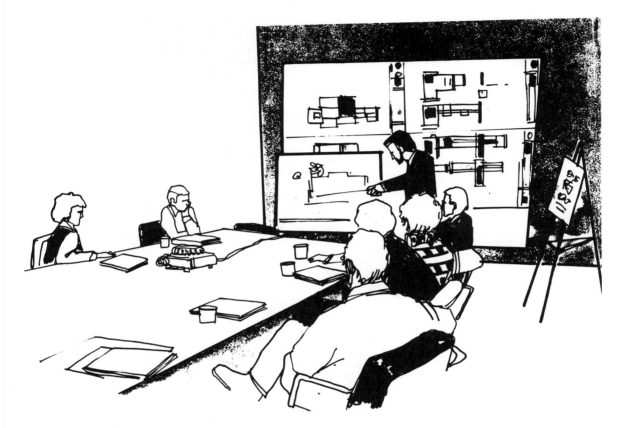

Working groups can meet periodically to provide design criteria, respond to design alternatives, and make recommendations for change.

design will reflect a unique mode of functioning and may be immediately obsolete if the individual leaves the organization. As a result, other working-group members may feel that their efforts have been wasted.

Working groups progress most smoothly when they are run by a skilled, neutral leader. The leader can be responsible for scheduling, setting agendas, procuring necessary documents, guiding discussions, recording, and distributing results. Because working-group discussions can become quite heated, the leader's neutrality can maximize the group's productivity.

Systematic Research

Systematic research is another approach to user participation. A large group of users, such as obstetrics and gynecology clinic patients, can be sampled to obtain a reasonably accurate representation of user characteristics and viewpoints through a number of research techniques including face-to-face and telephone interviews, written surveys, and simulation, such as evaluation of scale models.

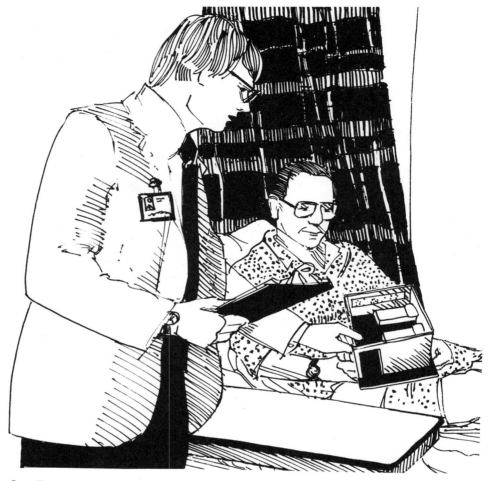

Small room models can be used for interviewing patients about their room design preferences.

Participation through research may be useful on both small and large-scale projects. It would be a cost-effective and time-effective way for obstetrics and gynecology patients and companions to voice their needs and preferences about a clinic renovation, for example. It would also be a practical way to involve house officers, staff nurses, housekeeping and maintenance staff, clerical staff, and patients and visitors in the design of a new teaching hospital.

Users' needs and preferences might be tapped in a single study, such as a study of responses to models showing different designs for obstetrics and gynecology examination rooms and waiting areas. Or, a number of different studies might be needed to optimize user participation in the design of a teaching hospital, such as a study of patients' comfort and nurses' ease of operation of different beds, a study of visitors' preferences about the location of bathrooms in relation to waiting areas, and a study of clerical staffs' preferences for different office landscape systems.

Consultants

Attention to users' design needs can also be provided by behavioral consultants. This approach may be appropriate when the time schedule and budget do not allow for either direct participation or systematic research or when users are neither known nor available. Consultants can contribute information from previous research on similar facilities, can act as user advocates, may have skill at interpreting and reviewing design documents from a behavioral point of view, and can offer a clear perspective on the whole design process that "insiders" might not have.[1]

Techniques for Information Gathering

Gathering information can be considered a two-phase process. The first phase consists of becoming knowledgeable about the relevant issues. During the second phase, information about use, needs, and preferences is gathered from users themselves.

For example, let's say a private inpatient room is being designed. First, codes and regulations could be examined. Next might come a literature review to discover what is already known about users' design needs. This could be supplemented by unobtrusive observations of patients, families, nurses, and physicians as they use a patient room. Minutes of meetings and other organization records might be perused to learn about the history of the project, in order to see whether some informal decisions have already been made or whether certain decision makers favor certain design approaches. The initial learning period could be supplemented by visits to other hospitals for a brief overview about how well their patient rooms function. Finally, an expert or two might be consulted.

With this background knowledge, it is easier and more efficient to plan user participation. The issues worth focusing on, the realistic alternatives, and how this situation compares with others become more apparent. To gather information in a way that will be useful to design decision makers and satisfying to users, there must be choices users can react to. These choices must be easily understood, and users' responses should be something they can do readily and competently.[5]

For example, showing a floor plan of a private room to a group of nurses and asking them what they think of it is not necessarily a useful approach. They do not have alternatives to compare, they may not be able to make sense of a two-dimensional floor plan, and they may feel that they don't have the expertise to comment. They would not be likely to contribute much and would probably end up feeling frustrated.

However, if these same nurses were shown several different three-dimensional models of shoebox size, with movable parts, the participation would probably be more successful. They could assess the different design alternatives, could manipulate the beds, walls, and other features in the models, and could more easily visualize how different activities would be accommodated. This approach is more fun, generates useful design ideas, and leaves the participants feeling satisfied that they have made a contribution.

Selecting the appropriate information-gathering technique for a specific situation is part of the art of managing user participation. In addition to the considerations we have already mentioned, you should also consider the expertise available, the amount of time allowed in the schedule, the numbers of users who need to be involved, the relevance, quantity, and quality of information needed, and the budget. Figure 1 describes some techniques that can be used to provide background information about the design problem at hand.[3,13-19]

Figure 1. Some Techniques for Gathering Background Information

Literature Reviews. These are searches for relevant articles, books, reports, codes, standards, and other materials that may bear on the project at hand. Once initial relevant titles are identified (often by computer), articles need to be located, read, and their bibliographies examined, until the reviewer is satisfied that sufficient relevant information has been uncovered.

Review of Project History and Related Archival Documents. Certain types of archival records may help in piecing together a project's history and thus may contribute useful insights to the design process. Some of the types of records that may be helpful are position papers; meeting notes; correspondence; reports; design documents; maintenance and repair records; purchase records; health, safety, or medical records; and employee and consumer surveys.[3]

Facility Visits. Much can be learned about how new or renovated facilities should work by observing existing environments and behavior in similar organizations. In order to prepare for a facility visit, identify the specific environmental features and policies you want to investigate, line up a knowledgeable person within the facility to act as your guide, learn how to recognize telling "physical traces" (actual evidence that environments may not be working as intended, such as hand-lettered, taped-up signs)[3,17,19] and set realistic time estimates for the visit (you'll probably remember more if you cover the territory slowly). It is useful to document the visit with notes and photographs or slides, both as a way to refresh your memory about what you learned and as a way of sharing the information with others who did not make the trip.

Consultants. Consultation with experts can be costly but may save money in the long run because consultants may be able to quickly identify relevant design and behavior issues, resources, performance criteria, and other useful information.[1]

Recommended reading:

Brill, M., with Margulis, S., Konar, E., and BOSTI. *Using Office Design to Increase Productivity*, Vol. 2. Buffalo, NY: Workplace Design and Productivity, Inc., 1985.

Madge, J. *The Tools of Social Science*. Garden City, NY: Doubleday, 1965.

Michelson, W. M., editor. *Behavioral Research Methods in Environmental Design*. Stroudsburg, PA: Dowden, Hutchinson and Ross, 1975.

Reizenstein, J. E., Simmons, D. A., and others. *Hospital Design and Human Behavior: A Bibliography*. Architectural Series, A673. Monticello, IL: Vance Bibliographies, 1982.

Stern, P. C. *Evaluating Social Science Research*. New York: Oxford University Press, 1979.

Webb, E. J., Campbell, D. T., and others. *Unobtrusive Measures*. Chicago: Rand McNally, 1966.

Wohlwill, J. F., and Weisman, G. D. *The Physical Environment and Behavior: An Annotated Bibliography and Guide to the Literature*. New York: Plenum Press, 1981.

Zeisel, J. *Inquiry by Design: Tools for Environment Behavior Research*. Monterey, CA: Brooks Cole, 1981.

Although every information-gathering technique has its strengths, there are always corresponding weaknesses. For example, guided interviews with open-ended questions can produce large amounts of data that are rich in detail, yet these are extremely time-consuming to code or quantify. Selecting more than one technique, however, can compensate for the weaknesses of each.

Timing and Scheduling Participation

In order to have real impact on the design of health care facilities, user participation must occur during most stages of the design process, from conceptualization through post-occupancy evaluation. The ways in which participation occurs, however, may vary at the different stages. Figure 2 describes some techniques that can be used to enable users to participate in design.[5,13,19-24]

Figure 2. Some Techniques that Enable Users to Participate in the Design Process

Interviews and Surveys. Users can be asked about existing design features and can express their preferences for realistic alternatives for future design. They can be asked these things individually or in groups (often called "focus groups" because they focus on a particular issue). They can be asked these questions in person, on the telephone, or through a self-administered questionnaire handed out or sent in the mail. Interviews and surveys can be structured in different ways: some have fixed questions in a fixed order and others have open-ended or flexibly ordered questions. Despite these general parameters, there are enormous complexities in managing survey research, including issues of how respondents are sampled, how a questionnaire is designed, and how data can be analyzed and presented most usefully. It would be wise to seek some expert involvement if these techniques are being considered.

Simulation. Proposed environments can be simulated in many different ways in order to obtain useful feedback about how well they function. Drawings produced by hand or with the aid of a computer, three-dimensional scale models, full-scale mock-ups, photographs, videotape simulation, and other techniques have been successfully used to elicit user responses to various design options.

Design Review. Users can participate in design review—the assessment of a proposed design scheme—by comparing the scheme with stated or implied performance criteria. Comments can be noted in annotations made directly on design documents.

Recommended reading:

Frey, J. H. *Survey Research by Telephone.* Beverly Hills, CA: Sage, 1984.

Kaplan, S., and Kaplan, R. *Cognition and Environment: Functioning in an Uncertain World.* New York: Praeger, 1983.

King, J., Marans, R. A., and Solomon, L. A. *Pre-Construction Evaluation: A Report on the Full Scale Mock-Up and Evaluation of Hospital Rooms.* Ann Arbor: Architectural Research Laboratory, University of Michigan, 1982.

Lawrence, R. J. Designers' dilemma: participatory design methods. In: Bart, P., Chen, A., and Francescato, G., editors. *Knowledge for Design: Proceedings of EDRA 13.* Washington, DC: Environmental Design Research Association, 1982.

Madge, J. H. *The Tools of Social Science.* Garden City, NY: Doubleday, 1965.

Moser, C. A., and Kalton, G. *Survey Methods in Social Investigation.* 2nd ed. New York: Basic Books, 1972.

Sanoff, H. *Methods of Architectural Programming.* Stroudsburg, PA: Dowden, Hutchinson and Ross, 1977.

Zeisel, J. *Inquiry by Design: Tools for Environment Behavior Research.* Monterey, CA: Brooks Cole, 1981.

User concerns should be made apparent during the formulation of the project's mission and role. They should be reflected in a statement of the types and sizes of spaces needed. And their needs and preferences should be represented in a series of performance criteria.

Once the actual designing begins, users or behavioral consultants should be involved in the review process. They can help assess the probable performance of the proposed design according to previously established (and periodically updated) criteria based on users' needs, preferences, and behaviors. Design progress can be reviewed using annotated floor plans, written comments, verbal exchange, and the like. If the phase of the design process and types of issues being examined are appropriate, one particularly effective way to involve users is to have them respond to three-dimensional simulation, such as scale models or full-scale mock-ups.[5,21,25]

Participation needs to occur even during the construction phase of a project when last-minute design changes are made. Within a realistic framework of cost, code, and other constraints, users are in the best position to assess the eventual functioning of the space. However, there should be a mechanism in place so users' input can be immediately evaluated by design decision makers. This way, informed decisions about design changes and materials substitutions can be transmitted speedily to the construction site.

Post-occupancy evaluation (POE), assessing how new or renovated facilities actually perform, is another stage of the design process in which user participation is valuable.[19,25-27] User participants can contribute to the planning of the evaluation by helping to identify which aspects of the design should be evaluated. They can give feedback on the performance of the design features they regularly use. And, they can make recommendations about changes in design and related policies.

Early in the participation effort, users who will be directly involved need to have an overview of the design process for their area. This mental road map helps clarify where their contribution fits in. They will know when certain types of functional information is most useful, enabling them to work productively and to use meeting time efficiently.[1]

Another key aspect of timing is the scheduling of the participation process itself. The recommendations growing out of the participation process must be geared to key milestone dates in the design project's schedule. In fact, user participation should be planned and some information gathered even before the design process begins. In this way, certain information will be available as it is needed, without costly delays.

Managing User Participation

Whether users participate in the design of a small scale project or a large one, participation requires management, either by in-house staff members or by outside consultants. These managers should be familiar with the behavioral design needs of health care facility users, with the ways in which design decisions are made within their organization, with the timing of these decisions, and with the role that user information plays in this process. A manager should also be a skilled researcher, advocate, meeting facilitator, interpreter of design graphics, and project manager.[28]

A manager's biggest challenge is likely to be handling competing design needs. Users themselves may disagree, users and design decision makers may disagree, or external constraints, such as a fixed budget or fire code, may make a user group's needs impossible to meet. As a result, user participants must be made aware of the often extensive negotiations that go on among the affected parties and of the likelihood that users' recommendations will not always sway design decisions.

Implementing Recommendations That Result from User Participation

When users and design decision makers come together in working groups, users have the opportunity to lobby for their own recommendations. They might argue from personal experience, bring in relevant data, or report the consensus of their colleagues. In addition to a recommendation's objective merit, other factors may play a role in influencing a design decision, such as timing, cost, political power, values, personality, personal relationships, organizational norms, and others.[29]

When users participate in design through systematic research, results and recommendations may reach design decision makers through slide presentations, reviews of documents and design graphics, written reports, and meetings. The results of a detailed study of participation through research in a large-scale design project (the Patient and Visitor Participation Project of the University of Michigan Hospitals) indicate that multiple, face-to-face contacts between users' representatives and design decision makers were the most effective way of influencing design decisions.[29] On this large-scale project, periodic design reviews were important, and written reports that documented research findings promoted credibility, but neither one was sufficient to ensure utilization. The advantage of face-to-face settings, like meetings, is the opportunity for two-way conversation. Troublesome issues can be clarified, and recommendations can be elaborated on and reinforced using visual aids. In addition, alliances can be formed, and compromises can often be worked out.

Documenting the User Participation Process___

It is important to document user participation, because it may be the source of many recommendations reflected in the final design. If this process and the resulting recommendations are not documented, important information may be lost and the design may not function as intended. For example, two sets of elevators might be built in a large hospital, one for staff and the other for public use. If staff members are not aware of this distinction and use the public elevator, they might inadvertently discuss patient care information in the presence of worried visitors.

Users who are not involved in design decision making are almost always curious about why certain decisions were made. Documentation of the user participation process will offer them at least some of these rationales. Documentation will also provide a record of design intentions that will be important to understand when the relationship between the facility's design and performance is assessed in a post-occupancy evaluation.

Conclusion___

Participation is not always successful, but when it is, everyone benefits—the institution, design decision makers, and users themselves. Examples of successful participation are sprinkled throughout the book. We hope that this material will encourage more people to become involved with health care facility design through a well-planned, systematic participatory process, so that the design of future facilities directly reflects the needs of all the people who use them.

References

1. Sommer, R. *Social Design: Creating Buildings with People in Mind.* Englewood Cliffs, NJ: Prentice Hall, 1983.

2. Brubaker, T., editor. Design and construction project manual. Unpublished report, Office of the Replacement Hospital Program, University of Michigan, Ann Arbor, 1985.

3. Brill, M., with Margulis, S., Konar, E., and BOSTI. *Using Office Design to Increase Productivity,* Vol. 2. Buffalo, NY: Workplace Design and Productivity, Inc., 1985.

4. Becker, F. D. *Housing Messages.* Stroudsburg, PA: Dowden, Hutchinson and Ross, 1977.

5. Kaplan, S., and Kaplan, R. *Cognition and Environment: Functioning in an Uncertain World.* New York: Praeger, 1983.

6. Reizenstein, J. E. Hospital design and human behavior: a review of the recent literature. In: Baum, A., and Singer, J., editors. *Advances in Environmental Psychology.* Vol. 4, *Environment and Health.* Hillsdale, NJ: Erlbaum Press, 1982.

7. Carpman Associates. St. Joseph Mercy Hospital emergency department behavioral design program. Unpublished report, Carpman Associates, Ann Arbor, 1984.

8. Carpman, J. R., Grant, M. A., and Simmons, D. A. Hospital design and wayfinding: a video simulation study. *Environment and Behavior.* 1985 May. 17(3).

9. Becker, F. D. *User Participation, Personalization and Environmental Meaning: Three Field Studies.* Ithaca, NY: Program in Urban and Regional Studies, Cornell University, 1977.

10. Reizenstein, J. E. *Social Research and Design: Cambridge Hospital Social Service Offices.* Springfield, VA: National Technical Information Service, 1976.

11. Falick, J. Humanistic design sells your hospital. *Hospitals.* 1981 Feb. 16. 55(4):68-74.

12. Carpman, J. R., and Trester, K. Marketing implications of consumer-responsive health facility design. In: Cooper, P., editor. *Responding to the Challenge: Proceedings of the Sixth Annual Health Services Marketing Symposium.* Chicago: American Marketing Association, 1986.

13. Madge, J. H. *The Tools of Social Science.* Garden City, NY: Doubleday, 1965.

14. Michelson, W. M., editor. *Behavioral Research Methods in Environmental Design.* Stroudsburg, PA: Dowden, Hutchinson and Ross, 1975.

15. Reizenstein, J. E., Simmons, D. A., and others. *Hospital Design and Human Behavior: A Bibliography.* Architectural Series, A673. Monticello, IL: Vance Bibliographies, 1982.

16. Stern, P. C. *Evaluating Social Science Research.* New York: Oxford University Press, 1979.

17. Webb, E. J., Campbell, D. T., and others. *Unobtrusive Measures.* Chicago: Rand McNally, 1966.

18. Wohlwill, J. F., and Weisman, G. D. *The Physical Environment and Behavior: An Annotated Bibliography and Guide to the Literature.* New York: Plenum Press, 1981.

19. Zeisel, J. *Inquiry by Design: Tools for Environment Behavior Research.* Monterey, CA: Brooks Cole, 1981.

20. Frey, J. H. *Survey Research by Telephone.* Beverly Hills, CA: Sage, 1984.

21. King, J., Marans, R. A., and Solomon, L. A. *Pre-Construction Evaluation: A Report on the Full Scale Mock-Up and Evaluation of Hospital Rooms.* Ann Arbor: Architectural Research Laboratory, University of Michigan, 1982.

22. Lawrence, R. J. Designers' dilemma: participatory design methods. In: Bart, P., Chen, A., and Francescato, G., editors. *Knowledge for Design: Proceedings of EDRA 13.* Washington, DC: Environmental Design Research Association, 1982.

23. Moser, C. A., and Kalton, G. *Survey Methods in Social Investigation.* 2nd ed. New York: Basic Books, 1972.

24. Sanoff, H. *Methods of Architectural Programming.* Stroudsburg, PA: Dowden, Hutchinson and Ross, 1977.

25. Reizenstein, J. E., and Grant, M. A. *From Hospital Research to Hospital Design.* Patient and Visitor Participation Project. Office of Hospital Planning, Research and Development, University of Michigan, Ann Arbor, 1982.

26. Zimring, C. M., and Reizenstein, J. E. Post-occupancy evaluation: an overview. *Environment and Behavior.* 1980 Dec. 12(4):429-50.

27. Zimring, C. M., and Reizenstein, J. E. A primer on post-occupancy evaluation. *American Institute of Architects Journal.* 1981 Nov. 70(13):52-58.

28. Fiedler, J. *Field Research: A Manual for Logistics and Management of Scientific Studies in Natural Settings.* San Francisco: Jossey-Bass, 1978.

29. Carpman, J. R. Influencing design decisions: an analysis of the impact of the Patient and Visitor Participation Project on the University of Michigan Replacement Hospital Program. Ph.D. dissertation, University of Michigan, Ann Arbor, 1983. Available from UMI, 300 N. Zeeb Road, Ann Arbor, MI 48106.

Conclusion

In the face of increasingly sophisticated medical technology and the present focus of administrators and staff on reducing health care costs, the human needs of patients and visitors are often forgotten. Throughout this book, we have argued for a new approach to the design of health care facilities—design that not only cares *for* patients and visitors but design that also cares *about* them.

Our focus is on consumers—on patients and their companions. We recognize their compelling needs, their traditional lack of input into the design decisions that affect them, and their increasing power as the competition for their health care dollars increases.

We also recognize the inherent stress involved in visits to health care facilities and the relationship between facility design and stress. Caring is an objective that is appropriate for environmental design at all levels, from the basic building layout to the design of a door handle. All spaces within a health care facility should reflect such concern: outdoor spaces, parking areas, corridors, reception and waiting areas, examination and treatment rooms, inpatient rooms, food service areas, and public spaces.

The design guidelines presented in this book are drawn from many different, systematic studies of the needs and preferences of health care facility users. Although this information base is still in its infancy, it represents a solid beginning, one that can and should be built upon.

However, no set of general guidelines can be perfectly appropriate for a specific design project. User participation should be an integral part of the decision-making process of virtually any health care facility design. User participation offers the necessary link from the general to the specific and can result in a design that is attractive, functional, and cost-effective.

The set of informed design guidelines presented in this book is a start, but the work must continue. A tremendous amount of applicable design research is still needed on a wide variety of topics, such as ways to reduce the frightening ambience of medical procedure areas, the effects of color on patient morale, inpatient room designs that enable companions to stay at all times, design needs of visually-impaired users, comprehensible map design, and many others. In addition, a further understanding of the design decision-making process in health care organizations would prove useful to those who seek to influence such decisions.

More post-occupancy evaluations of health care facilities would also make a significant contribution to the information base. Findings and recommendations resulting from such evaluations would enable each new project to build on the experience of its forerunners.

This book offers the beginnings of a more humane, marketing-oriented, systematic, and participatory approach to the design of health facilities—facilities that patients and visitors recognize as caring places.

Bibliography ⎯⎯⎯⎯⎯⎯⎯⎯⎯⎯⎯⎯⎯⎯⎯⎯⎯⎯⎯⎯⎯⎯⎯⎯⎯⎯⎯

A slightly serious look at a serious problem: hospital design and policy versus patient comfort. *Medical Journal of Australia.* 1974 Aug. 2(8):301-2.

Abend, A., and Chen, A. Developing residential design statements for the hearing-impaired elderly. *Environment and Behavior.* 1985 July. 17(4): 475-500.

Alcock, A., Goodman, J., and others. Environment and waiting behaviors in emergency waiting areas. *Children's Health Care: Journal of the Association for the Care of Children's Health.* 1985 Spring. 13(4):174-80.

Alcock, D. Developing an outdoor playground. *Dimensions in Health Service.* 1978. 55:32-37.

Alexander, C., Ishikawa, S., and Silverstein, M. *A Pattern Language.* New York: Oxford University Press, 1977.

Alexander, M. E. No windows. *Lancet.* 1973 Mar. 10. 1(7802):549.

Altman, W. CAT scanning and patient inconvenience. *New England Journal of Medicine.* 1977 July 28. 297(4):226-27.

American Hospital Association. *Signs and Graphics for Health Care Facilities.* Chicago: AHA, 1979.

American Institute of Architects Foundation. *Design for Aging: An Architect's Guide.* Washington, DC: AIA Press, 1986.

American National Standards Institute. *American National Standards Specifications for Making Buildings and Facilities Accessible to and Usable by Physically Handicapped People.* (A117.1-1980) New York: ANSI, 1980.

Appleyard, D. Why buildings are known: a perspective tool for architects and planners. *Environment and Behavior.* 1969 Dec. 1(2):131-56.

Barker, M. People-oriented design. *Hospitals Forum.* 1985 July-Aug. pp. 35-36.

Baron, J. H., and Greene, L. Art in hospitals. *British Medical Journal.* 1984 Dec. 289(22):1731-37.

Becker, F. D. *Housing Messages.* Stroudsburg, PA: Dowden, Hutchinson and Ross, 1977.

⎯⎯⎯. *User Participation, Personalization and Environmental Meaning: Three Field Studies.* Ithaca, NY: Program in Urban and Regional Studies, Cornell University, 1977.

Beckman, R. Getting up and getting out: progressive patient care. *Progressive Architecture.* 1974 Nov. 55(11):64-68.

Berkeley, E. P. More than you want to know about the Boston City Hall. *Architecture Plus.* 1973 Feb. 1(1):72-77, 98.

Bibliography

Berkowitz, M., and others. *Reading with Print Limitations: Executive Summary.* Prepared for the National Library Service for the Blind and Physically Handicapped. New York: American Foundation for the Blind, 1979.

Best, G. Direction-finding in large buildings. Master's thesis, University of Manchester, Manchester, England, 1967.

Birren, F. Human response to color and light. *Hospitals.* 1979 July 16. 53(14):93-96.

Block, L. F., editor. *Marketing for Hospitals in Hard Times.* Chicago: Teach'em, Inc., 1981.

Bobrow, M. L., and Thomas, J. Achieving quality in hospital design. *Hospital Forum.* 1976 Sept. 19(4):4-6.

Boyce, P. R. *Human Factors in Lighting.* New York: Macmillan Publishing Co., 1981.

Brill, M., with Margulis, S., Konar, E., and BOSTI. *Using Office Design to Increase Productivity,* Vol. 2. Buffalo, NY: Workplace Design and Productivity, Inc., 1985.

Brubaker, T., editor. Design and construction project manual. Unpublished report, Office of the Replacement Hospital Program, University of Michigan, Ann Arbor, 1985.

Burgun, J. A. Construction considerations for ambulatory care facilities. *Hospitals.* 1976 Feb. 1. 50(3):79-84.

Burling, T., Lentz, E., and Wilson, R. *The Give and Take in Hospitals.* New York: G. P. Putnam's Sons, 1956.

Calderhead, J., editor. *Hospitals for People.* London: King Edwards's Hospital Fund for London, 1975.

Cambridge Research Institute. *Trends Affecting the U.S. Health Care System.* Washington, DC: U.S. Dept. of Health, Education, and Welfare, 1975 Oct.

Canter, D., and Canter, S. Creating therapeutic environments. In: Canter, D., and Canter, S., editors. *Designing for Therapeutic Environments.* New York: Wiley, 1979.

Carpman Associates. St. Joseph Mercy Hospital emergency department behavioral design program. Unpublished report, Carpman Associates, Ann Arbor, MI, 1984.

Carpman, J. R. Influencing design decisions: an analysis of the impact of the Patient and Visitor Participation Project on the University of Michigan Replacement Hospital Program. Ph.D. dissertation, University of Michigan, Ann Arbor, 1983. Available from UMI, 300 N. Zeeb Road, Ann Arbor, MI 48106.

———. Description of the wayfinding training program for the new University of Michigan Hospital and Health Care Center. Unpublished report, Ann Arbor, 1985 Oct.

———. *You Can Get There from Here: Wayfinding System for the New University Hospital and Health Care Center.* Booklet, Office of Planning and Marketing, Office of Human Resource Development, University of Michigan Hospitals, Ann Arbor, 1985 Nov.

Carpman, J. R., and Grant, M. A. Outdoor seating evaluation. Unpublished research report #22, Patient and Visitor Participation Project, Office of Hospital Planning, Research and Development, University of Michigan, Ann Arbor, 1983.

————. Executive summary: color, cubicle curtains, handrails. Unpublished research report #23, Patient and Visitor Participation Project, Office of Hospital Planning, Research and Development, University of Michigan, Ann Arbor, 1983.

————. TVs in hospitals: behavior and preferences. Unpublished research report #11, Patient and Visitor Participation Project; Office of Hospital Planning, Research and Development; University of Michigan, Ann Arbor, 1984.

————. Hospital patient room furnishings mock-ups. Unpublished research report #25, Patient and Visitor Participation Project, Office of Hospital Planning, Research and Development, University of Michigan, Ann Arbor, 1984.

————. Evaluation of waiting room seating. Unpublished research report #27, Patient and Visitor Participation Project, Office of Hospital Planning, Research and Development, University of Michigan, Ann Arbor, 1984.

————. Executive summary: design of interior "you-are-here" maps. Unpublished research report #29, Patient and Visitor Participation Project, Office of the Replacement Hospital Program, University of Michigan, Ann Arbor, 1984.

————. Inpatient preferences for hospital room artwork. Unpublished research report #32, Patient and Visitor Participation Project, Office of the Replacement Hospital Program, University of Michigan, Ann Arbor, 1984.

Carpman, J. R., Grant, M. A., and Norton, C. Needs of the hearing impaired in a hospital setting. Unpublished research report #30, Patient and Visitor Participation Project, Office of the Replacement Hospital Program, University of Michigan, Ann Arbor, 1984.

Carpman, J. R., Grant, M. A., and Simmons, D. A. *No More Mazes: Research About Design for Wayfinding in Hospitals.* Patient and Visitor Participation Project, Office of the Replacement Hospital Program, University of Michigan, Ann Arbor, 1984.

————. Wayfinding in the hospital environment: the impact of various floor numbering alternatives. *Journal of Environmental Systems.* 1984 May. 13(4):353-64.

————. Overnight accommodations for visitors and outpatients: a nationwide study. *Health Care Strategic Management.* 1984 June. 2(6):9-14.

————. Hospital design and wayfinding: a video simulation study. *Environment and Behavior.* 1985 May. 17(3).

Carpman, J. R., and Trester, K. Marketing implications of consumer-responsive health facility design. In: Cooper, P., editor. *Responding to the Challenge: Proceedings of the Sixth Annual Health Services Marketing Symposium.* Chicago: American Marketing Association, 1986.

Chaikin, A., Derlega, V., and Miller, S. Effects of room environment on self-disclosure in a counseling analogue. *Journal of Counseling Psychology.* 1976 Sept. 23(5):479-81.

Bibliography

Chaney, P. S. Decor reflects environmental psychology. *Hospitals.* 1973 June 1. 47(11):61-66.

Cheek, F. E., Maxwell, R., and Weisman, R. Carpeting the ward: an exploratory study in environmental psychology. *Mental Hygiene.* 1971 Jan. 55(1):109-18.

Christensen, K. An impact analysis framework for calculating the costs of staff disorientation in hospitals. Unpublished report, University of California at Los Angeles, Los Angeles, no date.

Clipson, C. W., and Wehrer, J. J. *Planning for Cardiac Care: A Guide to the Planning and Design of Cardiac Care Facilities.* Ann Arbor, MI: Health Administration Press, 1973.

Collins, B. L. *Windows and People: A Literature Survey.* Washington, DC: U.S. Government Printing Office, 1975.

Conway, D. J., Zeisel, J., and others. Radiation therapy centers: social and behavioral issues for design. Unpublished research report, Engineering Design Branch, National Institutes of Health, Bethesda, MD, 1977 July.

Corlett, E. N., Manenica, I., and Bishop, R. P. The design of direction-finding systems in buildings. *Applied Ergonomics.* 1972 June. 3(2):66-69.

Daniel, E. H. Signs and the school media center. In: Pollet, D., and Haskell, P., editors. *Sign Systems for Libraries.* New York: R. R. Bowker Co., 1979.

Deschambeau, G. L. More effort needed to move cart on carpet than tile, study finds. *Modern Hospital.* 1965 July. 105(1):30.

Devlin, A. Housing for the elderly: cognitive considerations. *Environment and Behavior.* 1980 Dec. 12(4):451-66.

Downs, R. Mazes, minds, and maps. In: Pollet, D. and Haskell, P., editors. *Sign Systems for Libraries.* New York: R. R. Bowker Co., 1979.

Drader, D. The design of geriatric assessment units: psychosocial considerations. Consulting report, Department of National Health and Welfare, Ottawa, Canada, 1982.

Drury, L. R., and Rosen, P. Multiple use, flexibility key to emergency department planning. *Hospitals.* 1977 July 16. 51(14):201-11.

Edwards, K. The environment inside the hospital. *Practitioner.* 1979 June. 222(1332):746-51.

English Tourist Board. *Providing for Disabled Visitors.* Pamphlet, English Tourist Board, 1983.

Facilities for the Elderly in Canada: Design and Environmental Considerations. Vol. 1, *Geriatric Units in Hospitals.* Ottawa, Canada: Department of National Health and Welfare, 1984.

Falick, J. Humanistic design sells your hospital. *Hospitals.* 1981 Feb. 16. 55(4):68-74.

Fiedler, J. *Field Research: A Manual for Logistics and Management of Scientific Studies in Natural Settings.* San Francisco: Jossey-Bass, 1978.

Fisher, T. Enabling the disabled. *Progressive Architecture.* 1985 July. pp 13-18.

Flourney, R. L. Gardening as therapy: treatment activities for psychiatric patients. *Hospital and Community Psychiatry.* 1975 Feb. 26(2):75-76.

Follis, J., and Hammer, D. *Architectural Signing and Graphics.* New York: Watson Guptill, 1979.

Fowles, D. G. *A Profile of Older Americans, 1984.* Washington, DC: American Association of Retired Persons, U.S. Department of Health and Human Services, Administration on Aging, 1984.

Frey, J. H. *Survey Research by Telephone.* Beverly Hills, CA: Sage, 1984.

Fusillo, A. E., Kaplan, S., and Whitehead, B. Human environmental considerations in health facility design. Unpublished report, Systems Science Institute, University of Louisville, Louisville, no date.

Genensky, S. M. Design sensitivity: the partially sighted. *Building Operating Management.* 1981 June. 28(6):50-54.

Goldish, L. *Braille in the United States: Its Production, Distribution, and Use.* New York: American Foundation for the Blind, 1967.

Goldsmith, S. *Designing for the Disabled.* London: RIBA Publications, Ltd., 1977.

Gowan, N. J. The perceptual world of the intensive care unit: an overview of some environmental considerations in the helping relationship. *Heart and Lung.* 1979 Mar.-Apr. 8(2):340-44.

Grant, M. A. Structured participatory input. Master's thesis, University of Michigan, Ann Arbor, 1979.

Greco, J. T. Carpeting vs. resilient flooring. *Hospitals.* 1965 June 16. 39(2):55-58, 102-10.

Green, A. Changes in care call for design flexibility. *Hospitals.* 1976 Feb. 1. 50(3):67-69.

Hamilton, D. N. Patient lounge study. Unpublished research report #1, Saskatoon Hospital Evaluation Project, University of Saskatchewan, Canada, 1983.

————. Lobby study. Unpublished report #2-A, Saskatoon Hospital Evaluation Project, University of Saskatchewan, Canada, no date.

Harkness, S. P., and Groom, J. N. *Building without Barriers for the Disabled.* New York: Watson Guptill, 1976.

Hayward, C., and members of the AIA Committee on Architecture for Health, Programming Subcommittee. *A Generic Process for Projecting Health Care Space Needs.* Washington, DC: AIA Committee, 1985 Oct.

Hayward, D. G. Psychological factors in the use of light and lighting in buildings. In: Lang, J., Burnette, C., and others, editors. *Designing for Human Behavior: Architecture and the Behavioral Sciences.* Stroudsburg, PA: Dowden, Hutchinson and Ross, Inc., 1974.

————. Working notes, Office of Hospital Planning, Research and Development, University of Michigan, Ann Arbor, 1982.

Hayward, D. G., and Gates, L. B. Lighting affects the social character of a space. Working paper, Environmental Institute, University of Massachusetts, Amherst, 1981.

Henneberry, J., and Robertson, P. Free in the sun: an outdoor program in a health care setting. *Children's Health Care.* 1983 Summer. 12(1):37-40.

Hiatt, L. G. Architecture for the aged: design for living. *Inland Architect.* 1978 Nov.-Dec. 23:6-17.

————. The color and use of color in environments for older people. *Nursing Homes.* 1981 May-June. 30(3):18-22.

Hickler, F. D. Symposium on design and function of the operating room suite and special areas. *Journal of Anesthesiology.* 1969 Aug. 31(2):103-6.

Hoover, M. J. Intensive care for relatives. *Hospitals.* 1979 July 16. 53(14):219-22.

Hopf, P., and Raeber, J. *Access for the Handicapped: The Barrier-Free Regulations for Design and Construction in All 50 States.* New York: Van Nostrand Reinhold, 1984.

Howell, S., Epp, G., Reizenstein, J., and Albright, C. *Shared Spaces in Housing for the Elderly.* Cambridge, MA: Massachusetts Institute of Technology, Department of Architecture, 1976.

Hughes, E. F., and Bryden, M. C. The development of an occupational therapy program in a solarium area. *Canadian Journal of Occupational Therapy.* 1983 Feb. 50(1):15-19.

Hunt, M. Environmental learning without being there. *Environment and Behavior.* 1984 May. 16(3):307-34.

Institute of Signage Research. Technical and psychological considerations for sign systems in libraries. In: Pollet, D., and Haskell, P., editors. *Sign Systems for Libraries.* New York: R. R. Bowker Co., 1979.

Johnson, B. Hospital "hotels": the time has come. *Michigan Hospitals.* 1985 Aug. pp. 5-11.

Johnson, E., and Johnson, R. *Hospitals in Transition.* Rockville, MD: Aspen Systems Corp., 1982.

Kamisar, H. Signs for the handicapped patron. In: Pollet, D., and Haskel, P., editors. *Sign Systems for Libraries.* New York: R. R. Bowker Co., 1979.

Kaplan, R. The role of nature in the urban context. In: Altman, I., and Wohlwill, J. F., editors. *Human Behavior and Environment: Advances in Theory and Research,* Vol. 6. New York: Plenum Press, 1983.

Kaplan, S. Adaptation, structure, and knowledge. In: Moore, G., and Golledge, R., editors. *Environmental Knowing: Theories, Research and Methods.* Stroudsburg, PA: Dowden, Hutchinson and Ross, Inc., 1976.

Kaplan, S., and Kaplan, R. *Cognition and Environment: Functioning in an Uncertain World.* New York: Praeger, 1983.

————, editors. *Humanscape: Environments for People.* Belmont, CA: Duxbury Press, 1978.

Kebart, R. C. Innovative designs for a diagnostic radiology department. *Radiologic Technology.* 1974 Jan.-Feb. 45(4):260-66.

Keep, P. J. Stimulus deprivation in windowless rooms. *Anesthesia.* 1977 July-Aug. 32(7):598-602.

Keep, P. J., James, J., and Inman, M. Windows in the intensive therapy unit. *Anesthesia.* 1980 Mar. 35(3):257-62.

Kenny, C., and Canter, D. Findings from the development of USEP. Report, Department of Psychology, University of Surrey, Guildford, Surrey, 1978 Sept.

King, J., Marans, R. A., and Solomon, L. A. *Pre-Construction Evaluation: A Report on the Full Scale Mock-Up and Evaluation of Hospital Rooms.* Ann Arbor: Architectural Research Laboratory, University of Michigan, 1982.

Kira, A. *The Bathroom.* New York: Bantam Books, 1977.

Koncelik, J. A. *Designing the Open Nursing Home.* Stroudsburg, PA: Dowden, Hutchinson and Ross, 1976.

————. *Aging and the Product Environment.* Stroudsburg, PA: Hutchinson and Ross, 1982.

Kornfeld, D. S. The hospital environment: its impact on the patient. *Advances in Psychosomatic Medicine.* 1972. 8:252-70.

Lam, W. M. C. *Perception and Lighting as Formgivers for Architecture.* New York: McGraw-Hill, Inc., 1977.

Langan, J., Wagner, H., and Buchanan, J. Design concepts of a nuclear medicine department. *Journal of Nuclear Medicine.* 1979 Oct. 20(10):1093-94.

Lawrence, R. J. Designers' dilemma: participatory design methods. In: Bart, P., Chen, A., and Francescato, G., editors. *Knowledge for Design: Proceedings of EDRA 13.* Washington, DC: Environmental Design Research Association, 1982.

Lawton, M. P. Therapeutic environments for the aged. In: Canter, D., and Canter, S., editors. *Designing for Therapeutic Environments.* New York: John Wiley and Sons, 1979.

Levine, M. You-are-here maps: psychological considerations. *Environment and Behavior.* 1982 Mar. 14(2):221-37.

Levine, M., Marchon, I., and Hanley, G. The placement and misplacement of you-are-here maps. *Environment and Behavior.* 1984 Mar. 16(2):139-57.

Lindell, M. The human hospital. *Dimensions in Health Service.* 1983 May. 60(5):27-29.

Lindheim, R. *Uncoupling the Radiology System.* Chicago: Hospital Research and Educational Trust, 1971.

Madge, J. H. *The Tools of Social Science.* Garden City, NY: Doubleday, 1965.

Marks, B. The language of signs. In: Pollet, D., and Haskel, P., editors. *Sign Systems for Libraries.* New York: R. R. Bowker Co., 1979.

Mathews, R. The psychological and social effects of design. *World Hospitals.* 1976 Mar. 12(1):63-68.

McDuffie, R. F. The greening of interiors. *Interior Landscape Industry.* 1984 June. 1(6):29-31.

McLaughlin, H. The monumental headache: overtly monumental and systematic hospitals are usually functional disasters. *Architectural Record.* 1976 July. 160(1):118.

Mehrabian, A., and Diamond, S. G. Seating arrangements and conversation. *Sociometry.* 1970. 34:281-89.

Mehrabian, A., and Diamond, S. G. Effects of furniture arrangement, props and personality on social interaction. *Journal of Personality and Social Psychology.* 1971 Oct. 20(1):18-30.

Michael, D. *On Learning to Plan and Planning to Learn: The Social Psychology of Changing Toward Future-Responsive Societal Learning.* San Francisco: Jossey-Bass Books, 1973.

Michelson, W. M., editor. *Behavioral Research Methods in Environmental Design.* Stroudsburg, PA: Dowden, Hutchinson and Ross, 1975.

Michigan Department of Labor. *Barrier-Free Design Codes.* Lansing: Michigan Department of Labor, 1985.

Miller, D. B., and Goldman, L. Selecting paintings for the nursing home. *Nursing Homes.* 1984 Jan.-Feb. pp. 12-16.

Milner, M. Breaking through the deafness barrier: environmental accommodations for hearing impaired people. Unpublished report, Division of Public Services and Design and Construction Department, Washington, DC: Gallaudet College, 1981.

Molter, N. C. Needs of relatives of critically ill patients: a descriptive study. *Heart and Lung.* 1979 Mar.-Apr. 8(2):332-39.

Moore, G., Cohen, U., and McGinty, T. *Planning and Design Guidelines: Child Care Centers and Outdoor Play Environments.* (7 vols.) Milwaukee: University of Wisconsin, Milwaukee, Center for Architecture and Urban Planning Research, 1979.

Moore, G., Cohen, U., and others. *Designing Environments for Handicapped Children.* New York: Educational Facilities Laboratory, 1979.

Moser, C. A., and Kalton, G. *Survey Methods in Social Investigation.* 2nd ed. New York: Basic Books, 1972.

Murtha, D. M. Environmental requirements for a community room on a patient care unit: recommendations. Unpublished report, Nurse Utilization Project, St. Mary's Hospital, Milwaukee, WI, 1970.

Naisbitt, J. *Megatrends: Ten New Directions Transforming Our Lives.* New York: Warner Books, 1982.

Nelson-Shulman, Y. Information and environmental stress: report of a hospital intervention. *Journal of Environmental Systems.* 1983-1984. 13(4):303-16.

Newman, O. *Design Guidelines for Creating Defensible Space.* Washington, DC: U.S. Government Printing Office, 1975.

Nicklin, W. M. The role of the family in the emergency department. *Canadian Nurse.* 1979 Apr. 75(4):40-43.

Noble, A., and Dixon, R. Ward evaluation: St. Thomas Hospital. Unpublished report, Medical Architecture Research Unit, Polytechnic of North London, London, 1977 Dec.

Oberlander, R. Beauty in a hospital aids the cure. *Hospitals.* 1979 Mar. 16. 53(6):74-75.

Olds, A. Psychological considerations in humanizing the physical environment of pediatric outpatient and hospital settings. In: Gellert, E., editor. *Psychosocial Aspects of Pediatric Care.* New York: Grove and Stratton, 1978.

Olds, A., and Daniels, P. *Child Health Care Facilities: Design Guidelines and Literature Review.* Washington, DC: Association for the Care of Children's Health, forthcoming.

Olsen, R. V. A user evaluation of a hospital park. Unpublished report, Environmental Design Program, Bellevue Hospital Center, New York, no date.

Olsen, R. V., and Pershing, A. Environmental evaluation of the interim entry to Bellevue Hospital. Unpublished report, Environmental Psychology Department, Bellevue Hospital, New York, 1981.

Olsen, R. V., Pershing, A., and Winkel, G. A patient and staff evaluation of the Scanmural lounges. Unpublished research report, Environmental Design Program, Bellevue Hospital Center and Environmental Psychology Program, City University of New York, New York, 1984.

Paine, R. Design guidelines for hospital open space: case studies of three hospitals. Master's thesis, University of California, Berkeley, 1984.

Panther, R. E. Hospital design in the year 2015. In: Lasdon, G. S., and Gann, J. S., editors. *The Future of Hospital Design: A Discussion Among Experts.* Washington, DC: U.S. Department of Health and Human Services, 1984.

Parston, G. Hospital buildings and consumer needs. *Consumer Health Perspectives.* 1983 Sept. 9(5):1-7.

Passini, R. Wayfinding: a study of spatial problem-solving with implications for physical design. Ph.D. dissertation, Pennsylvania State University, University Park, 1977. Available from UMI, 300 N. Zeeb Road, Ann Arbor, MI 48106.

Pendell, S. D., Coray, K. E., and Veneklasen, W. D. Architectural/behavioral correlates of hospital lobbies. Architectural Psychology Symposium, Rocky Mountain Psychological Association, Salt Lake City, 1975 May.

Petersen, R. W. Behavioral design in OPD architecture: considerations for reception and waiting areas. In: *Proceedings of the Symposium on Pediatric Clinic and Emergency Architecture, 1981 June 26-28*. Chicago: American Academy of Pediatrics, Chicago, 1981.

————. Behavioral design criteria: patient and companion needs for reception and waiting areas. Unpublished report, R. W. Petersen and Associates, McMinnville, OR, 1981 July 31.

Petrie, R. E. Patient well-being is designers' first concern. *Michigan Hospitals*. 1980 Sept. 16(9):12-13.

Pierce, G. Carpeting cuts maintenance costs. *Canadian Hospital*. 1973 Apr. 50(4):55-60.

Popkin, S. Form must follow function. *Michigan Hospitals*. 1980 Sept. 16(9):9-11.

Prototype hospital room provides privacy and amenities. *Contract*. 1985 Feb. pp. 92-93.

Rabin, M. Medical-facility colors reduce patient stress. *Contract*. 1981 Feb. 23(2):78-83.

Radiation unit improves patient access and comfort. *Hospitals*. 1980 Sept. 16. 53(18):57-58.

Reizenstein, J. E. *Social Research and Design: Cambridge Hospital Social Service Offices*. Springfield, VA: National Technical Information Service, 1976.

————. Hospital design and human behavior: a review of the recent literature. In: Baum, A., and Singer, J., editors. *Advances in Environmental Psychology*. Vol. 4, *Environment and Health*. Hillsdale, NJ: Erlbaum Press, 1982.

Reizenstein, J. E., and Grant, M. A. Schematic design of the inpatient room. Unpublished research report #1, Patient and Visitor Participation Project, Office of Hospital Planning, Research and Development, University of Michigan, Ann Arbor, 1981.

————. Patient activities and schematic design preferences. Unpublished research report #2, Patient and Visitor Participation Project, Office of Hospital Planning, Research and Development, University of Michigan, Ann Arbor, 1981.

————. Patient and visitor issues: currently unmet needs and suggested solutions. Unpublished research report #4a, Patient and Visitor Participation Project, Office of Hospital Planning, Research and Development, University of Michigan, Ann Arbor, 1981.

————. Spontaneous design suggestions by patients and visitors. Unpublished report #6, Patient and Visitor Participation Project, Office of Hospital Planning, Research and Development, University of Michigan, Ann Arbor, 1981.

————. Executive summary: patient hair care and storage. Unpublished research report #9, Patient and Visitor Participation Project, Office of Hospital Planning, Research and Development, University of Michigan, Ann Arbor, 1981.

————. Patient and visitor preferences for outdoor courtyard design. Unpublished research report #10, Patient and Visitor Participation Project, Office of Hospital Planning, Research and Development, University of Michigan, Ann Arbor, 1981.

————. *From Hospital Research to Hospital Design.* Patient and Visitor Participation Project, Office of Hospital Planning, Research and Development, University of Michigan, Ann Arbor, 1982.

————. Visitor preferences for overnight accommodations. Unpublished research report #13, Patient and Visitor Participation Project, Office of Hospital Planning, Research and Development, University of Michigan, Ann Arbor, 1982.

————. Outdoor seating evaluation. Unpublished research report #22, Patient and Visitor Participation Project, Office of Hospital Planning, Research and Development, University of Michigan, Ann Arbor, 1983.

————. Color, cubicle curtains, handrails. Unpublished research report #23, Patient and Visitor Participation Project, Office of Hospital Planning, Research and Development, University of Michigan, Ann Arbor, 1983.

Reizenstein, J. E., Grant, M. A., and Vaitkus, M. A. Visitor activities and schematic design preferences. Unpublished research report #4, Patient and Visitor Participation Project, Office of Hospital Planning, Research and Development, University of Michigan, Ann Arbor, 1981.

Reizenstein, J. E., Simmons, D. A., and others. *Hospital Design and Human Behavior: A Bibliography.* Architectural Series, A673. Monticello, IL: Vance Bibliographies, 1982.

Reizenstein, J. E., and Vaitkus, M. A. Hospital visitors and environmental stress. Patient and Visitor Participation Project, Office of the Replacement Hospital Program, University of Michigan, Ann Arbor, in progress.

Reizenstein, J. E., Vaitkus, M. A., and Grant, M. A. Patient belongings. Unpublished research report #9, Patient and Visitor Participation Project, Office of Hospital Planning, Research and Development, University of Michigan, Ann Arbor, 1982.

Relf, P. D. Horticulture as a recreational activity. *Journal—American Health Care Association.* 1978 Sept. 4(5):68-71.

Remen, S. Physical surroundings serve as therapeutic catalyst for patients. *Michigan Hospitals.* 1982 Apr. 18(4):20-25.

Ringoir, S. Design and function of a hospital artificial kidney centre. *International Journal of Artificial Organs.* 1980 May. 3(3):134-35.

Robinette, G. *Barrier-Free Exterior Design.* New York: Van Nostrand Reinhold, 1985.

Rose, J. C. Marketing new food services. *Hospitals.* 1983 Aug. 1. 57(15):64-66.

Rosenfeld, N. Indirect lighting improves outlook for everyone. *Modern Hospital.* 1971 Aug. 117(2):78-80.

Rueter, L. Providing room to care. *Hospitals.* 1974 Feb. 16. 48(4):62-65.

Sanoff, H. *Methods of Architectural Programming.* Stroudsburg, PA: Dowden, Hutchinson and Ross, 1977.

Schultz, J. K. Plants in OR harbor potential contaminants. *Association of Operating Room Nurses Journal.* 1979 Apr. 29(5):898-99.

Selfridge, K. M. Planning library signage systems. In: Pollet, D., and Haskel, P., editors. *Sign Systems for Libraries.* New York: R. R. Bowker Co., 1979.

Shaw, H. Anti-stress art. *Nursing Times.* 1976 June 24. 72(25):960-61.

Shumaker, S., and Reizenstein, J. E. Environmental factors affecting inpatient stress in acute care hospitals. In: Evans, G. W., editor. *Environmental Stress.* New York: Cambridge University Press, 1982.

Simmons, D. A., Reizenstein, J. E., and Grant, M. A. Considering carpets in hospital use. *Dimensions in Health Service.* 1982 June. 59(6):18-21.

Simple, efficient departmental design suits functions, growth of nuclear medicine. *Hospitals.* 1977 May 16. 51(10):30-32.

Snyder, J. Carpeting in the modern hospital. *Canadian Hospital.* 1966 Apr. 43(4):56-68.

Solomon, L. A., and Gaudette, R. Adult general hospital bed and furniture evaluation. Unpublished report, Office of Hospital Planning, Research and Development, University of Michigan, Ann Arbor, 1984.

Sommer, R. The distance for comfortable conversation: a further study. *Sociometry.* 1962. 25:111-16.

————. *Social Design: Creating Buildings with People in Mind.* Englewood Cliffs, NJ: Prentice Hall, 1983.

Special Committee on Aging of the U.S. Senate. *America in Transition: An Aging Society,* 1984-85 edition. Serial no. 99-B. Washington, DC: U.S. Government Printing Office, 1985.

Spelfogel, B., and Modrzakowski, M. Curative factors in horticultural therapy in a hospital setting. *Hospital and Community Psychiatry.* 1980 Aug. 31(8):572-73.

Spivak, M. Sensory distortions in tunnels and corridors. *Hospital and Community Psychiatry.* 1967 Jan. 18(1):12-18.

Spreckelmeyer, K. F. Designing for health care in the twenty-first century. In: Heyer, O., and Graybow, S., editors. *Proceedings of the International Conference of the Association of Collegiate Schools of Architecture.* Washington, DC: ACSA, 1984.

Stern, P. C. *Evaluating Social Science Research.* New York: Oxford University Press, 1979.

Sturdavant, M. Intensive nursing service in circular and rectangular units compared. *Hospitals.* 1960 July 16. 34(14):46-48, 71-78.

Sullivan, M. E. Horticultural therapy: the role gardening plays in healing. *Journal—American Health Care Association.* 1979 May 5(3):3-8.

Templer, J. A., Mullet, G. M., and Archea, J. *An Analysis of the Behavior of Stair Users.* Springfield, VA: National Technical Information Service, 1978.

Tetlow, K. Healing research. *Interiors.* 1984 Oct. pp. 140-52.

———. New design for physical fitness. *Interiors.* 1985 Oct. pp. 168-76.

Toffler, A. *The Third Wave.* New York: Bantam Books, Inc., 1981.

U.S. Department of Health and Human Services. *Guidelines for Construction and Equipment of Hospital and Medical Facilities.* Washington, DC: U.S. Government Printing Office, 1984.

———. Health Care Financing Administration. Telephone interview, Washington, DC, 1985 Mar.

Ulrich, R. S. Visual landscapes and psychological well-being. *Landscape Research.* 1979 Spring. 4(1):17-23.

———. Natural versus urban scenes: some psychological effects. *Environment and Behavior.* 1981 Sept. 13(5):523-56.

———. Aesthetic and affective response to natural environment. In: Altman, I., and Wohlwill, J. F., editors. *Human Behavior and Environment: Advances in Theory and Research,* Vol. 6. New York: Plenum Press, 1983.

———. View through a window may influence recovery from surgery. *Science.* 1984 Apr. 27. 224(4647):420-21.

Valenta, A. L. Human behavioral needs in hospital admissions management: some architectural implications. Ph.D. dissertation, University of Illinois at the Medical Center, Chicago, 1981. Available from UMI, 300 N. Zeeb Road, Ann Arbor, MI 48106.

Verderber, S. F. Windowness and human behavior in the hospital rehabilitation environment. Ph.D. dissertation, University of Michigan, Ann Arbor, 1982. Available from UMI, 300 N. Zeeb Road, Ann Arbor, Michigan 48106.

Vestal, A. J. Analysts discuss pros and cons of carpeting in hospitals. *Hospital Topics.* 1972 Feb. 50(2):45-48.

Wasserman, B. Greening the corner where you are. *Dental Management.* 1974 Dec. 14(12):65-71.

Webb, E. J., Campbell, D. T., and others. *Unobtrusive Measures.* Chicago: Rand McNally, 1966.

Wechsler, S. Perceiving the visual message. In: Pollet, D., and Haskel, P., editors. *Sign Systems for Libraries.* New York: R. R. Bowker Co., 1979.

Weisman, G. D. Way-finding in the built environment: a study in architectural legibility. Ph.D. dissertation, University of Michigan, Ann Arbor, 1979. Available from UMI, 300 N. Zeeb Road, Ann Arbor, MI 48106.

———. Way-finding in the built environment. *Environment and Behavior.* 1981 Mar. 13(2):189-204.

————. Way-finding and architectural legibility: design considerations in housing environments for the elderly. In: Regnier, V., and Pynoos, J., editors. *Housing for the Elderly: Satisfaction and Preferences.* New York: Garland Publishing, Inc., 1982.

Welch, P. Hospital emergency facilities: translating behavioral issues into design. Report, Department of Architecture, Harvard University, Cambridge, MA, 1977.

Wener, R. E., and Kaminoff, R. D. Improving environmental information: effects of signs on perceived crowding and behavior. *Environment and Behavior.* 1983 Jan. 15(1):2-20.

Wilt, L., and Maienschien, J. Symbol signs for libraries. In: Pollet, D., and Haskell, P., editors. *Sign Systems for Libraries.* New York: R. R. Bowker Co., 1979.

Winkel, G., Olsen, R., and others. The museum visitor and orientational media: an experimental comparison of different approaches in the Smithsonian Institution, National Museum of History and Technology. Environmental Psychology Program, City University of New York, no date.

Wohlwill, J. F. The concept of nature: a psychologist's view. In: Altman, I., and Wohlwill, J. F., editors. *Human Behavior and Environment: Advances in Theory and Research,* Vol. 6. New York: Plenum Press, 1983.

Wohlwill, J. F., and Weisman, G. D. *The Physical Environment and Behavior: An Annotated Bibliography and Guide to the Literature.* New York: Plenum Press, 1981.

Wyatt, H. J. You and your deaf patients. Seminar materials, National Academy of Gallaudet College, Washington, DC, 1983.

Zeisel, J. *Inquiry by Design: Tools for Environment Behavior Research.* Monterey, CA: Brooks Cole, 1981.

Zilm, F., Brimhall, D., and Ryan, D. Ambulatory care survey paves way to the future. *Hospitals.* 1978 June 1. 52(11):79-83.

Zimring, C. M. The built environment as a source of psychological stress: impacts of buildings and cities on satisfaction and behavior. In: Evans, G. W., editor. *Environmental Stress.* New York: Cambridge University Press, 1982.

Zimring, C. M., Carpman, J. R., and Michelson, W. Designing for special populations: mentally retarded persons, children, hospital visitors. In: Stokols, D., and Altman, I., editors. *Handbook of Environmental Psychology.* New York: John Wiley and Sons. In press.

Zimring, C. M., and Reizenstein, J. E. Post-occupancy evaluation: an overview. *Environment and Behavior.* 1980 Dec. 12(4):429-50.

————. A primer on post-occupancy evaluation. *American Institute of Architects Journal.* 1981 Nov. 70(13):52-58.

Zimring, C. M., and Templer, J. Wayfinding and orientation by the visually impaired. *Journal of Environmental Systems.* 1983-1984. 13(4):333-52.

Zubatkin, A. D. Psychological impact of medical equipment on patients. *Journal of Clinical Engineering.* 1980 July-Sept. 5(3):250-55.

Index _____

Certain topics are the subject of brief, self-contained reports of research projects called *research boxes*, indicated here by a page number followed by *(b)*. The Index refers only to the text and not to the Design Review Questions.

Accessibility codes and standards, 220
Acute care inpatient rooms, 156-74
    artwork in, 170, 171*(b)*
    bathrooms in, 175-78, 235
    clocks in, 171
    elderly users of, 234
    furnishings for, 163
    lighting in, 172
    mock-ups of, 157*(b)*
    number of occupants in, 158
    overnight visitors and, 174, 256-59
    privacy in, 158-62
    size of, 156
    sound travel in, 161
    storage in, 164-68
    television in, 169
    visitors in, 173
    windows in, 162
Admitting department, 43-46, 45*(b)*
Aging. *See also* Elderly users
    changes accompanying, 225
Architectural cues, wayfinding and, 29,
    31*(b)*, 61
Artwork
    high-stress waiting and, 122
    in inpatient rooms, 170, 171*(b)*
    in treatment areas, 142

Banners, wayfinding and, 76*(b)*
Bathrooms, 175-78. *See also* Rest rooms
    for elderly users, 235
    privacy in, 158

Beds
    for elderly users, 234
    in inpatient rooms, 163
Bedside stands, 168
Benches in outdoor areas, 206
Blindness. *See* Visual
        impairments
Block plans, 2
Buildings
    layout of, 60
    names of, 27*(b)*
Bus systems, 35

Cafeterias, 254
Carpeting
    in corridors, 83
    in waiting areas, 112
Cars, 26-35
    parking and, 31*(b)*
    signs and, 26-29
Chairs. *See also* Seating
    elderly users and, 231
    in inpatient rooms, 164
    in waiting areas, 111*(b)*
Chapels, 255
Checkout, 247
Child care, 259
Children, waiting areas and,
    114
Clocks
    in inpatient rooms, 170
    waiting areas and, 119

Clothing, 43
    storage areas for, 137, 165
    waiting areas and, 115
Color
    elderly users and, 229
    in inpatient rooms, 172
Color coding
    elderly users and, 229
    wayfinding and, 76
Companions of patient, 146. *See also*
        Visitors
Confidentiality, admitting department and,
        45*(b)*
Construction documents, 3
Construction phase of design process, 3
Consultation rooms, 246
Control panel for elevators, 86
Conversations in admitting department
        and, 45*(b)*
Corridors in facilities, 82-85
    elderly users and, 233
    unplanned use of, 87
Courtyards. *See* Outdoor areas
Curtains, cubicle, 160

Deafness. *See* Hearing impairments
Decision points in wayfinding, 71, 73*(b)*
Demographic trends, 11
    elderly users and, 224
Design development documents, 3
Design phase of design process, 2
    user participation in, 272
Design process, 2-4
    user participation in, 203*(b)*, 271-85
Design review, 4
Design review questions, 48, 89, 124, 147,
        185, 213, 237, 261
Diagnostic and treatment areas, 133-46
    patient comfort in, 141
    patient companions in, 146
    privacy in, 141
    rooms in, 140-44
Directional signs, 29
Disabled persons. *See* Handicapped
        persons
Documents for design process, 3
Dressing, areas for, 135
Drop-off points, wayfinding and, 31*(b)*, 33

Eating. *See also* Meals
    and waiting areas, 107, 118
Educational activities in waiting areas, 113
Elderly users, 12, 224-36
    bathrooms for, 235
    environmental accommodations for,
        228
    inpatient rooms for, 234

physiological changes in, 225
    safety for, 227
    wayfinding and, 233
Elevators, 85
    in parking facility, 39
    unplanned use of, 87
Emergency department, 246-49
Entrance areas, 36-47
    handicapped persons and, 38
    special users and, 40
    waiting areas and, 41, 102
Environment
    elderly users and, 226
    stress and, 19
Equipment, patient comfort and, 142
Examination rooms, 140. *See also*
        Diagnostic and treatment areas
    patient comfort and, 142

Family members. *See* Visitors; Companions
        of patient
Family planning, health care and, 14
Flooring materials
    elderly users and, 231
    waiting areas and, 112
Floors in facilities
    numbering of, 62, 63*(b)*
    traveling between, 85
Food service areas, 254
Furnishings
    for elderly users, 234
    for inpatient rooms, 163
    for waiting areas, 110

Gowns, hospital, 138, 139*(b)*
Grieving rooms, 246

Hair care, 259
Handicapped persons, 219-24
    facility access for, 38
    outdoor areas and, 204
    parking for, 35
    signage for, 29
    dressing areas for, 136
Handrails
    in corridors, 83
    in outdoor walkways, 204
    in stairways, 87
Health care
    economics of, 15
    trends in, 11
Hearing impairments, 220
    aging and, 225, 228
    facility access and, 39
High-stress waiting areas, 121
Hospital building names, 27*(b)*
Hospital gowns, 138, 139*(b)*

Information desk, 42, 43(b)
Information gathering, 279
Inpatient lounges, 249-253
    evaluation of, 250(b)
    unusual, 252(b)
Inpatients. See also Patients
    rooms for. See Acute care inpatient
        rooms
    waiting areas for, 145
Intensive care units, 178-84
    privacy in, 179
    stress and, 180
    visitors and, 183
    windows in, 181(b)
Interior design, design process and, 3

Landmarks, wayfinding and, 60
Landscape architecture. See also Outdoor
        areas
    design process and, 4
Language choice for signage, 66
Libraries, 253
Life span, health care and, 12
Lighting
    in corridors, 83
    for elderly users, 228
    in inpatient rooms, 172
    in waiting areas, 112
Lights, colored, wayfinding and, 76(b)
Lobby, main, 120
Lockers, 137
Lounge, inpatient. See Inpatient lounges

Main lobby, 120
Maps, 36, 77-81
    design of, 78(b), 79(b)
    interior, 77
    You-Are-Here, 36, 77-81
Meals
    food service areas and, 254
    inpatient rooms and, 173
Medical equipment
    design process and, 4
    in inpatient rooms, 156
    patient comfort and, 141
Medical staff, design needs of, 15
Medical terminology on signs, 67
Memory, aging and, 226
Mobility impairments, 220
    aging and, 225
    facility access and, 39
Mock-ups of inpatient rooms, 157(b)
Multilingual signs, 66

Names of hospital buildings, 27(b)
Nonsmoking areas, 119
Numbering schemes, 62-65

Outdoor areas
    access to, 197-212
    design of, 200-203, 203(b)
    evaluation of, 199(b)
    location of, 204
    seating in, 205-9, 208(b)
    walkways in, 204
Outpatients, waiting areas for, 145
Overnight accommodations, 175, 256-259,
        258(b)
    visitor preferences for, 257(b)

Park and ride facilities, 34
Parking
    handicapped persons and, 35, 38
    rates for, 33
    wayfinding and, 31(b), 33
Parking facilities
    elevators in, 39
    safety and security in, 38
Parks. See Outdoor areas
Participation. See User participation, design
        process and
Patient and Visitor Participation (PVP)
        Project, 1, 27, 68(b), 284
Patients
    activities for distraction of, 143
    comfort of, 141
    communication with staff by, 145
    companions of, 146
    design needs of, 17
    dressing areas for, 135
    hospital gowns for, 138, 139(b)
    personal belongings of, 137
    room design and, 140
    inpatient and outpatient separation,
        145
    self-disclosure of, 143(b)
    special needs of, 134
Personal belongings
    patients', 137
    storing of, 43, 164-68
    waiting areas and, 115
Pictographs on signs, 69
Plants, indoor use of, 210
Play areas for children, 114
Population changes, 12
Post-occupancy evaluation, 4, 283
Predesign phase of design process, 2
Privacy
    acoustical, 161
    admitting department and, 44
    in bathrooms, 158
    hospital gowns and, 138
    inpatient rooms and, 158
    in intensive care unit, 179
    reception areas and, 105

Index

Privacy (*continued*)
    treatment rooms and, 141
    undressing and, 136
    windows and, 162, 163*(b)*
Private rooms. *See* Acute care inpatient
    rooms
Public transit, 35

Reception areas, 101-23. *See also* Waiting
    areas
    design of, 104
Recovery, windows and, 212*(b)*
Refreshments, waiting areas and, 118
Registration desk, 104. *See also* Waiting
    areas
    emergency department and, 247
Renovation
    room numbers and, 65
    signage and, 71
Research, user participation in, 277
Rest rooms. *See also* Bathrooms
    waiting areas and, 107, 118
Review stage of design process, 4
Room design, patient communication and,
    143*(b)*
Rooms
    consultation and grieving, 246
    for diagnosis and treatment, 140-44
    inpatient. *See* Acute care inpatient
        rooms
    numbering of, 62, 64

Safety precautions
    in admitting departments, 45*(b)*
    for elderly users, 227
    in outdoor areas, 209
    in parking facilities, 38
Schematic design, 3
Seating. *See also* Chairs
    elderly users and, 231
    in hallways, 85
    in outdoor areas, 205-9, 208*(b)*
    in waiting areas, 109-12, 111*(b)*
Security precautions
    in admitting departments, 45*(b)*
    in outdoor areas, 209
    in parking facilities, 38
Semiprivate rooms. *See* Acute care
    inpatient rooms
Senior citizens. *See* Elderly users
Sexual segregation, hospital gowns and,
    139*(b)*
Showers in inpatient bathrooms, 176
Shuttle bus systems, 34
Sight, impaired. *See* Visual impairments
Signs, 70-75
    decision points and, 73*(b)*

    location of, 71
    parking and, 31*(b)*
    pictographs on, 69
    placement of, 29
    terminology of, 66-69, 68*(b)*
    typeface for, 70
    waiting areas and, 103
    wayfinding and, 26
    visibility of, 28
Sinks
    for elderly users, 235
    in inpatient bathrooms, 175
Smoking, waiting areas and, 119
Snacks, waiting areas and, 118
Social contact in facility, 19
Stairways, 86
    unplanned use of, 87
    for visually impaired users,
        223
Storage areas
    for outerwear, 43, 137, 165
    for personal belongings, 164-68
    in waiting areas, 115
Stress, 18
    admitting department and,
        45*(b)*
    environment and, 19
    intensive care unit and, 180
    waiting areas and, 121
    wayfinding and, 59
Symbols on signs, 69

Table, overbed, 168
TDDs (telecommunications devices for the
    deaf), 220
Telephones
    for elderly users, 235
    enclosures for, 116*(b)*
    in waiting areas, 115
Television
    in inpatient rooms, 169
    for patient distraction, 143
    in waiting areas, 108
Terminology of signs, 66-69, 68*(b)*
Toilets
    for elderly users, 235
    in inpatient bathrooms, 177
Transportation to facility, 25
    public, 35
Treatment areas. *See* Diagnostic and
    treatment areas
Triage areas, 247
Typeface for signs, 70

Undressing, areas for, 135
University of Michigan Replacement
    Hospital Program, 1, 208*(b)*

User participation, design process and, 16, 271-85
User groups, design process and, 275

Vegetation, indoor, 210. *See also* Outdoor areas
Vending machines, 107, 118
Visitor information centers, 46
Visitors, 146
    design needs of, 17
    emergency department and, 248
    inpatient rooms and, 173
    intensive care unit and, 183
    overnight accommodations for, 175, 256-59
    waiting areas and. *See* Waiting areas
    wayfinding and. *See* Wayfinding
Visual cues, wayfinding and, 29, 31(b)
Visual impairments, 222
    aging and, 225
    facility access and, 39

Waiting areas, 101-23. *See also* Reception areas
    behavior in, 108(b)
    children and, 114
    clocks and, 119
    eating and, 118
    educational activities in, 113
    emergency department and, 248
    entrances and, 41, 102
    information in, 103(b)
    inpatient, 145
    interior design of, 112
    location of, 107
    main lobby and, 120
    rest rooms and, 118
    seating in, 109
    size of, 106
    smoking and, 119
    telephones in, 115
Walkways in outdoor areas, 204
Wall coverings, in waiting areas, 112
Wardrobes, 168
Wayfinding, 57-88
    architectural features and, 31(b)
    building layout and, 60
    color coding and, 76
    decision points in, 71
    elderly users and, 233
    emergency department and, 247
    entrance areas and, 36, 40
    information desk and, 43(b)
    oral directions and, 82
    parking and, 31(b), 33
    problems with, 58
    signage and, 26-29
    stress and, 19, 59
    visual cues and, 29, 31(b)
    waiting areas and, 103
    You-Are-Here maps and, 36, 77-81, 78(b), 79(b)
Wheelchairs, 38, 220. *See also* Handicapped persons
Windows, 211
    in inpatient rooms, 159, 162, 163(b)
    in intensive care unit, 181(b)
    recovery and, 212(b)
    in waiting areas, 107

You-Are-Here maps, 36, 77-81
    design of, 78(b), 79(b)
    interior, 77